FAST FACTS
for the
ER NURSE

Alexander Menard, DNP, AGACNP-BC, is an assistant professor at the University of Massachusetts Chan Medical School, Tan Chingfen Graduate School of Nursing, where he coordinates the Adult-Gerontology Acute Care Nurse Practitioner (AGACNP) program. Dr. Menard has worked in critical care as a nurse and nurse practitioner for more than 10 years.

He is a member of the American Association of Critical Care Nurses (AACN), where he volunteers his time to develop new offerings for critical care nurses and nurse practitioners, and is also a member of the National Organization of Nurse Practitioner Faculties (NONPF).

Sarah Berry, RN, BSN, CEN, PHRN, TNCC, is a registered nurse at Geisinger Medical Center in Danville, Pennsylvania. She has been in the emergency department for 7 years, working in various roles until January 2020, when she became an RN at a rural level one trauma center. She watched the fields of bedside nursing and emergency medicine change and evolve in the face of a historic pandemic.

She received caregiver of the year for 2023 in the ED. She is a member of the Emergency Nursing Association (ENA) and the Society of Trauma Nursing (STN) and is currently working as a flight nurse for the prestigious Geisinger Life Flight program.

OTHER *FAST FACTS* BOOKS

Fast Facts on ADOLESCENT HEALTH FOR NURSING AND HEALTH PROFESSIONALS: A Care Guide (*Herrman*)

Fast Facts for the ADULT-GERONTOLOGY ACUTE CARE NURSE PRACTITIONER (*Carpenter*)

Fast Facts for the ANTEPARTUM AND POSTPARTUM NURSE: A Nursing Orientation and Care Guide (*Davidson*)

Fast Facts Workbook for CARDIAC DYSRHYTHMIAS AND 12-LEAD EKGs (*Desmarais*)

Fast Facts for the CARDIAC SURGERY NURSE, Fourth Edition (*McLaughlin*)

Fast Facts for CAREER SUCCESS IN NURSING: Making the Most of Mentoring (*Vance*)

Fast Facts for the CATH LAB NURSE, Second Edition (*McCulloch*)

Fast Facts for the CLASSROOM NURSING INSTRUCTOR: Classroom Teaching (*Yoder-Wise, Kowalski*)

Fast Facts for the CLINICAL NURSE LEADER (*Wilcox, Deerhake*)

Fast Facts for the CLINICAL NURSE MANAGER: Managing a Changing Workplace, Second Edition (*Fry*)

Fast Facts for the CLINICAL NURSING INSTRUCTOR, Fourth Edition (*Kan, Stabler-Haas*)

Fast Facts on COMBATING NURSE BULLYING, INCIVILITY, AND WORKPLACE VIOLENCE: What Nurses Need to Know (*Ciocco*)

Fast Facts About COMPETENCY-BASED EDUCATION IN NURSING: How to Teach Competency Mastery (*Wittmann-Price, Gittings*)

Fast Facts for the CRITICAL CARE NURSE, Third Edition (*Hewett*)

Fast Facts About CURRICULUM DEVELOPMENT IN NURSING: How to Develop and Evaluate Educational Programs, Second Edition (*McCoy, Anema*)

Fast Facts for DEMENTIA CARE: What Nurses Need to Know, Second Edition (*Miller*)

Fast Facts for DEVELOPING A NURSING ACADEMIC PORTFOLIO: What You Really Need to Know (*Wittmann-Price*)

Fast Facts About DIVERSITY, EQUITY, AND INCLUSION IN NURSING: Building Competencies for an Antiracism Practice (*Davis, O'Brien*)

Fast Facts for DNP ROLE DEVELOPMENT: A Career Navigation Guide (*Menonna-Quinn, Tortorella Genova*)

Fast Facts About EKGs FOR NURSES: The Rules of Identifying EKGs (*Landrum*)

Fast Facts for the ER NURSE, Fifth Edition, (*Menard, Berry*)

Fast Facts for EVIDENCE-BASED PRACTICE IN NURSING, Fourth Edition (*Godshall*)

Fast Facts for the FAITH COMMUNITY NURSE: Implementing FCN/Parish Nursing (*Hickman*)

Fast Facts About FORENSIC NURSING: What You Need to Know (*Scannell*)

Fast Facts on GENETICS AND GENOMICS FOR NURSES: Practical Applications (*Subasic*)

Fast Facts for the GERONTOLOGY NURSE: A Nursing Care Guide (*Eliopoulos*)

Fast Facts About GI AND LIVER DISEASES FOR NURSES: What APRNs Need to Know (*Chaney*)

Fast Facts About the GYNECOLOGICAL EXAM: A Professional Guide for NPs, PAs, and Midwives, Second Edition (*Secor, Fantasia*)

Fast Facts in HEALTH INFORMATICS FOR NURSES (*Hardy*)

Fast Facts for HEALTH PROMOTION IN NURSING: Promoting Wellness (*Miller*)

Fast Facts for Nurses About HOME INFUSION THERAPY: The Expert's Best Practice Guide (*Gorski*)

Fast Facts for the HOSPICE NURSE: A Concise Guide to End-of-Life Care, Second Edition (*Wright*)

Fast Facts for the L&D NURSE: Labor and Delivery Orientation, Third Edition (*Groll*)

Fast Facts About LGBTQ+ CARE FOR NURSES: How to Deliver Culturally Competent and Inclusive Care (*Traister*)

Fast Facts for the LONG-TERM CARE NURSE: What Nursing Home and Assisted Living Nurses Need to Know (*Eliopoulos*)

Fast Facts to LOVING YOUR RESEARCH PROJECT: A Stress-Free Guide for Novice Researchers in Nursing and Healthcare (*Marshall*)

Fast Facts for MAKING THE MOST OF YOUR CAREER IN NURSING (*Redulla*)

Fast Facts for MANAGING PATIENTS WITH A PSYCHIATRIC DISORDER: What RNs, NPs, and New Psych Nurses Need to Know (*Marshall*)

Fast Facts About MEDICAL CANNABIS AND OPIOIDS: Minimizing Opioid Use Through Cannabis (*Smith, Smith*)

Fast Facts for the MEDICAL OFFICE NURSE: What You Really Need to Know (*Richmeier*)

Fast Facts for the MEDICAL–SURGICAL NURSE: Clinical Orientation (*Ciocco*)

Fast Facts for the OPERATING ROOM NURSE: An Orientation and Care Guide, Third Edition (*Criscitelli*)

Fast Facts for PATIENT SAFETY IN NURSING: How to Decrease Medical Errors and Improve Patient Outcomes (*Hunt*)

Fast Facts for PSYCHOPHARMACOLOGY FOR NURSE PRACTITIONERS (*Goldin*)

Fast Facts for the SCHOOL NURSE, Fourth Edition (*Loschiavo*)

Fast Facts About STROKE CARE FOR THE ADVANCED PRACTICE NURSE, Fourth Edition (*Morrison, McLaughlin*)

Fast Facts for TRAUMA NURSING (*Carpenter, Menard*)

Fast Facts for WOUND CARE NURSING: Practical Wound Management, Second Edition (*Myers*)

FAST FACTS
for the ER NURSE

Fifth Edition

Alexander Menard, DNP, AGACNP-BC

Sarah Berry, RN, BSN, CEN, PHRN, TNCC

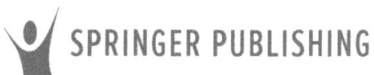

Copyright © 2026 Springer Publishing Company, LLC
All rights reserved.

First Springer Publishing edition 978-0-8261-0521-9, 2009; subsequent editions 2013, 2017, 2021

No part of this publication may be reproduced, stored in a retrieval system, used for text and data mining, machine learning, artificial intelligence model training, or any other automated processing or analysis, or transmitted in any form or by any means, electronic, mechanical, photocopying, recording, or otherwise, without the prior permission of Springer Publishing Company, LLC, via our website at https://www.springerpub.com/permission-requests, or authorization through payment of the appropriate fees to the Copyright Clearance Center, Inc., 222 Rosewood Drive, Danvers, MA 01923, 978-750-8400, fax 978-646-8600, info@copyright.com or at www.copyright.com.

Springer Publishing Company, LLC
902 Carnegie Center/Suite 140, Princeton, NJ 08540
www.springerpub.com
connect.springerpub.com

Acquisitions Editor: John Zaphyr
Compositor: Transforma
Production Editor: Claire Kramer

ISBN: 978-0-8261-8919-6
eBook ISBN: 978-0-8261-4859-9
DOI: 10.1891/9780826148599

25 26 27 28 / 5 4 3 2 1

Medicine is an ever-changing science. Research and clinical experience are continually expanding our knowledge, in particular our understanding of proper treatment and drug therapy. The authors, editors, and publisher have made every effort to ensure that all information in this book is in accordance with the state of knowledge at the time of production of the book. Nevertheless, the authors, editors, and publisher are not responsible for any errors or omissions or for any consequence from application of the information in this book and make no warranty, expressed or implied, with respect to the content of this publication. Every reader should examine carefully the package inserts accompanying each drug and should carefully check whether the dosage schedules therein or the contraindications stated by the manufacturer differ from the statements made in this book. Such examination is particularly important with drugs that are either rarely used or have been newly released on the market.

The work is provided, "as is," and the publisher disclaims any and all warranties, express or implied, including any warranties as to accuracy, comprehensiveness, or currency of the content of this work or any information that can be accessed through the work via a hyperlink or otherwise, the persistence and accuracy of which is hereby disclaimed. Neither the publisher nor its licensors shall be liable to you or anyone else for any inaccuracy, error or omission, regardless of cause, in the work or for any damages resulting therefrom.

Library of Congress Control Number: 2025947691

Publisher's Note: **New and used products purchased from third-party sellers are not guaranteed for quality, authenticity, or access to any included digital components.**

Printed in the United States of America by Gasch Printing.

This book is dedicated to all nurses who care for patients and families in the ED. We are inspired by your commitment and dedication to the nursing profession.

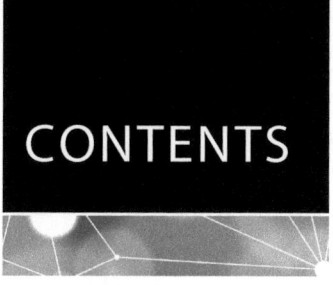

CONTENTS

Contributors — *ix*
Foreword   Dawn Carpenter, DNP, ACNP-BC, CCRN, FAANP — *xi*
Preface — *xiii*
Acknowledgments — *xv*

SECTION I ED BASICS

1. Introduction to ED Nursing — 3
2. Triage — 11
3. Acid–Base Imbalances — 27
4. Fluid and Electrolyte Emergencies — 33

SECTION II SYSTEM-BASED ED NURSING CARE

5. Neurological Emergencies — 43
6. Cardiovascular Emergencies — 53
7. Respiratory Emergencies — 69
8. Gastrointestinal Emergencies — 89
9. Dental and Ear, Nose, and Throat Emergencies — 99
10. Ocular Emergencies — 113
11. Endocrine Emergencies — 119
12. Genitourinary Emergencies — 131
13. Hematologic Emergencies — 137
14. Musculoskeletal and Wound Care Emergencies — 149
15. Infectious Disease Emergencies — 159
16. Shock Emergencies — 179
17. Traumatic Emergencies — 189
18. Substance Abuse and Toxicologic Emergencies — 203

SECTION III SPECIAL POPULATIONS IN ED NURSING CARE

19. Geriatric Emergencies — 221
20. OB/GYN Emergencies — 227
21. Mental Health Emergencies — 249
22. Pediatric Emergencies — 255

SECTION IV UNIQUE CIRCUMSTANCES IN ED NURSING

23. Disaster Management — 269
24. Safety in the ED — 279
25. Tips for Success for ED Nurses — 283

SECTION V ANSWERS AND RATIONALES

26. Answers and Rationales — 289

Index — *297*

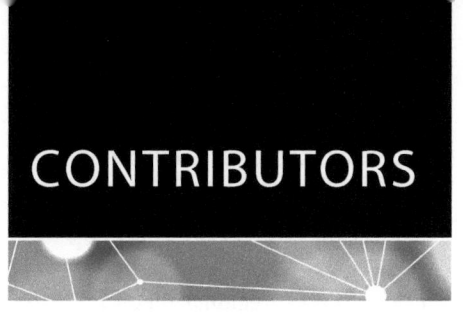

CONTRIBUTORS

Kristen Bauman, RN, ADN, Registered Nurse, Emergency Department, Robert Packer Hospital, Sayre, Pennsylvania

Dawn Carpenter, DNP, ACNP-BC, CCRN, FAANP, Trauma & Surgical ICU Nurse Practitioner, Guthrie Healthcare System, Robert Packer Hospital, Sayre, Pennsylvania; Associate Professor, Faculty Doctor of Nursing Practice Program, Tan Chingfen Graduate School of Nursing, UMass Chan Medical School, Worcester, Massachusetts

Henry Ellis, DNP, AGACNP-BC, Trauma & Surgical ICU Nurse Practitioner, Surgical ICU Group, UMass Memorial Medical Center, Worcester, Massachusetts; Assistant Professor, Tan Chingfen Graduate School of Nursing, UMass Chan Medical School, Worcester, Massachusetts

Johnny Isenberger, DNP, ACNP-BC, CCRN, Assistant Professor, Tan Chingfen Graduate School of Nursing, UMass Chan Medical School, Worcester, Massachusetts; Surgical Critical Care Nurse Practitioner, UMass Memorial Medical Center, Worcester, Massachusetts

Michael Konetzny, BSN, RN, CEN, CCRN, CFRN, NR-P, FP-C, Assistant Clinical Manager–Emergency Department, UMass Memorial Medical Center, Worcester, Massachusetts; Flight Nurse/Paramedic, Air Methods–Life Flight 2, Fitchburg, Massachusetts

Melissa Snyder, RN, BSN, CEN, TCRN, PHRN, Critical Care Nurse Educator, ER, ICU, Cath Lab, IR, Observation, Robert Packer Hospital, Sayre, Pennsylvania

Raymond St. Péter, MSN, RN, CCRN, NeuroTrauma Critical Care Registered Nurse, UMass Memorial Medical Center, Worcester, Massachusetts; Clinical Instructor, Graduate Entry Pathway, Tan Chingfen Graduate School of Nursing, UMass Chan Medical School, Worcester, Massachusetts; Adjunct Professor, Department of Nursing Education, Quinsigamond Community College, Worcester, Massachusetts

Jessica Valentine, MSN, RN, CEN, CPEN, CCRN, Nurse Education Safety Specialist, University Campus Emergency Department, UMass Memorial Health, Worcester, Massachusetts

Nicole Zuidema-Ellis, RN, BSN, Registered Nurse, Emergency Department, UMass Memorial Health-Milford Regional Medical Center, Milford, Massachusetts

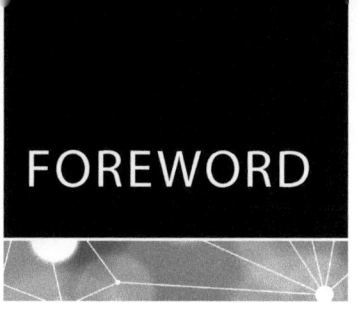

FOREWORD

Nobody wakes up saying I'm going to meet an ED nurse today. Patients unexpectedly seek expert care for a diverse set of acute, urgent, and emergent conditions. And they expect to receive care by highly knowledgeable, skilled, efficient, and compassionate nurses. *Fast Facts for the ER Nurse* provides a concise review of a variety of topics for which patients seek care in the ED. This book provides resources to enable the ED nurse to meet patient and family needs. This book is distinctive in that it specifically emphasizes the unique needs of critically ill and injured patients who are routinely boarding in the ED while awaiting an ICU bed. Additionally, special sections on workplace safety, disaster response to mass casualties, and tips for success make this a must-have book for all ED nurses. Bad things happen quickly, and when they do, the ED nurses are there to administer expert nursing care, which improves patient outcomes and retains quality of life for their patients. This book is an essential tool to enhance all ED nurses' knowledge and practice.

Dawn Carpenter, DNP, ACNP-BC, CCRN, FAANP
*Nurse Practitioner, SICU and Trauma, Guthrie Clinic, Sayre, Pennsylvania;
Associate Professor, Tan Chingfen Graduate School of Nursing,
UMass Chan Medical School, Worcester, Massachusetts; Adjunct Associate
Clinical Professor of Surgery, Surgery Institute,
Geisinger College of Health Professions, Scranton, Pennsylvania*

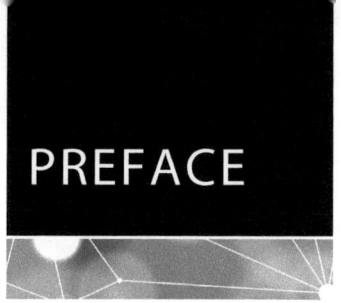

PREFACE

Welcome to the fifth edition of *Fast Facts for the ER Nurse*. This book was created specifically for new nurses, nurses new to the ED, and nursing students. This book presents critical information at the nurses' fingertips for quick reference in the clinical setting.

This book is designed to fit in the pocket for daily use. This pocket resource puts vital information at your fingertips with succinct, easy-to read bullet points, tables, and figures. It is designed to be used by nurses in the ED but has helpful information for any nurse working in areas where nursing meets the community.

This book is unique in that it provides large amounts of data in a condensed format. Given the expansive knowledge that ED nurses must know, it was impossible to include everything and yet be small enough for the pocket; thus, selective components were chosen for inclusion.

KEY FEATURES

- Quick access guide—written by experienced ED and critical care nurses
- Organized in a clinical system-based approach
- Streamlines complex information into easily understandable language
- Includes evidence-based treatments and nursing interventions for best practice and patient care

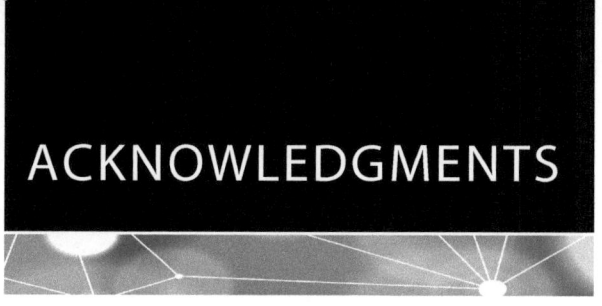

ACKNOWLEDGMENTS

We want to extend sincerest gratitude to all our colleagues at Guthrie Healthcare System, Robert Packer Hospital Level 1 Trauma Center, the University of Massachusetts Chan Medical School, Tan Chingfen Graduate School of Nursing, UMass Memorial Medical Center, and Geisinger Medical Center for providing encouragement through this process.

Thank you to John Zaphyr and Brenna Croker at Springer Publishing Company for providing the opportunity to publish this book. You have been excellent partners on this journey. We sincerely appreciate your guidance and unwavering support. You have been crucial to making this project come to fruition. It is an honor to work with both of you!

We would also like to acknowledge Jennifer R. Buettner, RN, BSN, CEN, HHP, who has developed and written the previous editions of this important book.

Alex: This book would not have been possible without the support from my wife, Heather, and two children, Madelynn and Isabelle. I am most grateful for their support and encouragement.

Sarah: I would like to take the time to thank my husband, Chris, our cat, Tippy, and my parents, Deborah and Robert, for their support. I am forever grateful for their patience, love, and encouragement through not just this process but in my career and every aspiration I have.

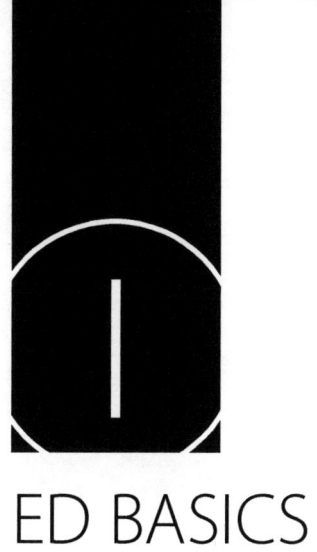

ED BASICS

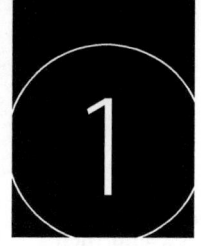

Introduction to ED Nursing

Sarah Berry

> *For 22 years and counting, nursing has been named the most trusted profession in the United States (Brenan, 2024). Nursing is esteemed in this poll for its honesty and ethics. According to the U.S. Bureau of Labor (2024), there are an estimated 3.1 million nurses in the United States, with approximately 789,000 of them being ED nurses (Zippia, 2024). Comprising roughly 25% of the nursing profession, ED nursing is a specialty like no other. It allows nurses to care for a variety of patients that are differentiated by demographics, medical problems, acuity, and complexity. Being an ED nurse is a challenge that will teach you as much as it will reward you.*

In this chapter, you will learn to:
1. Identify the key characteristics of a great ED nurse
2. Articulate the purpose of this book
3. Engage in self-care

INTRODUCTION

Congratulations on deciding to become an ED nurse! The ED is one of the most versatile, yet challenging departments in the hospital. ED nurses get to do a lot and see even more. They may be the first person a patient interacts with when they come into the hospital and may be the last person to hold their hand. Being an ED nurse is an honor and a privilege.

First, we will discuss characteristics that make a great ED nurse. Some of these are characteristics that nurses already possess because of being a nurse in general, while other characteristics are developed over time and through experiences working in the ED. Every day nurses should strive to cultivate and refine each of these traits.

Compassion
Compassion is the feeling that arises when a person is confronted with another's suffering and feels motivated to relieve that suffering. Some might think this would go without saying. In the ED, staff see people and their families on what could be one of the worst days of their lives. The patients are sick, vulnerable, and scared. They do not know what is going on yet, why they are sick, or what their outlook is after their illness or injury. ED nurses bear witness to this fear and must remember that although this is just another day for those at work, it is not for the patients and their loved ones.

Flexibility
Being an ED nurse requires being flexible and adaptable to anything. In the ED environment, nurses care for a variety of patients of different races, ethnicities, religions, genders, and identities, as well as age groups, all who present with diverse acuity levels of various stages of different diseases. Many patients may have physical or intellectual disabilities, cognitive impairment, and/or varied health literacy. At one moment, the nurse could be caring for an older medical-surgical overflow patient, and the next, they could be the primary nurse for a pediatric patient who is in cardiac arrest. In the ED, being a little bit of every type of nurse at once is necessary because there is no way of knowing what type of patient will present next.

Teachability
Nursing school was a good foundation, but it does not teach nurses everything, and that is okay. Part of being a good nurse is recognizing limitations and knowing who to go to when help is needed. No one knows everything. Knowing limitations and resources will save time and will affect the patient's outcomes. Being an ED nurse is a team sport. Coworkers teach each other things they do not know or a new or different way to do something almost every day. Hospital staff have varied backgrounds and experiences, including different hospitals or other areas of specialty, before joining the ED, and they can be a wealth of knowledge, experience, tips, and tricks. As a new ED nurse, take everyone's advice and determine which best fits into practice. Having a "know it all" attitude is going to sell any nurse short in the long run. No one will ever know everything, and they are not supposed to.

Focus
The ED has a soundtrack entirely of its own. Call bells are going off; monitors and pumps are beeping; ventilators, in some cases, are sending off alarms; and, not to mention, coworkers, the patients, and their visitors all engaged in their own conversations. The stimulation can be constant. In high-acuity situations like a resuscitation, cardiac arrest, or trauma activations, there are often many people in the room. This is especially true in academic centers where staff are encouraged to respond to these activations as learning opportunities. In these situations, being able to focus is crucial.

Being task oriented is a critical part of ED nursing. Tuning out all the extra chatter and unnecessary noise is important to be able to accomplish the ED nurse role while still being an active member in the patient's care.

Problem-Solving and Troubleshooting

Troubleshooting is generally defined as the process of identifying, diagnosing, and resolving problems or issues. In the ED, that means solving problems such as finding equipment that has not been returned to its storage location, dealing with a supply being out of stock, or finding out the stock in hand is not working properly. A good ED nurse may have to troubleshoot by putting several things together just to make the one thing that is needed or, if that is not possible, making a call to other departments of the hospital to find that missing supply. Every hospital has different challenges and different equipment that a nurse will have to become familiar with during their time there.

FAST FACTS

- **Active listening:** To give someone your undivided attention; to make a conscious effort to understand and empathize with the person speaking.
- **Therapeutic silence:** Silence that allows the speaker to process their emotions and voice their thoughts at their own pace without the need to maintain the cadence of regular conversation.
- **Therapeutic touch:** "A form of complementary and alternative medicine based on the belief that vital energy flows through the human body. This energy is said to be balanced or made stronger by practitioners who pass their hands over, or gently touch, a patient's body" (National Cancer Institute [NCI], n.d.).
- **Closed-loop communication:** When the person receiving instructions or information repeats the information back to the speaker to ensure understanding.

Listening and Not Just Hearing

Listening is a huge part of being a nurse and not just in the ED. Active listening and therapeutic silence are important to incorporate in professional relationships both with colleagues and with patients and their families. Understanding why someone feels the way they do or noting small details in a patient's story can make all the difference in diagnosing and treating someone. Also allowing someone to just vent is important. When people come to the ED, they are often having a terrible time. Now this is not to say this is every case, but staff frequently are meeting people and their families on some of the hardest, most trying, most painful days of their lives. They are sick, they are scared, and they do not know what is happening or what to expect. Allowing someone to express those anxieties and concerns without feeling like they are being brushed off or not heard can make all the difference. With active listening comes closed-loop responses, therapeutic silence, and sometimes therapeutic touch when appropriate. Closed-loop responses help the other person to understand that they are being heard and the listener is processing it in a meaningful way. Sometimes, even more importantly, is just knowing when to be quiet and listen. There is not always something to say or a need to respond. Nodding and making direct eye contact when the other person participates will help to establish a safe space for them to speak. Holding someone's hand, offering them a hug, or placing a reassuring hand on their shoulder can help to build that connection between the nurse and a patient or their family member.

ADVOCACY

Being an advocate is something that is true throughout the entire hospital, not just the ED. Advocacy is such a large part of nursing that it will have to be broken down into sections. A nurse advocates for themselves, their patients, their families, and their coworkers.

Nurse

Part of advocating is knowing the nurse's scope of practice and hospital policies. Despite a nurse's scope of practice within their respective states, hospital policy varies by institution. It is important to know an individual's scope within their healthcare system and be sure to abide by this. Additionally, the nurse needs to understand if there are appropriate nurse-to-patient ratios that they need to abide by. If someone is asking for the ED nurse to take an assignment characterized by an unsafe nurse-to-patient ratio, the nurse must know what those ratios are and how to ensure the ratio is enforced. Making sure the nurse takes adequate breaks to have a glass of water, to have a snack, or to use the restroom is another form of advocacy that the nurse has to ensure for themselves in order to meet their personal needs.

Patient

When the nurse is at the bedside, they are the ones updating the provider on changes in the patient's condition. When a patient first arrives in the ED, staff often know minimal information. Information gathered from emergency medical services (EMS), as well as the report if it was called from another facility, and from the patient or family themselves is where most of the background comes from. If the patient has been to the facility before, providers can sometimes gather past medical history or a medication list from their chart. If the patient is unable to communicate or deteriorating rapidly, the initial presentation to the ED is crucial. While the team is working to get the patient settled, take a moment to glance over their medical history. Look for cues like congestive heart failure (CHF), chronic kidney disease, pulmonary diseases, and sepsis. If a provider is asking for fluid resuscitation on a patient because they are hypotensive from presumed sepsis but they have a history of CHF and edema, that would be an opportunity for the nurse to advocate for the patient and ask the provider to consider the volume of fluids. Ultimately, the nurse is the final safety check between an order and the patient. Over time, and with knowledge and experience, nurses develop a "gut instinct" that tells them whether something is appropriate. At work in a hospital with residents, there will be interns. After being a nurse for 4 years, a nurse will officially have been in the field longer than interns have been in medical school and have been doctors. This is not to say they are not knowledgeable and cautious about their orders. But everyone is human, and all make mistakes and have oversights. This experience will allow the nurse to advocate for their patient and themselves with the provider and have that interdisciplinary relationship. Knowing a patient's wishes or advance directives before they clinically deteriorate is critical. Advance directives are legally binding documents that outline the patient's wishes regarding medical decisions (House et al., 2023). There are several types of advance directives, and they can vary from state to state. Advance directives also may assign a person or several people the permission to enforce or make additional decisions for the patient in the event that the patient cannot make decisions for themselves (House et al., 2023). Establish the patient's wishes with them and the provider before situations become too drastic or intense. If the paitent has legal documentation regarding their wishes, have this either scanned into the chart and updated or readily available at the bedside. Make sure the patient has full mental capacity and is making fully informed decisions. Sometimes, this may require the nurse to ask the patient if they understand what is being asked of them or if they understand their impending procedure or the direction their care seems to be heading. "Do you understand the plan?" "Does what is happening make sense?" "Do you understand what you are agreeing to or what the provider is talking about?" "What questions do you have about x, y, and z?" Asking these questions is not only appropriate but is a huge part of advocating for the patient as a nurse. It is important to remember that patients have varying degrees of health literacy. Depending on geographic area or the population being served, patients may not have any higher education. Providers often use technical terms and can get lost in the nitty-gritty details of information. That is the opportunity as a nurse to take that technical information and translate it in a way that the patient can comprehend and understand.

Families

Advocating for families can be challenging. If a patient is not able to advocate for themselves, the responsibility falls to the next of kin or appointed person. If the patient has a large family, the shifting opinions and wishes of everyone can easily drown out the patient and/or their appointed healthcare proxy. Be available to the patient's appointed healthcare proxy or next of kin. It is important to answer questions to the best of the nurse's ability, and when the nurse reaches their extent of knowledge, call the provider to the bedside to answer any remaining questions. Much like making sure patients understand their circumstances, families or friends need to understand as well.

Coworkers

Nursing coworkers are each other's strongest allies and loudest cheerleaders. Being an ED nurse is a team sport. And that means that coworkers are each other's team members. This includes fellow nurses, nursing assistants or ED technicians, physicians, advanced practice providers, and everyone in between. Advocating for coworkers is part of being a team member. If there is a patient, family member or friend, or another coworker who is not being a good teammate, supporting coworkers in that situation can make a world of difference. Many hospitals are initiating a zero-tolerance policy for harassment and violence in the workplace. This goes for everyone who enters the hospital. No one has the right to harass, berate, abuse, belittle, or be condescending toward a nurse or their coworkers.

PURPOSE OF AND HOW TO USE THIS BOOK

ED nursing has evolved over the years, placing increased demands on the healthcare system. These demands have been rapidly and largely exacerbated by COVID-19. Primary care providers are sometimes difficult to find and hard to get in to see, leaving people to use the ED in their place. Flow issues that trickle down from increased lengths of stay on inpatient units, decreased outpatient resources for quicker discharge, and lack of staffing have put a strain on the ED by boarding admitted patients. ED nursing has evolved over the years, leading to increasing complexity of patient care, increased acuity of patients, and increased length of stay in the department, especially for critical patients.

This book is going to break down the different systems into chapters and talk about the emergencies that can arise from each of those systems. Signs and symptoms, characteristics, assessment findings, and treatment of many emergencies are reviewed. This book also touches on special populations and other special issues that are commonly seen in the ED. Each chapter has resources based on common topics or low-volume/high-risk conditions. At the end of the book is a section for taking notes to ask department educators questions to clarify understanding. Remember nurses will not know everything, but hopefully this book can fill in the gaps of knowledge they may have.

Lastly, after taking care of other people all day, self-care can often be overlooked. The ED can be tough some days. It can be dirty, loud, overstimulating, and taxing. ED staff are going to see people and their families on some of the worst days of their lives. There will be days where ED nurses feel like they did not do any emergency nursing, and there will be days where it will feel like they did nothing but emergency nursing. This can be a traumatic environment for patients and healthcare workers alike. It is crucial to remember to take care of oneself. Find healthy outlets for the situations encountered. Nurses constantly pour from their cup for others. They pour into their patients' cups and their patients' families' cups. They pour into their coworkers' cups. But they cannot pour from an empty cup; thus they must do things to fill their own cup. They cannot take care of others if they do not take care of themselves.

In the movie *A League of Their Own*, Tom Hanks said, "It's supposed to be hard. If it wasn't hard, everyone would do it. It's the hard that makes it great" (Marshall, 1992). And being an ED nurse? It is the greatest job in the world.

REVIEW QUESTIONS

1) What is the primary purpose of an advance directive?
    a. To identify a durable power of attorney for financial decisions only
    b. To outline a patient's wishes regarding medical care
    c. To authorize the hospital to make decisions on behalf of the patient
    d. To provide discharge instructions after a hospital stay
2) The ED nurse knows that repeating verbal orders back to the ordering provider is an example of:
    a. Open communication
    b. Active listening
    c. Closed-loop communication
    d. Therapeutic communication

REFERENCES

Brenan, M. (2024, February 7). *Nurses retain top ethics rating in U.S., but below 2020 high*. Gallup.com. https://news.gallup.com/poll/467804/nurses-retain-top-ethics-rating-below-2020-high.aspx

House, S. A., Schoo, C., & Ogilvie, W. (2023, August 8). *Advance directives*. In StatPearls [Internet]. StatPearls Publishing. Retrieved August 26, 2025, from https://www.ncbi.nlm.nih.gov/books/NBK459133/

Marshall, P. (1992, July 1). *A league of their own* [Film].Columbia Pictures.

National Cancer Institute. (n.d.). *NCI dictionary of cancer terms: therapeutic touch*. National Cancer Institute. https://www.cancer.gov/publications/dictionaries/cancer-terms/def/therapeutic-touch

U.S. Bureau of Labor Statistics. (2024, April 3). *Registered nurses*. U.S. Bureau of Labor Statistics. https://www.bls.gov/oes/current/oes291141.htm

Zippia. (2024, April 5). *Emergency room nurse demographics and statistics [2024]: Number of emergency room nurses in the* US. https://www.zippia.com/emergency-room-nurse-jobs/demographics/

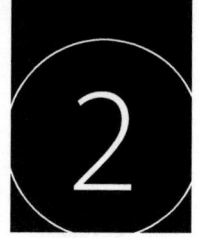

Triage

Sarah Berry

> *Triage is one of the most important skills an ED nurse must acquire. This is a skill that determines how sick someone is and how quickly they need to be evaluated by an advanced practitioner or physician. Experience and education are resources that will facilitate accurate triaging of patients. Over time, practice and comfort with triaging will increase your speed and improve your judgment.*

In this chapter, you will learn to:
1. Identify which patients can wait versus those who cannot wait by performing an "across-the-room" assessment
2. Identify different acuity systems and the emergency severity index (ESI) levels of triage
3. Differentiate between resources and nonresources to assign an ESI level
4. Conduct triage interventions and triage pediatric patients

INTRODUCTION

Although most EDs have a triage area, triage is not actually a place but a process. Triaging can take place anywhere, even starting in the parking lot. Triage is a French-derived word that means "to choose or to sort." Sorting sounds simple enough. So, what is the big deal? Well, the decisions made by the triage nurse determine the level of care and urgency in which a patient will be seen. For instance, a 21-year-old female presenting with severe right-sided abdominal pain is triaged as a level 3, or nonurgent. The triage nurse may think, "She is not that sick because she looks fine." The patient waits several hours while all the level 2, or urgent, patients are seen by the doctor. When the doctor finally sees the patient, she is now hypotensive and bleeding internally because her ectopic pregnancy ruptured. ED nurses are trained to hope for the best but anticipate the worst. With this anticipation, it can sometimes be hard to look at the objective and subjective information presented and not get carried away with the "what ifs." Additionally, the previous example is an excellent reason why reassessment of patients in the waiting room while they are waiting for evaluation is vital. Getting repeat vital signs on patients who are waiting for their initial evaluation, reevaluation, or a room in the department can indicate to the triage nurse a need to increase a patient's acuity to reflect their change in status. Studies show that repeating vital signs while in the waiting room could indicate impending deterioration in patients (Quinten et al., 2018). While wait times have increased in the ED, it leaves patients vulnerable in the waiting room. Notifying the charge nurse of any changes in patient acuity or status can also expedite their care. Decisions made in triage can directly affect patient outcomes. It sounds scary, but with the right training, experience, and critical thinking skills, ED nurses can master the art of triage.

It is important that ED nurses are well educated and comfortable with the facility-specific triage acuity system and documentation requirements. Triage protocols may vary from ED to ED, so knowing the institution-specific triage protocols is essential. All nurses must be aware of the Emergency Medical Treatment and Active Labor Act (EMTALA). EMTALA was essentially the first federal law that established that all people are entitled to a medical evaluation and basic treatment for medical emergencies, regardless of their ability to pay for treatment (Brown & Brown, 2019).

BEFORE A NURSE CAN TRIAGE

Additional education is required to work as a triage nurse. The weight of the decisions made by the triage nurse is heavy. Triage decisions require sound critical thinking skills, a strong nursing foundation, the ability to multitask, and excellent interpersonal skills. Most EDs require a triage nurse to have a certain amount of experience, specific certifications, and evidence of having taken a triage class or demonstrated competency. The Emergency Nurses Association (ENA) recommends that triage be conducted by an RN or nurse practitioner who has at least 1 year of experience and received formal triage training (Stone & Wolf, 2018). Additionally, certification as a board-certified emergency nurse (BCEN) and certification in pediatric, cardiac, and/or trauma care are also recommended. Take the initiative to find out what competencies are required and what triage classes are available at your facility, and sign up for them as soon as you are eligible. Speak with the unit educator about opportunities to better prepare for triage. In addition to education provided by the department, it can be beneficial to shadow an experienced triage nurse to understand their decision-making process.

SAFETY FIRST

While triage can occur anywhere, it commonly occurs at the entry points of the ED. Essentially, the triage nurse is the front line. Triage nurses must consider the safety of the patients and themselves first. For example, become familiar with the hospital's infection prevention policies regarding triage. Ask the appropriate travel screening questions at the designated time of the patient's arrival and document them. If a patient arrives with symptoms of a respiratory or airborne infection, initiate airborne precautions according to hospital policy. Have the patient wear a mask, and assign patients to a negative-pressure room where indicated. Another consideration for infection control are patients who present with specific types of rashes, such as shingles or measles. Initiating appropriate isolation precautions and making those of childbearing age aware of possible exposure is crucial. Especially with shingles, those who are pregnant, may be pregnant, or have special populations at home, such as immunocompromised, very young, or older family members, should be notified of possible exposure to patients with open lesions (Centers for Disease Control and Prevention, 2025). Failing to do so may result in spreading infections to others and themselves.

An additional safety concern to take into consideration is the proximity. Depending on where triage takes place in the ED, the "triage room" may be quite small. When in a small space with someone who is potentially angry or upset about the wait time, someone who is in pain and is having a hard time expressing themselves in a safe manner, someone who is being encouraged by family to be evaluated when they do not want to be or feel they need to be, or someone who is being brought in by police, there is an inherent risk for safety. It is critical for the nurse to be continuously aware of the space between them and the patient, the patient's body language, and their behavior. Open the door to the triage space and participate in verbal redirection. If the patient or their visitors continue to escalate, reach out for a coworker to be present until security can be notified.

TRIAGE ACUITY SYSTEMS

There are a variety of triage acuity systems. A triage acuity system is a rapid way for the nurse (or other qualified healthcare provider) to determine the severity of a patient's need for medical attention and any life-threatening conditions or injuries. It also helps to determine who needs treatment or attention first in the event that multiple people need to be evaluated, like in a busy ED waiting room (Yancey & O'Rourke, 2023). While one ED may use a five-level triage acuity system, one of the neighboring EDs may be using a three-level triage acuity system. The first thing the nurse must do is identify the triage system that is being using. Table 2.1 demonstrates some of the differences among the various systems.

Emergency Severity Index

Although there are many different triage systems, the latest evidence by the ENA supports the use of a five-level system such as the ESI. The ESI algorithm is used by approximately 94% of U.S. hospitals, making it the most used severity index (ENA, 2024). Similar five-level triage scales are the Canadian Triage and Acuity Scale, Australian Triage Scale, and Manchester Triage System.

TABLE 2.1

Comparing Triage Systems

Level	Five-Level Systems	Four-Level Systems	Three-Level Systems	Two-Level Systems
1	Resuscitation	Life threatening	Emergent	Emergent
2	Emergent	Emergent	Urgent	Nonemergent
3	Urgent	Urgent	Nonurgent	
4	Nonurgent	Nonurgent		
5	Referred			

Note: Level 1 or resuscitation: Requires immediate lifesaving interventions; *Level 2* or emergent: A high-risk situation, confused/lethargic/disoriented patient, in severe pain or distress, or has dangerously abnormal vital signs; *Level 3* or urgent: Requires many resources; *Level 4* or nonurgent: Requires just one resource; *Level 5* or referred: Requires no resources.

FAST FACTS

The triage process should take about 2 to 5 minutes per patient. With experience, confidence, accuracy, and speed will improve.

Choosing an Acuity Level

Now that the triage system has been established, the nurse will need specific information to select the appropriate acuity level. First, they will need an "across-the-room" assessment, followed by a chief complaint, interview with patient, vital signs, and focused physical exam.

- *Across-the-room assessment:* This is exactly as it reads. What does the nurse see when they look across the room as the patient approaches the triage desk? In order to do this well, the triage nurse must be in a position to view the entire waiting room. Things to assess include the following:
- *General appearance:* Is the patient(s) alert or unresponsive, crying, laughing, or talking and speaking with or without difficulty? Are there any obvious deformities or bloody clothing?
- *Work of breathing:* Is there labored or unlabored breathing, coughing, drooling, gasping, wheezing, rapid or slow respiratory rate, or use of accessory muscles?
- *Circulation:* Is the skin pink or pale, diaphoretic, cyanotic, ashen or gray, flushed, normal, or jaundiced?

If an unstable patient enters the waiting room, do not delay care. If they are unstable, bypass the triage area altogether and take the patient to a bed to begin treatment. For example, if a family member wheels a pale, diaphoretic, unresponsive patient into the waiting room, do *not* stop to take vital signs and interview the patient. The patient is unresponsive. Bring the patient back for treatment immediately. This patient would be given an acuity level of 1 because they require immediate resuscitation or lifesaving intervention.

Remember, triage is a process, not a place; it can be done simultaneously as the patient receives care.

Another important aspect of triaging is multitasking by hooking the patient up to the monitor and starting the interview simultaneously. "Hi, my name is [your name] I'm going to be your triage nurse. Tell me, what brings you to the ED today?" While obtaining vital signs and gathering their overall appearance, listen to their story and write the triage note. Use direct quotes when appropriate. Ask open-ended questions that elicit information about their issue. Has the patient been having this issue for weeks, months, or years? Do not be afraid to ask them, "So what made it an emergency today?" Asking this question is not meant to be insensitive or critical of their visit. Sometimes, the change in their symptoms that made them want to be seen today can make or break your acuity level or uncover information needed to make a more informed decision.

- *Elicit the chief complaint:* The first question to ask is, "What brought you in to see us today?" Certain chief complaints can carry higher risks than others. For example, chest pain would be a higher-risk chief complaint than toe injury. The patient with chest pain could be having a fatal myocardial infarction, whereas toe injuries, though painful, are not usually fatal.
- *Interview the patient:* Triage is not the time to conduct an entire head-to-toe assessment. Your goal in triage is to elicit the essential facts needed to make an acuity decision. You should be asking questions that relate to the chief complaint. Look over the triage document at your facility. Most ED triage screening tools include the following:
  - Duration of the chief complaint
  - Related symptoms
  - Mechanism of injury
  - Medical history
  - Current medications (prescription or nonprescription), including anticoagulants
  - Immunizations (tetanus, influenza)
  - Last menstrual period
  - Allergies
  - Height and weight
  - Department-specific screening questions
- *Obtain vital signs:* Vital signs can influence your final acuity selection. If the patient looks fine, has a normal exam result, and tells you, "I just feel anxious," you might not think too much of it. But once you take the patient's heart rate and it is 200, you will think differently. Be sure to memorize the different age-specific normal average vital signs shown in Table 2.2.
- *Conduct a focused physical assessment:* Now that you have collected your subjective data (what the patient says), it is time to document what you see (objective data). If the patient tells you, "I twisted my ankle," remove their socks and shoes and document what the ankle looks like: Is it swollen, obviously deformed, ecchymotic, and edematous? Is it tender upon palpation? Are distal pulses present? Is the patient ambulatory? Is sensation intact? Is motor intact?

TABLE 2.2
Age-Specific Normal Vital Signs

Age	Newborn	Infant	Toddler	Preschooler	School Age	Adolescent	Adult
Respirations	30–60	30–45	20–30	20–25	14–22	12–18	12–18
Heart rate	110–160	100–150	80–125	70–115	60–100	60–100	60–100
Systolic BP	65–85	70–100	90–105	95–110	100–120	100–120	90–120

BP, blood pressure.
Source: Adapted from Cleveland Clinic. (2024, April 30). *Pediatric vital signs & what they tell you.* https://health.clevelandclinic.org/pediatric-vital-signs.

TABLE 2.3

Resources Versus Nonresources

Resources	Nonresources
■ Laboratory tests (blood, urine, respiratory or specimen swabs) ■ EKGs, imaging (CT, x-ray, MRI, and ultrasound) ■ IV fluids ■ IV, IM, or nebulized medications ■ Specialty consultation ■ Simple procedure—one resource 　■ Laceration repair, Foley insertion ■ Complex procedure—two resources 　■ Requiring conscious sedation	■ History and physical 　■ Including pelvic exam or MSE ■ Point-of-care testing 　■ Glucose, HCG, PT/INR, blood gases, electrolytes, and blood composition ■ IV insertion with saline lock ■ PO medications, metered-dose inhalers ■ Tetanus immunization (IM injection) ■ Prescription refills ■ Phone call or message to PCP ■ Simple wound care 　■ Dressing or wound check ■ Crutches, splints, or slings

HCG, human chorionic gonadotropin; IM, intramuscular; MSE, medical screening exam; PCP, phencyclidine; PO, by mouth; PT/INR, prothrombin time/international normalized ratio.
Source: Adapted from Wolf, L., Ceci, K., McCallum, D., & Brecher, D. (2023). Emergency severity index handbook (5th ed.). Emergency Nurses Association.

Resources

The next question asked is, "What exactly is a resource?" Resources consist of laboratory tests, imaging, specialty consults, simple procedures, IV fluids or medications, intramuscular (IM) medications, and inhaled medications. Complex procedures such as moderate sedation count as two resources. However, do not be fooled! Some interventions do *not* actually count as a resource. These include simple IV access, pelvic exam, point-of-care testing, by mouth (PO) medications, a consult to the patient's primary physician, simple dressings, slings, crutches, and splints. Point-of-care testing varies greatly by facility of what tests are available, situations in which they are used, and staff who are competent to perform them. Oftentimes, when patients are assigned a higher ESI level, how many resources the triage nurse is anticipating that they require plays a large role in that assignment. When patients are sicker, they require more resources, leading to a higher ESI level. Therefore, one could conclude that patient is going to require more care, leading to a heavier lean on that nurse's assignment. See Table 2.3.

TRIAGE INTERVENTIONS

Triage simply means to sort, but at times you will need to implement some basic interventions. These interventions may include basic life support, cervical immobilization, isolation procedures, some medications (e.g., aspirin for chest pain), EKG (should precede the triage of a patient with chest pain), point-of-care blood glucose, and simple wound care (e.g., splinting or ice packs).

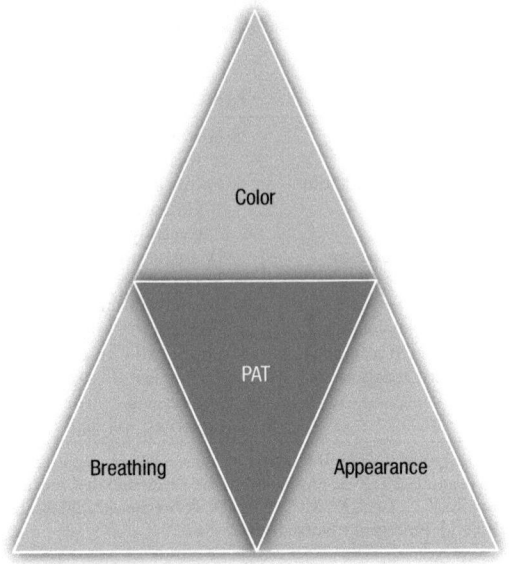

Figure 2.1 Pediatric assessment triangle (PAT).

Pediatrics

Performing triage with pediatric patients is different from performing triage with adults. Treat the patient and the family as one unit. Use of the pediatric assessment triangle (PAT) will help you quickly determine which child is the sickest (see Figure 2.1). If all components of the PAT are stable, the child is sick on the basis of concerns of the caregiver. Disruption in one component of the PAT means the child is sicker. Disruption in two or more components of the PAT indicates that this is the sickest child. Typically, it is best to start with the least invasive assessment and interventions and end with the most invasive. For example, a rectal temperature may cause the infant to cry, interfering with observational assessments. Provide honest answers with kid-friendly words. Be familiar with the normal vital signs for each age group. Obtain actual weights rather than the parent's report of the weight at the last provider visit.

Children who are grunting, stridorous, using accessory muscles, have sunken or bulging fontanels, or have any petechial or purpuric rashes especially with mental status changes, are pediatric red flags. Fevers could be caused by multiple sources and therefore often require more resources to rule out potential causes.

FAST FACTS

Pediatric medications and fluids are weight based. An accurate weight is crucial for dosing.

Infants

To best assess an infant, the nurse must inspect their skin. When weighing the infant on the baby scale, the nurse should get them down to their diaper and take the opportunity to assess their skin and work of breathing. Obtain a rectal temperature at this time and note if their diaper is wet or dry. Allow the caregiver to hold the infant or child throughout the triage process to decrease stress and anxiety. Remember, you are a stranger, and you are poking at them when they do not feel well.

A good way to quickly triage an infant or toddler is by assessing their general appearance. Begin by waking the child to determine if they are sleeping or unconscious. Assess muscle **T**one, **I**nteractivity, **C**onsolability, **L**ook or gaze, and **S**peech or cry, using the mnemonic **TICLS** (Foley & Dodge, 2023). While assessing for TICLS, watch for neonate red flags (addressed in Box 2.1).

Box 2.1 RED FLAGS FOR TRIAGING NEONATES

- Lethargy
    - A baby who is not awake enough to interact is not awake enough to feed or feed well.
    - Increased sleepiness or lethargy might indicate infection, high bilirubin, or congenital heart defects (CHDs).
- Decreased PO intake
    - Poor feeding or poor sucking coordination can lead to hypoglycemia or be a sign of current hypoglycemia; check a blood glucose if you are concerned about hypoglycemia.
- Bilious vomiting
    - A midgut volvulus is most common in infants, although it can occur at any age.
    - Ninety-seven percent of infants diagnosed with malrotation report bilious or green vomit as the primary symptom.
    - A volvulus could lead to decreased circulation in the mesenteric artery.
- Hypothermia
    - Hypothermia activates the hypothalamus, causing a release of norepinephrine.

(continued)

> **Box 2.1 (continued)**
>
> - This release causes an increase in oxygen consumption and respiratory rate to meet an increase in metabolic demand, which leads to glucose consumption.
> - Hypothermia is more common than fever in the setting of infection or sepsis.
> - Fevers
>   - Like hypothermia, fever causes a release of norepinephrine, breaking down brown fat to create heat.
>   - Nonshivering thermogenesis is used to maintain body heat and follows hypothermia.
> - Jaundice
>   - Increased bilirubin causes jaundice, a yellowing of skin and eyes, usually seen in the conjunctiva first.
>   - Acceptable jaundice levels can be calculated and are displayed on a curve based on bilirubin level and exact age.
>   - Jaundice that is noticeable within the first 24 hours of life is a significant cause for concern; additionally, appearance after 2 weeks of age or worsening jaundice at any age is a red flag.
> - CHD
>   - Common signs of CHDs are weight loss or poor weight gain, poor feeding, and poor breathing (retractions and tachypnea).
>   - Perform pulse oximetry on the right hand, then compare it to either foot; this is a fast tool to determine possible CHDs that have not been diagnosed yet.
> - Seizures
>   - Normal symptoms of seizures are not present in neonates because their brains are not fully developed yet.
>   - The most common signs are lip smacking, horizontal eye movement, sustained eye deviation, abnormal tongue movements, pedaling, and apnea.
>   - Approximately 60% of seizures are caused by hypoxia.
>
> *Source*: Modified from Foley, A., & Dodge, T. (2023). Neonatal triage red flags. *Journal of Emergency Nursing, 49*(6), 811–813. https://doi.org/10.1016/j.jen.2023.08.007

Additional assessments of children include observing how the child is interacting with their environment. Are they curious about what you are doing? Are they playful or withdrawn? Are they behaving ageappropriately? Are they disinterested or lethargic? You can tell a lot about a child, at any age, by how they interact with their environment. Use kid-friendly terms and explanations: "Listen for the birdy" when taking their temperature; "Look at the red light; it is like Rudolph's nose" when measuring a pulse oximetry and heart rate; "This is going to give you a big hug, hold as still as a statue" when obtaining a blood pressure (BP). Children also mimic their environment. Play the statue game with the child to obtain their BP if they are not in immediate, acute distress.

As children age, it is important to make them an active member of their care team. Toddlers and older children are generally able to tell broad information that becomes more specific depending on the age of the child. Ask the patient directly, "What hurts? How do you feel? or Point to where it hurts," and then ask the parents to supplement information as needed. Allowing this independence helps the child feel involved and more in control of the situation. As children get older, hold them accountable for their care. School-age children to teenagers should be given more independence in the description of their signs and symptoms, because they are the ones who are feeling and experiencing it. If you notice that you have a patient who is school age or older, be cognizant that part of your triage may include asking sensitive questions like menstrual cycle, chances of pregnancy or sexual activity, drugs and alcohol consumption, domestic violence issues, or thoughts of suicide. Statements and questions such as, "I have some questions to ask you that might be a little personal. Are you okay with [parent or caregiver] staying for them, or would you like them to step out for a moment?" allow the patient the opportunity to have their parents or caregivers leave the room to maintain their privacy in these instances.

LEGAL ISSUES

As the triage nurse, "hospitality" is your middle name. By law, any healthcare professional cannot turn any patient away or even discourage them from seeking emergency medical care. The EMTALA is known as the federal "antidumping" law. It was enacted in 1986 to prohibit hospitals from refusing to see or to transfer financially "undesirable" patients. Prior to this law, patients died in the back of ambulances driving from hospital to hospital, seeking an accepting facility. Under EMTALA, hospitals are obligated to provide a nondiscriminatory medical screening exam (MSE) to any patient seeking care within 250 yards of the hospital. Understand that a triage assessment is not typically the same as an MSE unless a provider is at triage. If a medical emergency condition exists, the hospital is obligated to provide stabilizing interventions and appropriate transfers when indicated. Failure to uphold this law can result in a fine of $50,000 or more. These laws also apply to any pregnant person in active labor.

Additionally, keep in mind that any person who presents to the hospital seeking medical care must be screened and have an MSE completed by a qualified provider. This also includes minors and those seeking help for mental health or substance abuse. An essential component of being a great triage nurse is knowing your local and state regulations regarding emancipation and care of minor patients and those individuals with decreased mental capacities. Take the time to look up your state or governing authority's laws regarding legal age for consent. Some exceptions may include emergency medical conditions, minors seeking mental health treatment versus medical treatment, emancipated minors, reproductive issues, sexually transmitted infections, drug abuse, or abortion.

Language barriers can cause miscommunications in triage. Be sure to only use hospital-approved translators or language phone services. The patient's family members are *not* legal translators, do not allow patient privacy, and may not translate correctly. Document any use of a translator or language phone service.

One of the patient's rights is the right to privacy and confidential care. Be sure to interview patients in as private an area as possible. This may mean pulling the curtain closed or closing the door. It is important that the nurse notifies the patient that they will be asking personal questions and ask if they would like any visitors to leave during the interview. Make sure the volume of conversation is appropriate.

FAST FACTS

When screening for domestic violence, be mindful of those who are with the patient. If you are concerned about possible safety issues, find a way to ask the patient about their safety in private.

COMMON PITFALLS OF TRIAGE

After spending some time in triage, the nurse may think to themselves, "Oh, this is not so hard, I've got this." But tread carefully; even the most experienced ED nurse can be fooled. Following is a list of everyday chief complaints or issues that at first glance appear simple or vague. However, these might actually be much more emergent than they appear. In triage, you must always assume the worst-case scenario and ask questions to rule out that "worst-case" possibility:

- "I feel weak" or "I am dizzy."
  - *What the nurse might be thinking:* This is a vague complaint. It could just be the flu, a virus, heat exhaustion, or a fever.
  - *What they should be thinking*: What are the worst things that could make someone feel weak or dizzy? Hypoglycemia, hyperglycemia, dehydration, hypotension or hypertension, hypoxia, sepsis, myocardial infarction, stroke, or arrhythmias are possibilities.
- "I have a headache."
  - *What the nurse might be thinking*: So do I. Are you sensitive to lights or sounds? Is this "the worst headache of your life"?
  - *What they should be thinking*: What is the worst thing this could be? Hypertensive emergency, meningitis, intracerebral bleed, brain tumor, head injury, or concussion. What is the patient's neurological status? What is their BP? How suddenly did this headache start, and

what associated symptoms do they have? Any nausea, vomiting, or photophobia?
- The patient does not look very sick.
  - *What the nurse might be thinking*: If the patient looks fine, it cannot be that bad.
  - *What they should be thinking*: Legally, their opinion does not matter. Look at the subjective and objective data. Is this a high-risk situation?

Example: A seasoned triage nurse once performed triage with a 65-year-old male with no significant medical history and a short daily medication list that consisted primarily of vitamins and supplements. He came in with intermittent feelings of fluttering in his chest that went away with rest. It had been ongoing for a few weeks, so they asked him, "If this has been going on for a few weeks, what made today an emergency?" He went on to tell her that the episodes were lasting longer, not going away with rest, and he was feeling tired and a little anxious. He was not one to experience anxiety, and this was concerning to him. The pulse oximeter read a heart rate of 200. It was later discovered he was going into supraventricular tachycardia. He was otherwise well appearing. He had good color, no increased work of breathing, or diaphoresis. He drove himself and walked into the ED. Making him an acuity level 1 was appropriate because shortly after he got to an exam room, he became hypotensive.

- "I fell."
  - *What the nurse might be thinking*: Treat the injury. If the bleeding is controlled, everything is okay. Ground-level falls are not dangerous.
  - *What they should be thinking*: Why did the patient fall? Syncope, hypoglycemia, stroke, hypotension, sepsis, medication related, or arrhythmia. Was the patient dizzy or weak before the fall, or did they trip and fall? Did the patient lose consciousness? If so, which came first: the fall and then the loss of consciousness (LOC) or LOC and then the fall? Is a head or C-spine (cervical spine) injury involved? Is the patient taking anticoagulants? What is the neurological status? Did the patient consume any alcohol or drugs beforehand? Does the patient have a heart condition?
- "My doctor told me to come here."
  - *What the nurse might be thinking*: Those primary care doctors send all their patients here with no information and likely before they finished their office or call note, so I also have no idea why they are here.
  - *What they should be thinking*: What is the phone number to the primary physician? What tests were performed at the office? What symptoms made the patient call their doctor today? Why did they see their primary care provider in the first place to have something done to land them in the ED? Some patients go to the doctor when they should come to the ED.
- The patient is not telling you the whole story.
  - *What the nurse might be thinking*: This does not make any sense. The symptoms do not align with what the patient is saying.
  - *What they should be thinking*: What is the patient's neurological status? Why does this person think they cannot tell me what is really

wrong? Are they fearful of the person accompanying them to the ED? Did the patient consume any alcohol or drugs? Do they think I will call the police? Perhaps they think insurance will not pay, or they may be too embarrassed.

- "I feel anxious."
  - *What the nurse might be thinking*: Oh, she has a history of panic attacks; it is just a panic attack. Slam dunk.
  - *What they should be thinking*: Anxious people get sick too. Is this a normal anxious feeling, or is it different? Hypoxia, anaphylaxis, a cardiac event, a cerebrovascular accident, and even things that are very painful such as bowel obstruction or kidney stones can cause a person to appear "anxious."
- "I have back pain."
  - *What the nurse might be thinking*: Another patient with back pain. I bet it has been hurting for years.
  - *What they should be thinking*: Kidney stones, shingles, pyelonephritis, dissecting renal or thoracic aneurysm, or a spinal injury are possibilities Has the patient lost control of their bowels or bladder? Does the pain radiate to the groin or leg? Are there any urinary problems? Is paralysis noted on assessment? Did the pain occur suddenly or gradually?
- "I have been vomiting."
  - *What the nurse might be thinking*: They just need some Zofran and ginger ale and they can go home. It is just another stomach flu.
  - *What they should be thinking*: What is the worst-case scenario of what this could be? Diabetic ketoacidosis, chemotherapy, bowel obstruction, increased intracranial pressure, cardiac problem, food poisoning, or pregnancy are possibilities. Consider how many times the patient vomited. What is the result of too much vomiting? Electrolyte imbalance and dehydration.
- "My throat is really sore."
  - *What the nurse might be thinking*: It is just strep throat or tonsillitis. I do not really need to look at their tonsils; the doctor will do that. This is a young, healthy patient.
  - *What they should be thinking*: What is the worst-case scenario of what this could be? Allergic reaction with swelling to the mouth and airway, toxic ingestion, foreign body ingestion, epiglottitis, or peritonsillar abscess are possibilities.

FAST FACTS

Excessive salivation could indicate epiglottitis or possible esophageal obstruction. If not acted on in a timely manner, the salivation could evolve into respiratory distress due to the inability to clear secretions, especially if the patient is altered.

SUMMARY

After reading this chapter, hopefully you have gained some of the tools necessary to triage effectively. When used properly, new triage skills provide communication of care needed across the entire ED. With practice, the ED nurse's triage skills will improve, and they will easily identify which patients can wait and which patients cannot wait, differentiate the levels of triage acuity, perform an across-the-room assessment, and list the common pitfalls of triage. Be sure to review each facility's triage requirements and policies. Stick to the facts and the triage algorithm; do not let opinions or biases sway the chosen ESI level. Just because something is common does not mean that it is normal. Although it may take time to qualify for triage training, the ED nurse may find it helpful to observe the triage operation and process during orientation and practice with an experienced preceptor.

REVIEW QUESTIONS

1) What is the most accurate way to obtain an infant weight?
    a. On an infant scale, after removing their clothes and diaper
    b. Have the caregiver hold the infant and obtain a weight; then remove the infant from the caregiver and obtain another weight; subtract them, and the result is the baby's weight.
    c. Lay the infant on the standard scale clothed because it is dirty from other patients' shoes.
    d. On an infant scale, in their onesie, because their caregiver reported fever and chills
2) Which patient should be assigned an acuity level of 2?
    a. A 58-year-old male who requires an artificial airway immediately
    b. A 65-year-old female with a history of coronary artery disease and hypertension presenting with crushing chest pain, diaphoresis, and nausea
    c. A 2-year-old male with rhinorrhea, cough, and an axillary temperature of 100.3°F
    d. A 14-year-old female with diffuse abdominal pain, nausea, vomiting, diarrhea, and stable vital signs
3) How long should triage take?
    a. Triage should take as long as needed to gather all the information required to make a diagnosis.
    b. Triage should be able to be completed without actually having to speak to the patient, on the basis of your "assessment from the door."
    c. Triage should be completed in about 10 to 15 minutes.
    d. Triage should be completed in about 2 to 5 minutes.

REFERENCES

Brown, H. L., & Brown, T. B. (2019, July). EMTALA: The evolution of emergency care in the United States. *Journal of Emergency Nursing, 45*(4), 411–414. Retrieved August 26, 2025, from https://doi.org/10.1016/j.jen.2019.02.002

Centers for Disease Control and Prevention (2025). *About shingles (herpes zoster).* https://www.cdc.gov/shingles/about/index.html

Emergency Nurses Association University: Triage. (2024). *ENA's triage offerings.* https://www.ena.org/enau/educational-offerings/triage?https%3A%2F%2Fwww.ena.org&gad_source=1&gclid=CjwKCAjwydSzBhBOEiwAj0XN4MAnv8eORb7QrekVycD0RW2wzRYplg0zueOKy2JSjHuf2g2cvisi8RoCB9gQAvD_BwE#esi

Foley, A., & Dodge, T. (2023). Neonatal triage Red flags. *Journal of Emergency Nursing, 49*(6), 811–813. https://doi.org/10.1016/j.jen.2023.08.007

Quinten, V. M., van Meurs, M., Olgers, T. J., Vonk, J. M., Ligtenberg, J. J., & ter Maaten, J. C. (2018). Repeated vital sign measurements in the emergency department predict patient deterioration within 72 hours: A prospective observational study. *Scandinavian Journal of Trauma, Resuscitation and Emergency Medicine, 26*(1), 57. https://doi.org/10.1186/s13049-018-0525-y

Stone, E., & Wolf, L. (2018, February). *Triage qualifications and competency position statement.* Emergency Nurses Association.

Yancey, C., & O'Rourke, M. (2023, August 28). *Emergency department triage.* StatPearls [Internet]. Retrieved August 26, 2025, from https://www.ncbi.nlm.nih.gov/books/NBK557583/

Acid–Base Imbalances

Alexander Menard

The body requires a delicate balance of acids and bases to maintain natural homeostasis. Many life-threatening illnesses affect the acid–base balance. As a nurse in the ED, you will come across acid–base imbalances daily. Therefore, recognizing any acid–base imbalance is crucial to improving outcomes and even saving someone's life.

In this chapter, you will learn to:
1. Discuss the pathophysiology behind acid–base disturbances
2. Interpret arterial blood gases (ABGs)
3. Anticipate interventions to address acid–base disturbances

ACID–BASE DISTURBANCES

Acid–base balance is controlled by two organ systems: the respiratory system and renal system.

Patients breathe in oxygen (O_2) and breathe out carbon dioxide (CO_2). In the bloodstream, CO_2 mixes with water (H_2O) to make carbonic acid (H_2CO_3). H_2CO_3 dissociates into a base, a bicarbonate (HCO_3^-), and an acid (H^+), which is excreted or conserved by the kidneys. Normal pH of plasma contains a ratio of 20 bicarbonates to 1 carbonic acid. The normal range for arterial blood is a pH of 7.35 to 7.45, a partial pressure of arterial carbon dioxide ($PaCO_2$) is 35 to 45, and an HCO_3^- is 22 to 26 (Yee et al., 2022). The pH of venous blood gases are typically 0.03 to 0.04 less than ANG values.

The oxyhemoglobin dissociation curve demonstrates how changes in pH and/or body temperature directly impact O_2 affinity for hemoglobin (Figure 3.1). Acidosis and hyperthermia reduce oxyhemoglobin affinity, whereas alkalosis and hypothermia increase the tight bonds of oxyhemoglobin instead of exchanging with the peripheral tissues. Alkalosis and hypothermia can result in poor O_2 exchange.

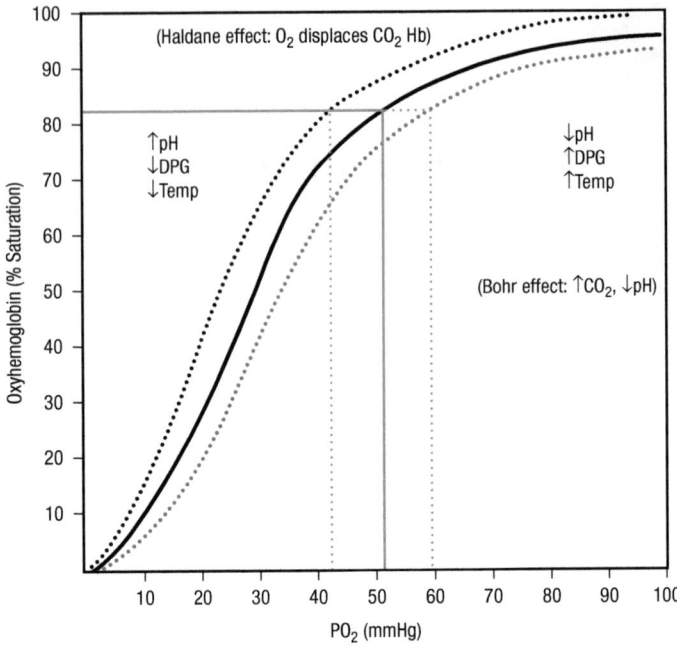

Figure 3.1 Oxyhemoglobin dissociation curve.

CO_2, carbon dioxide; DPG, diphosphoglycerate; O_2, oxygen; PO_2, partial pressure of oxygen.
Source: Ratznium. *Oxyhaemoglobin dissociation curve*.

RECOGNIZING AN IMBALANCE

An easy way to remember whether your patient has a respiratory or metabolic imbalance is with the simple mnemonic **ROME**. **R**espiratory is **O**pposite (pH and CO_2), **M**etabolic is **E**qual (pH and HCO_3^-). The arrows in Table 3.1 for respiratory pH and $PaCO_2$ are in opposite directions from each other, and the arrows for metabolic pH and HCO_3^- point in the same direction.

Every acid–base imbalance is described with three words, such as uncompensated respiratory acidosis. To determine which imbalance the patient has, follow these three simple steps:

- Step 1: Evaluate the pH. If it is normal (7.35–7.45), it is *compensated*. If it is out of range, it is *uncompensated*.
- Step 2: A pH <7.35 is *acidosis*. A pH >7.45 is *alkalosis*.
- Step 3: Evaluate the $PaCO_2$ and HCO_3^-. Abnormal $PaCO_2$ = respiratory. Abnormal HCO_3^- = metabolic. If both are abnormal, it is both respiratory and metabolic.

Common acid–base disorder patient presentations are described in Table 3.2.

TABLE 3.1
Interpreting Values From an ABG

Acid–Base Disorder	pH (7.35–7.45)	CO_2 (35–45 mmHg)	HCO_3^- 22–26 mEq/L
Respiratory acidosis	<7.35	↑	Normal or ↑
Respiratory alkalosis	>7.45	↓	Normal or ↓
Metabolic acidosis	<7.35	Normal or ↓	↓
Metabolic alkalosis	>7.45	Normal or ↑	↑

ABG, arterial blood gas; CO_2, carbon dioxide; HCO_3^-, bicarbonate.

TABLE 3.2
Common Acid–Base Disorder Patient Presentations

Acid–Base Disorder	Classic Presentation
Respiratory acidosis	A 53-year-old female presents with family to the ED due to excessive sleepiness. The family confirms that she had a recent surgery and has been taking narcotics frequently for uncontrolled pain. Her ABG reveals pH 7.21, $PaCO_2$ 75 mmHg, PaO_2 52 mmHg, and HCO_3^- 26.
Respiratory alkalosis	A 23-year-old male presents to the ED after a motor vehicle crash resulting in multiple lower extremity fractures. He reports his pain is 10/10. He is hyperventilating. His ABG reveals pH 7.55, $PaCO_2$ 23 mmHg, PaO_2 110 mmHg, and HCO_3^- 23.
Metabolic acidosis	A 72-year-old female presents for evaluation of shortness of breath, fever, and productive cough. She is found to be hypotensive with a lactic acid of 5.6 mmol/L. Her ABG reveals pH 7.17, $PaCO_2$ 22 mmHg, PaO_2 59 mmHg, and HCO_3^- 15.
Metabolic alkalosis	An 80-year-old female with a history of heart failure (ejection fraction of 35%) presents to the ED with a heart failure exacerbation. She underwent aggressive diuresis. Her ABG reveals pH of 7.54, $PaCO_2$ 55 mmHg, PaO_2 72 mmHg, and HCO_3^- 38.

ABG, arterial blood gas; HCO_3^-, bicarbonate; $PaCO_2$, partial pressure of arterial carbon dioxide; PaO_2, partial pressure of oxygen.

Respiratory Acidosis

In respiratory acidosis, pH is <7.35 because of inadequate ventilation. The primary driving factor is the buildup of CO_2. Poor ventilation can cause poor oxygenation and the patient to retain CO_2 (Patel & Sharma, 2024). That means O_2 cannot get in and CO_2 cannot get out. CO_2 builds up and mixes with H_2O, resulting in H_2CO_3 lowering pH. HCO_3^- is normal. This patient is at risk for hypoxia.

- *Causes:* Upper airway obstruction; pulmonary edema; hypoventilation; head trauma; chest trauma; pneumonia; chronic obstructive pulmonary disease (COPD); narcotic overdose; and muscle weakness.
- *Signs and symptoms:* Tachycardia; headache; decreased pulse oximetry reading; increased end-tidal carbon dioxide ($etCO_2$) >45 mmHg; confusion; weakness; coma; hyperkalemia; cyanosis; bradypnea; paralysis; and respiratory arrest.
- *Interventions:* Administer O_2; give nebulized breathing treatments; treat underlying condition; prepare for noninvasive ventilation or intubation for severe hypercarbia resulting in pH < 7.2; provide mechanical ventilation; measure pulse oximetry; monitor cardiac rhythm; and obtain IV access.
- *Caveat:* Patients with chronic hypercarbia from COPD should not be overcorrected. The goal is to normalize the pH for these patients. Check the chart to identify baseline CO_2.

Respiratory Alkalosis

In respiratory alkalosis, the pH is >7.45. When a person hyperventilates, they expel CO_2. There is no CO_2 left to mix with H_2O to make H_2CO_3 (Brinkman & Sharma, 2024). A reduction in acid will lead to alkalosis. HCO_3^- will be normal.

- *Causes:* Hyperventilation; pain; anxiety; pulmonary embolus; hypoxia; high altitude; drug toxicity (early salicylate adult overdose); third-trimester pregnancy; and fever.
- *Signs and symptoms:* Tetany or seizures from hypocalcemia; hypokalemia, diaphoresis; tingling of extremities; decrease in $etCO_2$ <35 mmHg; dizziness; altered mental status; anxiety; dyspnea; paresthesia; palpitations; tachycardia; and hyperventilation.
- *Interventions:* Treat the underlying condition. Encourage slower breathing. Manage anxiety with nonpharmacological interventions such as de-escalation techniques, guided imagery, family presence, and so forth.
- *Caveat:* Do not sedate these patients, as this can cause other sequelae.

FAST FACTS

Hyperventilation can cause respiratory alkalosis due to exhaling CO_2.

METABOLIC ACIDOSIS

In metabolic acidosis, the pH is <7.35 because of a decrease in HCO_3^- or increase in H^+ ions. $PaCO_2$ will be in the normal range. The kidneys compensate by excreting excess H^+ ions.

- *Causes:* Diabetic ketoacidosis; renal disease; starvation; hypothermia shock or sepsis; and loss of HCO_3^- in severe diarrhea.

- *Signs and symptoms:* Altered mental state; hypotension; abdominal pain; nausea, vomiting, and diarrhea; Kussmaul respirations; hyperventilation as a compensatory mechanism; tingling and numbness; decreased etCO$_2$ <35 mmHg; hyperkalemia; peaked T waves; flushed, warm skin; headache; bradycardia; and muscle weakness.
- *Interventions:* Treat the underlying problem, which may include administering fluids IV (lactated Ringer's). Treatments may include IV sodium HCO$_3^-$, IV dextrose, and IV regular insulin (to put potassium back in cells); assist ventilations; monitor cardiac rhythm; and perform serial basic metabolic panel (BMP).

Metabolic Alkalosis

In metabolic alkalosis, the pH is >7.45 because of elevated HCO$_3^-$ or decreased H$^+$. PaCO$_2$ is normal.
- *Causes:* Loss of stomach acid associated with vomiting or nasogastric tube (NGT) drainage; ingesting too many alkali substances (antacids, milk of magnesia, or baking soda); diuretics; hypokalemia; and Cushing syndrome.
- *Signs and symptoms:* Hypocalcemia (tetany, twitching, irritability, shaking, and seizures); confusion; nausea, vomiting, and diarrhea; coma; decreased ST segment on EKG; bradypnea; hypokalemia (muscle weakness and loss of reflexes); and polyuria.
- *Interventions:* Anticipate orders to prevent vomiting with antiemetics, avoid gastric suctioning, administer normal saline IV, perform BMP, provide potassium supplements for hypokalemia, and monitor cardiac performance and respirations.

FAST FACTS

Memory trick! With al**K**a**LO**sis, the serum **K** (potassium level) is **LO**w (hypokalemia).

The opposite is true in acidosis; the serum potassium is high (hyperkalemia).

SUMMARY

Although acid–base imbalances can be challenging to understand, they are critical to maintaining natural homeostasis. An ED nurse encounters acid–base imbalances in daily practice. The ED nurse should review the patient's arterial or venous blood gas results and be able to anticipate interventions. Practice the steps provided in this chapter to accurately interpret ABGs.

REVIEW QUESTIONS

1) The ED nurse is caring for a patient with the following ABG: pH 7.25, $PaCO_2$ 55, PaO_2 88, and HCO_3^- 24. What type of acid–base disturbance is this?
   a. Respiratory alkalosis
   b. Metabolic acidosis
   c. Respiratory acidosis
   d. Metabolic alkalosis
2) The ED nurse is caring for a patient with the following ABGs: pH 7.25, $PaCO_2$ 55, PaO_2 88, and HCO_3^- 24. What can the nurse expect as the next intervention?
   a. Place a nonrebreather mask over the patient's nose and mouth without O_2 flowing.
   b. Initiation of bilevel positive airway pressure (BiPAP) to increase ventilation.
   c. Initiation of BiPAP to decrease ventilation.
   d. No intervention needed at this time.

REFERENCES

Brinkman, J. E., & Sharma, S. (2024, January). *Respiratory alkalosis*. In StatPearls [Internet]. StatPearls Publishing. [Updated July 24, 2023]. Retrieved August 26, 2025, from https://www.ncbi.nlm.nih.gov/books/NBK482117/

Patel, S., & Sharma, S. (2024, January). *Respiratory acidosis*. In StatPearls [Internet]. StatPearls Publishing. [Updated June 12, 2023]. Retrieved August 26, 2025, from https://www.ncbi.nlm.nih.gov/books/NBK482430/#

Yee, J., Frinak, S., Mohiuddin, N., & Uduman, J. (2022, August 25). Fundamentals of arterial blood gas interpretation. *Kidney360*, *3*(8), 1458–1466. https://doi.org/10.34067/KID.0008102021

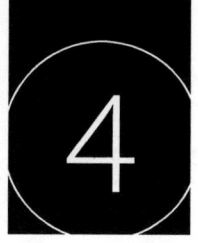

Fluid and Electrolyte Emergencies

Alexander Menard

> Fluid and electrolyte balance is essential to maintaining homeostasis within the body. It is important to understand the body's relationships between water and electrolytes. If not treated, interruptions to this balance can be fatal. Therefore, it is vital for the ED nurse to recognize the most common manifestations of fluid and electrolyte imbalances and how to correct them.

In this chapter, you will learn to:
1. Identify electrolyte disturbances
2. Assess the volume status
3. Anticipate the interventions to address electrolyte abnormalities

FLUIDS AND ELECTROLYTES

Elevations and deficiencies in electrolytes and intravascular volume status play a crucial role in the assessment and treatment of patients presenting to the ED. Understanding the normal values of electrolytes within the body is essential (see Table 4.1).

Furthermore, it is essential to know the common components of frequently used IV fluid within the ED. Commonly used IV fluid in the ED include lactated Ringer's, 0.9% sodium chloride, 0.45% sodium chloride, and dextrose (5%) in 0.9% sodium chloride or 0.45% sodium chloride (see Table 4.2).

VOLUME STATUS

Determining the volume status of a patient can be challenging and requires multiple assessments. Options for assessing a patient's volume status include trending weight over time, checking skin turgor, evaluating mucous membranes, and documenting intake and output. It is also important to note that a patient can be volume overloaded but intravascularly dry, meaning the fluid is not necessarily in the vasculature/circulating volume.

TABLE 4.1

Normal Value of Serum Electrolytes

Electrolyte	Normal Serum Value
Sodium	135–145 mEq/L
Potassium	3.5–5.5 mEq/L
Chloride	95–105 mEq/L
Calcium	Total = 8.6–10.2 mg/dL Ionized = 1.12–1.3 mmol/L
Magnesium	1.5–2.4 mg/dL
Phosphorus	2.5–4.5 mg/dL

TABLE 4.2

Common IV Fluid Compositions

	0.9% Sodium Chloride	0.45% Sodium Chloride	Lactated Ringer's	Dextrose (5%) in 0.9% Sodium Chloride	Dextrose (5%) in 0.45% Sodium Chloride
Tonicity	Isotonic	Hypotonic	Hypotonic	Hypertonic	Hypotonic
Sodium (mEq/L)	154	77	130	154	77
Potassium (mEq/L)	0	0	4	0	0
Chloride (mEq/L)	154	77	109	154	77
Osmolality (mOsm/L)	308		275	308	406

Overhydration

Overhydration is also known as "fluid overload."

- *Causes:* Drinking too much water or fluids; receiving too much IV fluid; long-term corticosteroid use; overproduction of antidiuretic hormone; and medical conditions such as congestive heart failure (CHF) and renal failure.
- *Signs and symptoms:* Pedal/pulmonary edema; nausea and vomiting; headache; anorexia; confusion; seizure; aphasia; or blurred vision.
- *Interventions:* Anticipate orders to restrict fluids, give diuretics, monitor and document intake and output, and document level of consciousness.

Dehydration

Dehydration is a lack of fluids.
- *Causes:* Inadequate fluid intake; diuretics; burns; third spacing (internal bleeding, crush injury); and vomiting or diarrhea. Fever and excessive sweating are not measurable but may result in excessive insensible fluid loss. Geriatric and pediatric patients are high-risk populations.
- *Signs and symptoms:* Confusion; disorientation; seizure; dry oral mucosa; dry skin; hyperthermia; weak, rapid pulse; orthostatic hypotension; lethargy; fever; thirst; sunken fontanelles and eyes in infants; lack of tears in crying children; concentrated urine; tachypnea; tachycardia; and decreased urine output.
- *Interventions:* Anticipate orders to give fluids IV or by mouth, administer antipyretics for fever, perform basic metabolic panel and EKG, document mental status, check orthostatic vital signs, and measure intake and output.

FAST FACTS

IV fluid memory trick:
Isotonic Fluids: Stay where **I** put them, **I**nside the vessel.
HypOtonic Fluids: Go **O**utside the vessel.
HypErtonic Fluids: **E**nter the vessel.

ELECTROLYTE ABNORMALITIES

Hyponatremia

Hyponatremia means that the sodium level in the blood is <135. Remember that sodium follows water and chloride. Where there is hyponatremia, there is also hypochloremia and dehydration.
- *Causes:* Syndrome of inappropriate antidiuretic hormone, medications (morphine sulfate, penicillin G, barbiturates, diuretics, mannitol, and oxytocin) and too much D5W (5% dextrose in water); nausea, vomiting, and diarrhea; gastrointestinal suction; excessive sweating; Addison disease; CHF; liver failure; renal failure; and extracellular fluid loss (burns, peritonitis, and bowel obstruction). Cerebral salt wasting, primary polydipsia due to psychosis, beer potomania, and renal disease are all potential causes as well.
- *Signs and symptoms for sodium <120:* Irritability; nausea and vomiting; fever; weakness; hypotension; headache; confusion; tachycardia; lethargy; abdominal cramps; and dry oral mucosa. Sodium levels <110: seizures, coma, and death.

- *Interventions:* Anticipate orders to correct fluid imbalances, administer IV normal saline 0.9% or 3% slowly if hyponatremia is severe, perform basic metabolic panel, and monitor closely. Goal is to change sodium levels at a rate ≤0.5 mEq/hr. Furosemide (Lasix) may be given to correct CHF.

Hypernatremia

Hypernatremia is a condition with a sodium level >145. Again, because sodium follows chloride, hypernatremia means hyperchloremia is present. Cellular dehydration is occurring.

- *Causes:* Diabetes insipidus; poor fluid intake in hot weather; fever; infections; renal disease; diarrhea; excessive sweating; diaphoresis; hyperventilation; overly effective diuretics; Cushing syndrome; and burns.
- *Signs and symptoms:* Anorexia; nausea; vomiting; agitation; thirst; oliguria; seizure; lethargy; coma; and muscle weakness/twitching.
- *Interventions:* Anticipate orders to obtain a basic metabolic panel, give water by mouth, or start an IV of D5W or hypotonic saline. The goal is a slow gradual correction to avoid cerebral edema and seizures.

Hypokalemia

Hypokalemia is a condition with a potassium level <3.5.

- *Causes:* Burns; gastrointestinal obstruction; acute alcoholism; diuretics; Cushing syndrome (adrenal hyperactivity); dialysis; vomiting and diarrhea; steroids; uncontrolled diabetes mellitus; excessive sweating; or gastrointestinal suctioning.
- *Signs and symptoms:* Lethargy; fatigue; muscle weakness and decreased/absent deep tendon reflexes; tachycardia; paresthesia; paralysis; paralytic ileus; weak, irregular pulse; tetany; orthostatic hypotension; and flatten/inverted T wave, U waves, and ST depression on an EKG. The U wave is an additional wave after the T wave.
- *Interventions:* Anticipate orders to correct alkalosis (no sodium bicarbonate, no vomiting, no diarrhea, and no gastrointestinal suctioning); administer potassium by mouth or IV; perform a basic metabolic panel; check magnesium; and give IV lactated Ringer's fluids.

Hyperkalemia

Hyperkalemia is a condition in which the potassium level is >4.5.

- *Causes:* Renal failure; diabetes mellitus; crush injury; early burn stages; aldosterone deficiency; excessive potassium intake; potassium-sparing diuretics; angiotensin-converting enzyme (ACE) inhibitor medications; hyponatremia; and respiratory/metabolic acidosis.
- *Signs and symptoms:* Muscle weakness, cramps, and pain; dyspnea; peaked T waves and widened QRS on EKG; nausea, vomiting, and diarrhea; paresthesia; irritability; dysrhythmias; sinus bradycardia; first-degree heart block; ventricular fibrillation; and asystole.

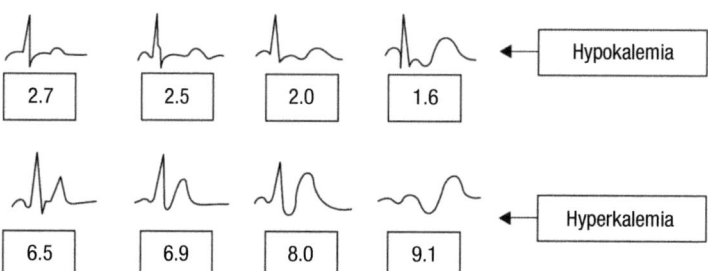

Figure 4.1 EKG changes in potassium imbalances.

- *Interventions:* Anticipate orders to monitor cardiac performance; restrict potassium intake (in food or medication); administer normal saline bolus IV; and give diuretics, sodium polystyrene (Kayexalate) by mouth or rectum, and possibly albuterol nebulizer. When IV medications are ordered, give calcium chloride or calcium gluconate via slow push over 5 to 10 minutes first to protect the heart, then IV glucose (dextrose 50% injection [D50]), then IV regular insulin, and finally IV sodium bicarbonate. If given too fast, the calcium bolus can cause hypotension.
Figure 4.1 illustrates EKG changes during hypokalemia and hyperkalemia. You can see how potassium directly affects the heart.

Hypocalcemia

Hypocalcemia is a condition in which the serum calcium level is <8.5 to 9 or an ionized calcium <4.5. It leads to increased neuromuscular excitability. Calcium counterbalances phosphate; therefore, hypocalcemia = hyperphosphatemia. Calcium follows magnesium; therefore, hypocalcemia = hypomagnesemia.

- *Causes:* Hypoparathyroidism; vitamin D deficiency; peritonitis; bone cancer; calcium channel blocker overdose; acute pancreatitis; burns; renal failure; sepsis; shock; citrate (anticoagulant used in blood transfusions); trauma; rhabdomyolysis; alcoholism; and malnutrition.
- *Signs and symptoms:* Just remember **CATS**: **C**onvulsions, **A**nxiety, **T**etany, and **S**pasms. Other symptoms include irritability; nausea, vomiting, and diarrhea; muscle cramps; muscle twitching; hyperactive deep tendon reflexes; numbness/tingling in toes, nose, fingers, lips, and earlobes; dysrhythmias (prolonged QT intervals); unconsciousness; and cardiac failure.
    - Chvostek sign: Facial muscle spasms when the facial nerve is tapped anterior to the external ear below the temporal bone.
    - Trousseau sign: Hand/carpal spasms when pumping up blood pressure cuff above systolic pressure for 3 minutes.
- *Interventions:* Anticipate orders to obtain repeat serum calcium and protein levels; administer normal saline IV, monitor cardiac performance, and document blood pressures; give slow IV calcium chloride or calcium gluconate bolus and correct magnesium deficit.

Hypercalcemia

Hypercalcemia is a condition with calcium level >10.6. It leads to decreased neuromuscular excitability. Phosphate counterbalances calcium. Therefore, hypercalcemia = hypophosphatemia. Calcium follows magnesium; therefore, hypercalcemia = hypermagnesemia.

- *Causes:* Renal disease; hyperparathyroidism; too much vitamin D; drinking too much milk; pancreatitis; peptic ulcers; Addison disease; thiazide diuretics; and prolonged immobilization.
- *Signs and symptoms:* Muscle weakness; decreased deep tendon reflexes; dehydration; nausea and vomiting; anorexia; constipation; ileus; kidney stones; polyuria; polydipsia; lethargy; headache; irritability; decreased level of consciousness; dysrhythmias (short QT interval); and cardiac arrest.
- *Interventions:* Anticipate orders to administer diuretics and 1 to 2 L of normal saline bolus IV; monitor cardiac rhythm; perform basic metabolic panel; measure magnesium level; measure intake and output; monitor for cardiac heart failure; and administer medications (glucocorticoids, diuretics, calcitonin, phosphate, or ethylenediaminetetraacetic acid).

Hypomagnesemia

Hypomagnesemia is a condition in which serum magnesium level is <1.5 mEq/L, and it can be commonly found in hospitalized patients. Magnesium follows calcium. Therefore, hypomagnesemia also results in hypocalcemia.

- *Causes:* May include malnutrition, alcoholism, cirrhosis, ulcerative colitis, diabetic ketoacidosis, diuretics, or renal disease.
- *Signs and symptoms:* Weakness; lethargy; hypotension; bradycardia or dysrhythmias (prolonged QT intervals, torsades de pointes, and ventricular fibrillation [V-fib]); increased deep tendon reflexes; nausea; vomiting; coma; and bradypnea and may lead to cardiac or pulmonary arrest.
- *Interventions:* Anticipate orders to administer magnesium by mouth or IV, apply cardiac monitor, monitor vital signs, obtain repeat serum magnesium levels, assess deep tendon reflexes, and monitor intake and output and magnesium levels. IV magnesium has multiple indications with various IV drip rates. Be sure to become familiar with the concentrations available to you; do not give IV magnesium too fast, or your patient could go into cardiopulmonary arrest.

FAST FACTS

Magnesium follows calcium. Therefore, hypomagnesemia also results in hypocalcemia.

Hypermagnesemia

Hypermagnesemia is a condition in which the serum magnesium level is >2.3 mEq/L.
- *Causes:* May include magnesium overdose, renal disease, or adrenocortical insufficiency.
- *Signs and symptoms:* Lethargy; nausea; headache; diminished or absent deep tendon reflexes; muscle weakness or paralysis; bradypnea or apnea; hypotension; hypocalcemia; EKG changes (atrioventricular blocks); and cardiac or respiratory arrest.
- *Interventions:* Anticipate orders to monitor cardiac rhythms, deep tendon reflexes, vital signs, and magnesium levels and to administer calcium gluconate or furosemide (Lasix) with saline diuresis. If severe, dialysis may be ordered.

SUMMARY

Fluids and electrolytes play a key role in health and homeostasis. The kidneys act as the gatekeeper for most fluids and electrolytes. It is critical that ED nurses understand this delicate balance, as a slight disturbance to this amazing balance can be fatal. Electrolytes typically affect the neuromuscular system. Make sure you learn the different lab values; you will need them every day in evaluating a wide variety of illnesses.

REVIEW QUESTIONS

1) The ED nurse has obtained a 12-lead EKG and notes there are peaked T waves across all leads. What electrolyte does the nurse suspect will be abnormal?
   a. Sodium
   b. Chloride
   c. Potassium
   d. Magnesium
2) Hypomagnesemia can result in a decrease in which electrolyte?
   a. Potassium
   b. Calcium
   c. Sodium
   d. Magnesium

REFERENCES

Castera, M. R., & Borhade, M. B. (2024, January). *Fluid management.* In StatPearls [Internet]. StatPearls Publishing. [Updated October 22, 2023]. Retrieved August 26, 2025, from https://www.ncbi.nlm.nih.gov/books/NBK532305/#

Hoorn, E. J. (2017, August). Intravenous fluids: Balancing solutions. *Journal of Nephrology, 30*(4):485–492. https://doi.org/10.1007/s40620-016-0363-9. Epub November 29, 2016. Erratum in: *Journal of Nephrology,* April 2020, *33*(2), 387. PMID: 27900717; PMCID: PMC5506238.

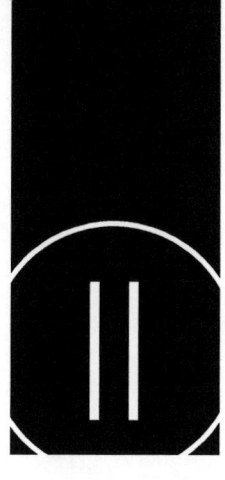

SYSTEM-BASED ED NURSING CARE

Neurological Emergencies

Alexander Menard

> *The neurological system is a critical piece of the human puzzle. It is fascinating and fragile. There are many different forms of neurological emergencies. In the ED, you may see anything from head trauma with grand mal seizures to Bell palsy. It is important to get a thorough history and a complete neurological assessment. This chapter will review major neurological emergencies and how to handle them.*

In this chapter, you will learn to:
1. Discuss the different presentations of neurological emergencies
2. Identify the signs and symptoms of neurological emergencies
3. Identify the interventions to address neurological emergencies

NEUROLOGICAL EMERGENCIES

The nervous system is complex, and the ED nurse must have a good foundation of the topics covered in this chapter. Neurological pathologies require the nurse to incorporate physical exam findings and good history taking to help patients.

Acute Stroke (Cerebrovascular Accident)

Cerebrovascular accident and "brain attack" are broad synonymous terms that refer to a stroke. Stroke can be further delineated into ischemic or hemorrhagic in origin. An acute stroke results in loss of or decreased blood flow to a certain part of the brain. Decreased blood flow reduces the delivery of oxygen and nutrients, which can result in neurological deficits. Prompt recognition, treatment, and rehabilitative programs have been shown to maximize meaningful recovery. Stroke is the second leading cause of death worldwide (Tadi & Lui, 2024).

Acute Ischemic Stroke

An ischemic stroke results from the interruption of blood flow to a particular area of the brain. Embolism is the most common cause of stroke. Most emboli originate from the heart (cardioembolic). With a stroke, the duration of symptoms will surpass 24 hours, whereas in contrast, with a transient ischemic attack (TIA), symptoms will resolve within 24 hours and usually within the first hour of onset (Henderson, 2017). Cardiac diseases that increase stroke risk include atrial fibrillation, valvular heart disease, cardiomyopathy related to myocardial infarction, and hypertension. Other diseases that increase the risk of ischemic stroke include hyperlipidemia, diabetes, and obesity.

- *Causes:* Clot; thrombus; embolus; compression; or spasm. Artery-to-artery embolism, paradoxical embolism (seen in right-to-left shunting), hypercoagulable states, arterial dissection, large and small vessel vasculitis, endocarditis.
- *Signs and symptoms:* Abrupt onset of neurological deficits. Symptoms will vary depending on location, magnitude, and duration of ischemic time. Symptoms include arm drift; pupillary changes; paralysis; facial droop; weakness; nausea and vomiting; hearing loss; headache; altered mental status; aphasia (expressive and/or receptive); dysphasia (language difficulty); dysphagia (swallowing difficulty); visual disturbances; vertigo; ataxia, paresthesia, and seizure.
- *Interventions:* It is imperative to activate and follow the hospital's stroke protocol. Interventions are time sensitive, and the American Heart Association (AHA) recommends time targets for assessment and interventions (Table 5.1). The AHA also recommends that the National Institutes of Health Stroke Scale (NIHSS) scoring system be used (Table 5.2). Maintain a patent airway; monitor cardiac rhythm and blood pressure (BP); insert two large-bore IVs; administer oxygen; activate the stroke team; and obtain emergent noncontrast CT scan of the head. Obtain a 12-lead EKG, accurate weight, blood glucose, and frequent neurological assessments per hospital protocol. Close communication with providers to ensure timely completion of orders, which may include blood sampling (complete blood counts, coagulation studies, type and screen, comprehensive metabolic panel, antihypertensive medications, and thrombolytic medications), is necessary.

TABLE 5.1

Key Time Intervals

Time	Intervention
<10 minutes of arrival to the ED	Perform initial patient assessment
<15 minutes of arrival to the ED	Notification of stroke team
<25 minutes of arrival to the ED	Initiate CT or MR scan
<45 minutes of arrival to the ED	Interpret CT or MR scan

TABLE 5.2

NIHSS Scale and Severity

Score	Severity
0	No stroke
1–4	Minor stroke
5–15	Moderate stroke
16–21	Moderate to severe stroke
21–42	Severe stroke

NIHSS, National Institutes of Health Stroke Scale.

Hemorrhagic Stroke

Acute intracerebral hemorrhage (ICH) is a type of stroke defined by acute bleeding into the brain parenchyma from a damaged or ruptured intracranial blood vessel. Acute ICH accounts for approximately 10% of the strokes per year in the United States and is associated with a 30% to 40% early-term mortality rate, with many survivors having long-term disability. Early identification, diagnosis, and intervention for acute ICH are essential. Older age, hypertension, cerebral amyloid angiopathy, and oral anticoagulant use are some of the most significant risk factors for acute ICH.

- *Causes:* See Box 5.1.
- *Signs and symptoms:* Often occurs suddenly, with symptom presentation varying depending on location and size. Symptoms include arm drift; pupil changes; paralysis; facial droop; weakness; nausea and vomiting; hearing loss; headache; altered mental status; aphasia (receptive and/

Box 5.1 CAUSES OF INTRACEREBRAL HEMORRHAGE

Causes
- Uncontrolled hypertension
- Cerebral amyloid angiopathy
- Arteriovenous malformation
- Ruptured aneurysm
- Brain tumors
- Hemorrhagic conversion of ischemic stroke
- Cavernous malformation
- Coagulopathies
- Sinus venous thrombosis
- Vasculitis
- Trauma
- Medication

or expressive); dysphasia (language difficulty); dysphagia (swallowing difficulty); visual disturbances; vertigo; ataxia; and seizure.
- *Interventions:* Adherence to institutional stroke protocols is essential to optimize care of the patient with a suspected stroke. Assessment of the airway, breathing, and circulation is required. Elevating the head of the bed, applying oxygen, and obtaining vital signs are nursing interventions that can be done immediately. A 12-lead EKG will need to be obtained; additionally, the nurse should be prepared to collect initial lab tests ordered by the provider, which are likely to include a point-of-care glucose, complete blood count, complete metabolic panel, coagulation studies, and a type and screen. A head CT will be obtained; further imaging will be ordered by the provider depending on the specifics of the patient presentation.

Transient Ischemic Attack

Approximately 240,000 individuals in the United States experience a TIA each year (Kleindorfer et al., 2021). A TIA is defined as a temporary blockage of blood flow to the brain. The clot usually dissolves or gets dislodged, and symptoms typically last for <5 minutes.
- *Causes:* The cause of a TIA is a temporary interruption in blood flow to a particular part of the brain. This can be caused by an embolus, a thrombus, or a vasospasm.
- *Signs and symptoms:* Usually last for only a few minutes and can include weakness, numbness, paralysis in the face, arms, or legs and typically will be unilateral. Dysarthria; aphasia; vision impairment, including blinding, blurred vision, or double vision; dizziness; and impairment to balance and coordination are all possible signs and symptoms.
- *Interventions:* Adherence to institutional stroke protocols is essential to optimize care of the patient with a suspected stroke. Assessment of the airway, breathing, and circulation is required. Elevating the head of the bed, applying oxygen, and obtaining vital signs are nursing interventions that can be done immediately. A 12-lead EKG will need to be obtained; additionally, the nurse should be prepared to collect initial lab tests ordered by the provider, which are likely to include a point-of-care glucose, complete blood count, complete metabolic panel, coagulation studies, and a type and screen. A head CT will be obtained; further imaging will be ordered by the provider depending on the specifics of the patient presentation.

FAST FACTS

With an acute ischemic stroke (AIS), the duration of symptoms will surpass 24 hours, whereas in contrast, with a TIA, symptoms will resolve within 24 hours and usually within the first hour of onset.

SEIZURES

Seizures involve sudden, temporary bursts of electrical activity in the brain that alter or disrupt the way messages are sent between neurons. These bursts have the potential to produce involuntary body movements and changes to sensation and awareness. When witnessing or recalling a seizure, inquire about the onset, duration, and characteristics that describe the seizure; urinary incontinence; and tongue biting.

- *Causes:* Aside from febrile seizures, the cause is not always known. Underlying conditions include brain tumor, cerebral infarct, head trauma, medication overdose, and alcohol abuse.
- *Signs and symptoms:* Each type of seizure, with specific signs and symptoms, is listed as follows:
    - *Generalized absence seizure (petit mal):* Characterized by staring or eyelid fluttering for 5 to 10 seconds.
    - *Tonic clonic (grand mal):* Generalized stiffening of extremities, followed by jerking movements; sweating; frothing at the mouth; incontinence; and amnesia.
    - *Partial (focal):* Affects only part of the brain. Symptoms vary according to location of the seizure. It is usually accompanied by an aura. Focal seizures may be the result of underlying problems (e.g., trauma, tumor, or infarct).
    - *Focal motor:* Starts with focal jerking that may persist or may spread to the entire body (grand mal).
    - *Febrile:* Common in infants and young children with high fever.
    - *Status epilepticus:* The seizure that never ends and is therefore an emergency. The patient keeps having one seizure after another, so it looks like one long seizure. The patient with status epilepticus may have increased temperature, BP, and pulse. The patient is at risk for hypoxic brain damage.
    - *Pseudo-seizures:* These appear to be seizures but do not involve abnormal electrical brain activity. Patient movements may be purposeful, but the patient is not postictal after a pseudo-seizure. This type of seizure is usually preceded by emotional upset and generally lasts longer than a true seizure, and the patient shows stable vital signs.
        - *Arm test:* Hold the patient's arm above their face and let go. A truly unconscious patient will hit their face with their arm. The patient with pseudo-seizures will avoid hitting the face.
        - *Wave ammonia in front of the patient:* Ammonia salts are often readily available in prehospital setups and inpatient settings. If it is a pseudo-seizure, the patient will suddenly be alert and oriented to person, place, and time.
- *Interventions:* Protect the patient from harm but do not restrain; assess and protect the airway; place in a recovery position afterward; administer oxygen; anticipate orders to obtain an IV access; give medications (lorazepam, diazepam, midazolam, and anticonvulsants); and reorient after postictal state.

BELL PALSY

Bell palsy is the most common condition in which there is a rapid and unilateral paralysis of cranial nerve VII, the facial nerve (Zhang et al., 2020). It usually resolves in several weeks to months.

- *Causes:* The cause of Bell palsy is unknown, but there is evidence of inflammation and swelling of cranial nerve VII. One possible trigger is a viral infection.
- *Signs and symptoms:* Mild weakness to complete paralysis to one side of the face (rarely does Bell palsy impact both sides of the face), drooling, headache, facial swelling, and inability to close one eye.
- *Interventions:* Medications, as prescribed by a provider, can help treat (steroids) and manage symptoms (pain and dry eyes) with analgesics and artificial tears. Once a diagnosis is made, reassuring the patient that these symptoms are not related to a stroke may be needed.

FAST FACTS

Bell palsy can mimic signs and symptoms of a stroke.

MYASTHENIA GRAVIS

Myasthenia gravis (MG) is an autoimmune neuromuscular disorder. It is the most common disorder affecting the neuromuscular junction (Beloor Suresh et al., 2023). The classic presentation is that of a patient with fluctuating weakness that is more evident later in the day. Additionally, the muscle weakness varies in severity, worsens with physical activity, and improves with rest. MG has several complications, including myasthenic crisis, respiratory paralysis, and opportunistic infections and lymphoproliferative malignancies related to long-term complications of medications used to treat MG.

- *Causes:* The cause of MG is a result of antibodies (immune proteins produced by the body's immune system) blocking, altering, or destroying the receptors for acetylcholine at the neuromuscular junction, which prevents the muscle from contracting.
- *Signs and symptoms:* Voluntary muscle weakness, especially of the face. Symptoms may improve with rest. The edrophonium (Tensilon) test is used to diagnose MG, as shown by the significant improvement of the patient after edrophonium is given IV.
- *Interventions:* These are made through neurological interventions, assessment of respiratory function, and immediate reporting of any sign of impairment (e.g., accessory muscle use, decreased negative inspiratory force).

MULTIPLE SCLEROSIS

Multiple sclerosis is a chronic autoimmune disorder that results in inflammation and damage to the central nervous system. The body attacks its own myelin sheaths, thereby damaging nerve impulses. The damage affects muscle coordination, strength, sensation, and vision. Multiple sclerosis is the most common nontraumatic cause of neurologic disability in persons <40 years of age (Olek, 2021).

- *Causes:* The cause of multiple sclerosis is multifactorial and is likely the cumulative impact of genetics and environmental factors. Geographic location of residence before adolescence also predicts risk, with increased rates in northern and southern latitudes compared with equatorial areas (Olek, 2021).
- *Signs and symptoms:* Patient presentations vary widely. The most common initial presenting symptom is subacute vision changes, most often in one eye, which is secondary to optic neuritis. Transient worsening of signs and symptoms with increased body temperature can occur as well; these are called flares or flare-ups. Focal muscle weakness and reduced sensation below the affected level are reported. In acute presentations of multiple sclerosis, muscles below the affected level can even present as flaccid.
- *Interventions:* The nurse can expect that the patient may need to get an MRI that will cover the head through the spine. Additionally, fever-reducing medications should be given as prescribed. Other medications that may be prescribed for patients with multiple sclerosis include disease-modifying therapies, immunomodulators, and steroids.

FAST FACTS

Transient worsening of signs and symptoms of multiple sclerosis can occur with increased body temperature.

HEADACHE

Headache is a frequent presenting symptom to the ED annually, accounting for 2.2% to 4.5% of all ED visits (Naik & Mollman, 2017). Notably <1% of those who present with headache have a life-threatening condition. Headache can be a result of inflammation, traction, displacement, or distension of pain-sensitive structures in the neck and above. It is possible that other disorders can cause headache pain, including scalp, ear, nasal, sinus, mouth, or dental disorders. Headache can be further broken into three categories: cluster, tension, and migraine (see Table 5.3).

TABLE 5.3
Types of Headaches

Headache	Signs and Symptoms	Interventions

Tension	Bilateral and gradual onset of headache. Often occipital or frontal in location and described as a tight band or pressure around the head. Nonthrobbing pain. They can be associated with nausea and photophobia but not often vomiting. Neurological exam remains normal.	■ Calm, quiet environment
		■ Pharmacological (acute attack)
		  ■ Sumatriptan
		  ■ Dihydroergotamine
		■ Pharmacological (transitional)
		  ■ Corticosteroids
		  ■ Naratriptan
		  ■ Ergotamine

Cluster	Severe unilateral headache with ipsilateral autonomic symptoms (ptosis, lacrimation, miosis, nasal congestion, or rhinorrhea). Often in the ocular, frontal, and temporal areas. Attacks build in intensity over 10–15 minutes and can last for a few hours. These can recur a couple of times a day. Attacks can be separated by headache-free periods of 6 months to 2 years.	■ Calm, quiet environment
		■ Oxygen via face mask
		■ Pharmacological
		  ■ NSAIDs
		  ■ Analgesics
		  ■ Combination medications with caffeine

Migraine	Headache pain is throbbing/pulsing and unilateral. Nausea, vomiting, photophobia, and phonophobia can be present. Can occur with or without aura. May have associated neurological symptoms (i.e., sensory symptoms or dysphasic speech.)	■ Calm, quiet environment
		■ Pharmacological
		  ■ NSAIDs
		  ■ Analgesics
		  ■ Aspirin
		  ■ Combination of medications with caffeine
		  ■ Antiemetics
		  ■ Steroids

NSAIDs, nonsteroidal anti-inflammatory drugs.

SUMMARY

In summary, neurological disorders will present to the ED, and the nurse must be prepared to evaluate and manage these patient presentations with the interdisciplinary team. Careful, detailed, and ongoing assessment of the patient with a neurological emergency is crucial. Many interventions for the patient with a neurological emergency are time sensitive.

REVIEW QUESTIONS

1) Bell palsy is paralysis of which cranial nerve?
    a. Cranial nerve V
    b. Cranial nerve III

c. Cranial nerve VII
d. Cranial nerve IX
2) The ED nurse is caring for a patient who presents with acute left-sided weakness. What should the nurse expect to do first?
   a. Place a nonrebreather mask over the patient's nose and mouth.
   b. Obtain IV access.
   c. Prepare the patient for an MRI of the brain.
   d. No intervention is needed at this time.

REFERENCES

Beloor Suresh, A., & Asuncion, R. M. D. (2023, August 8). *Myasthenia gravis*. In StatPearls [Internet]. StatPearls Publishing; 2024 January. Retrieved August 26, 2025, from PMID: 32644757.

Henderson, G. V. (2017). Transient ischemic attack and stroke. In S. C. McKean, J. J. Ross, D. D. Dressler, & D. B. Scheurer (Eds.), *Principles and practice of hospital medicine* (2nd ed.) (pp. 1681–1685). McGraw-Hill Education. https://accessmedicine-mhmedical-com.umassmed.idm.oclc.org/content.aspx?sectionid=146986657&bookid=1872#146986710

Kleindorfer, D. O., Towfighi, A., Chaturvedi, S., Cockroft, K. M., Gutierrez, J., Lombardi-Hill, D., Kamel, H., Kernan, W. N., Kittner, S. J., Leira, E. C., Lennon, O., Meschia, J. F., Nguyen, T. N., Pollak, P. M., Santangeli, P., Sharrief, A. Z., Smith, Jr., S. C., Turan, T. N., & Williams, L. S. (2021, July). Guideline for the prevention of stroke in patients with stroke and transient ischemic attack: A guideline from the American Heart Association/American Stroke Association. *Stroke, 52*(7), e364–e467. https://doi.org/10.1161/STR.0000000000000375. Epub 2021 May 24. Erratum in: (2021, July). *Stroke, 52*(7), e483–e484. https://doi.org/10.1161/STR.0000000000000383. PMID: 34024117.

Naik, P., & Mollman, M. (2017). Headache. In C. Stone & R. L. Humphries (Eds.), *CURRENT diagnosis & treatment: Emergency Medicine* (8th ed.). McGraw-Hill Education. Accessed October 30, 2024, from https://accessmedicine-mhmedical-com.umassmed.idm.oclc.org/content.aspx?sectionid=165060254&bookid=2172&Resultclick=2

Olek, M. J. (2021, June). Multiple sclerosis. *Annals of Internal Medicine, 174*(6), ITC81–ITC96. https://doi.org/10.7326/AITC202106150. Epub 2021 June 8. PMID: 34097429.

Tadi, P., & Lui, F. (2024, January). *Acute stroke*. In StatPearls [Internet]. StatPearls Publishing. [Updated 2023 August 17]. Retrieved August 26, 2025, from https://www.ncbi.nlm.nih.gov/books/NBK535369/

Zhang, W., Xu, L., Luo, T., Wu, F., Zhao, B., & Li, X. (2020, July). The etiology of Bell's palsy: A review. *Journal of Neurology, 267*(7), 1896–1905. https://doi.org/10.1007/s00415-019-09282-4. Epub 2019 March 28. PMID: 30923934; PMCID: PMC7320932.

Cardiovascular Emergencies

Sarah Berry

> Although the entire body is important, the heart is one of the most important organs. It pumps oxygen-rich blood throughout the whole body. It comprises two systems: the plumbing (the atria, ventricles, and vessels) and the electricity (the conduction pathway and its parts). Cardiovascular emergencies in the ED are a daily occurrence, and the nurse's knowledge and recognition of issues could be a make or break for that patient.

In this chapter, you will learn to:
1. Identify the common cardiac diseases and their treatments performed in the ED
2. Recognize the symptoms of acute myocardial infarctions (MIs)
3. Understand post–cardiac arrest treatment

CARDIOVASCULAR EMERGENCIES

In the ED, cardiovascular diseases are an everyday life-threatening occurrence. However, with proper assessment and fast treatment, they are managed every day in EDs across the country. After studying this chapter, the nurse will have a basic understanding of cardiovascular assessments and treatments. This chapter discusses congestive heart failure (CHF), acute MI (ST-elevation myocardial infarction [STEMI] and non-ST elevation myocardial infarction [NSTEMI]), arterial occlusions, endocarditis, cardiac tamponade, aortic injuries and dissection, arrhythmias, and cardiac arrest. This chapter does not replace EKG courses or the advanced cardiovascular life support (ACLS) certification required to work in the ED. Many nurses find keeping an ACLS handbook for study very helpful.

Acute Myocardial Infraction
Acute MI is the result of a blocked coronary artery supplying blood to the heart muscle. The patient's history often reveals hypertension, hyperlipidemia,

diabetes, coronary artery disease, smoking, and genetics. The primary nursing intervention for a patient with suspected heart attack is to obtain an EKG within 10 minutes of their arrival to the ED. See Figure 6.1 for goals of care for the patient experiencing an MI. There are two different types of MIs: NSTEMI and STEMI. Table 6.1 displays the different details between both etiologies and pathophysiologies.

- *Causes:* Atherosclerosis, thrombus, or, less common, coronary arterial spasm from cocaine use or other stimulants.
- *Signs and symptoms*: Anxiety; nausea and vomiting; diaphoresis; shortness of breath; fatigue; hypertension or hypotension; and chest pain (described often as pressure, squeezing, tightness, or vagueness) that may radiate to the left shoulder or jaw. Females may present with vague weakness, fatigue, and dyspnea. EKG may or may not reveal ST segment elevation.
- *Interventions:* The number one priority is to obtain an EKG within 10 minutes of a patient with chest pain arriving in the ED (Yiadom et al., 2017). The patient should undergo continuous cardiac monitoring, pulse oximetry, and frequent blood pressure checks. Consider attaching defibrillator pads in the event that the patient becomes unstable. Anticipate orders to obtain lab work consisting of coagulation panels, cardiac enzymes, a complete metabolic panel (CMP), and a complete blood count (CBC). Consider medication administration such as sublingual nitroglycerin, chewable aspirin, or heparin infusion. Arrange for chest x-ray and cardiologist consult. Prepare for possible cardiac catheterization lab and admission or, if in a non–percutaneous coronary intervention (PCI) facility, thrombolytics (alteplase), anticoagulant (heparin) therapy, and transfer.

FAST FACTS

According to the *Journal of the American Heart Association*, the standard "door to EKG time" is 10 minutes in patients who have a complaint of chest pain.

- MONA (morphine, oxygen, nitroglycerin, and aspirin) is no longer the standard of care for patients experiencing an MI.
  - *Morphine:* Studies show morphine could potentially delay activity of platelet inhibitor drugs in patients who are being treated for STEMI, therefore increasing their likelihood of a negative outcome (de Alencar Neto, 2018). Despite this negative impact, morphine is still a viable option for pain management in patients experiencing chest pain.
  - *Oxygen:* Oxygen use is only recommended in patients with an oxygen saturation of <90% on room air. Studies show that inappropriate administration of oxygen therapy in patients who are not hypoxic could potentially increase recurrent MIs (de Alencar Neto, 2018).

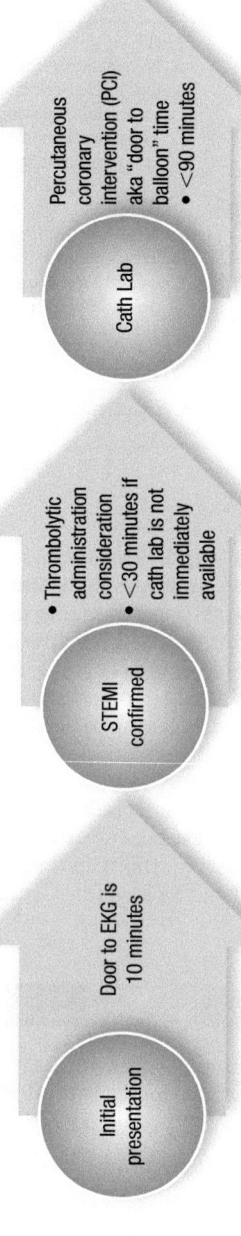

Figure 6.1 Timeline of care goals.

Source: Data from Yiadom, M. Y., Baugh, C. W., McWade, C. M., Liu, X., Song, K. J., Patterson, B. W., Jenkins, C. A., Tanski, M., Mills, A. M., Salazar, G., Wang, T. J., Dittus, R. S., Liu, D., & Storrow, A. B. (2017). Performance of emergency department screening criteria for an early ECG to identify ST-segment elevation myocardial infarction. *Journal of the American Heart Association, 6*(3), e003528. https://doi.org/10.1161/jaha.116.003528.

TABLE 6.1

STEMI Versus NSTEMI

STEMI	NSTEMI
■ Elevation in ST segment on EKG ■ Complete occlusion of a major vessel ■ Elevated cardiac enzymes ■ Treatment consists of thrombolytics if not at PCI facility, aspirin, anticoagulants, and PCI in cath lab. ■ TIME IS MUSCLE! Must be to cath lab in 90 minutes.	■ No elevation in ST segment on EKG ■ Complete occlusion of a minor vessel or partial occlusion of a major vessel, or due to demand ischemia from tachycardia or severe hypertension ■ Cardiac enzymes that trend up as time passes ■ New echo findings ■ Treatment consists of cardiology consult, anticoagulant infusion, and possible PCI in cath lab. *NSTEMIs have the capacity to evolve into STEMIs despite intervention.*

NSTEMI, non-ST elevation myocardial infarction; PCI, percutaneous coronary intervention; STEMI, ST-elevation myocardial infarction.

- *Nitrates:* Use of nitrates has been neither endorsed nor negated in studies regarding effectiveness and should be used subjectively. Be wary of using nitrates in patients experiencing inferior MIs. Patients who are experiencing inferior wall MIs are already at risk for losing significant preload because of the area of the damage. Nitroglycerin will further dilate the vessels, causing an even more profound decrease in preload, potentially leading to deadly hypotension (Ferguson et al., 1989).
- *Aspirin:* A study conducted in 1988 showed the benefits of administering 160 mg of aspirin (acetylsalicylic acid [ASA]) to patients in the acute phase of an MI. These benefits primarily consisted of a 23% decrease in cardiovascular mortality in the 5 weeks following patients with both NSTEMI and STEMI (de Alencar Neto, 2018).

FAST FACTS

Oxygen use is only recommended in patients with an oxygen saturation of <90% on room air. Studies show that inappropriate administration of oxygen therapy in patients who are not hypoxic could potentially increase recurrent MIs (de Alencar Neto, 2018).

Heart Failure

In CHF, the heart fails to pump blood effectively. It can be acute, chronic, or acute exacerbation on chronic. As a result of a weakened pump, blood backs up from the failing ventricle. It can back up to the body (right-sided heart failure) or the lungs (left-sided heart failure) or both. In systolic CHF, the heart is failing to pump, whereas in diastolic CHF, the heart is failing to relax. Systolic heart failure is characterized by the left ventricle being unable to push blood into circulation because of weakened muscle. Diastolic heart failure is noted when the ventricle is unable to relax normally because the muscle has stiffened over time. This causes the ventricle to not fill completely, preserving ejection fraction but increasing workload (Chatterjee & Massie, 2007).

- *Causes:* Other illnesses can, over time, lead to CHF. These include hypertension, arrhythmias, diabetes, coronary artery disease, valvular stenosis, cardiomyopathy, emphysema, obesity, pulmonary embolism, anemia, and thyroid disease.
- *Signs and symptoms:*
    - *Right-sided heart failure:* Pitting pedal edema, hepatojugular reflux, liver enlargement, nocturia, and jugular venous distention.
    - *Left-sided heart failure:* Usually develops first; crackles; shortness of breath; pulmonary edema (rales); tachypnea; left ventricular hypertrophy; tachycardia; S_3 or S_4 (if both S_3 and $S_{4,\,this}$ would be a ventricular gallop).
- *Interventions:* Anticipate management and monitoring of the patient's airway, respiratory status, possible cardiac arrhythmias, and urinary output.
    - *Airway:* Ensure adequate oxygenation, with monitoring through pulse oximetry. If the patient is lethargic or has an altered level of consciousness, initiate nasal end-tidal capnography to measure their ventilation status as well as oxygenation. Consider supplemental oxygen, starting conservatively with nasal cannula or nonrebreather based on the patient's presentation. Because the nurse at the bedside is caring for and monitors the patient continuously, it is their responsibility to report changes in patient status to the provider.
        - If the oxygen saturation fails to improve, the patient's work of breathing is unchanged or worsens, they become hemodynamically unstable, or the patient becomes more somnolent, more aggressive measures are required. At this point, the provider may consider noninvasive ventilation through continuous positive airway pressure (CPAP) or bilevel positive airway pressure (BiPAP) therapy or potentially intubation. Encourage the patient to be in an upright position as much as they can tolerate.
    - *Circulation:* Also establish IV access; anticipate administration of diuretics (furosemide, torsemide, or bumetanide) and vasodilators (nitroglycerin and nicardipine) in the hypertensive and fluid volume–overloaded patients. Nitroprusside used to be a first-line medication, but research shows other medication choices like

nitroglycerin and nicardipine are more easily titratable and have decreased risk of cyanide toxicity (Miller et al., 2020). There is a population of patients who can present in acute heart failure because of fluid volume overload but are hypotensive. These patients are at greater risk of brisk decompensation because their hypotension cannot be managed with normal fluid resuscitation.

- If a patient presents in this situation, anticipate conservative fluid administration and expect vasopressors to be administered. Single therapy or multitherapy may be initiated based on the patient's status. Norepinephrine, dobutamine, milrinone, and dopamine are all possible agents (Colucci, 2023). In these instances, establish a minimum of two IV access points, and be aware of IV compatibility for these medications. Continue to closely monitor cardiac performance and intake and output. Provide an external male catheter, external female catheter, urinal, bedside commode, or bedpan or discuss the use of a Foley catheter for frequent urination after diuretic administration.
- Closely monitor these patients for deterioration in respiratory status. Sometimes, patients require fluid resuscitation despite their current CHF condition. It is a fine line between fluid administration and restriction. Patients with CHF also run the increased risk of getting flash pulmonary edema, a life-threatening emergency that is discussed later in this book.

Acute Arterial Occlusion

Arterial occlusion is a blocked artery. These can occur in the extremities or the abdominal arteries such as the superior or inferior mesenteric artery that can cause acute mesenteric ischemia. The latter is discussed in Chapter 8.

- *Causes of acute extremity arterial occlusion:* Coronary artery disease, atherosclerosis, hypertension, smoking, hyperlipidemia, and diabetes. Atrial fibrillation is a common source of the emboli.
- *Signs and symptoms:* Pain has an abrupt onset; the patient will tell you the exact time the pain started. Pain is progressive and refractory to treatments by the patient. Pain worsens until they present with 10/10 pain. Pain typically presents as a single cool/cold (poikilothermia), pale (pallor) extremity that has a weak or absent pulse. The patient may have paresthesias and paralysis. Further discussions can reveal that the patient has limited ambulatory distance due to pain in the leg or buttock, known as claudication, that is present for weeks to months prior to presentation.
- *Interventions:* Maintain extremity in dependent position; anticipate possible anticoagulant infusion such as heparin; and assess pulses through Doppler ultrasound, a CT angiogram, and, if positive, a stat vascular consult. Begin to prepare the patient for emergency surgery by giving the patient nothing by mouth (NPO [nil per os]). Start IV access and draw labs, including coagulation studies, CBC, type and cross, CMP, and lactate level.

Endocarditis

Endocarditis is an infection of the inner lining of the heart and/or the heart valves.

- *Causes:* Endocarditis occurs in a person who has bacteremia. For example, a bacterial infection in the skin can travel through the bloodstream and attach to the heart valve, resulting in endocarditis, which can damage the valve and cause valvular disfunction. The origins of endocarditis are often poor dental hygiene, dental procedures, chronic skin disorders, infections, currently installed heart valves, burns, and IV drug use (American Heart Association, 2023; Schranz & Barocas, 2020).
- *Signs and symptoms:*
  - **P**etechiae
  - **S**hortness of breath
  - **F**ever and chills
  - **R**oth spots (red spots with white centers of varying translucency that appear on the retinas caused by hemorrhages)
  - **O**sler nodes (tender red or purple nodules typically found at the tips of the fingers and toes)
  - Systolic **M**urmur
  - **J**aneway lesions (red spots on soles of the feet)
  - **A**nemia
  - **N**ail bed splinter hemorrhaging
  - **E**mboli and chest pain
  - To remember these symptoms, just remember **PS: FROM JANE**.
- *Interventions:* Anticipate orders to obtain blood cultures from multiple sites, administer IV antibiotics, and draw a CBC. Anticipate admission and infectious diseases (ID) consultation.

Cardiac Tamponade

Cardiac tamponade is a medical emergency. This occurs when a substance (fluid, blood, pus, or air) accumulates in the pericardium and compresses the heart, causing inadequate cardiac output. The pericardial sac is the structure that surrounds the heart, normally containing a small amount of pericardial fluid for lubrication. This fluid allows the heart to move within the sac without causing friction. The sac protects the heart's outermost layer of muscle and vessels. Because the sac is minimally expansive and is mostly taken up by the heart and about 15 to 50 mL of pericardial fluid, there is little space for additional components or substances.

- *Causes:* Disease such as cancer, pericarditis, CHF, tuberculosis, or lupus; surgical procedures; penetrating chest trauma; cardiac or aortic rupture; and certain medications such as vasodilators and diuretics. These precursors can ultimately lead to compression of the heart chambers, which leads to hemodynamic instability, shock, cardiac arrest, and death.

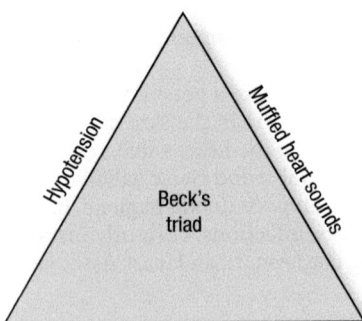

Figure 6.2 Beck triad.

- Signs and symptoms: Beck triad (Figure 6.2) can be remembered with the three Ds: distant heart sounds, decreased blood pressure (hypotension), and distended jugular veins. These do not all have to be present. Tachycardia, shortness of breath, anxiety, and pulsus paradoxus are also common signs and symptoms. Pulsus paradoxus is a decrease in the patient's blood pressure by >10 mmHg during inspiration. This decrease in pressure is caused by the left side of the heart filling less to compensate for the right side of the heart filling more during inspiration. As the pressure in the pericardial sac increases, it compresses all chambers of the heart, leading to cardiac arrest.
- *Interventions: P*rovide the patient with oxygen if indicated; avoid BiPAP or CPAP, if possible, because the additional pressure will further decrease venous return to the heart. Elevate the patient's legs. Prepare to transport the patient to a definitive treatment space for pericardiocentesis or pericardial window. If done at the bedside in the ED, anticipate use of a sterile field; ultrasonography; end-tidal capnography; and continuous cardiac, oxygen saturation, and frequent blood pressure monitoring. If the patient loses pulses or previous treatments are unsuccessful, anticipate an emergency ED thoracotomy (Stashko, 2023).

Aortic Injuries and Dissection

Aortic injuries and dissections may occur anywhere on the ascending aorta, aortic arch, descending thoracic aorta, or abdominal aorta. These can result in aneurysm, dissection, or complete rupture. Without immediate surgery, the patient can rapidly exsanguinate. So it is critical to identify an aortic injury early.

- *Causes:* A history of aortic injuries may reveal hypertension, coronary artery disease, CHF, or a recent chest/abdominal trauma.
- *Signs and symptoms (may vary depending on location):* Patients will describe a tearing chest or abdominal pain that radiates to the back. Unequal blood pressures between arms may be present, hypertension may occur in upper extremities, and a pulse that is stronger in the arms than in the legs may be present. Chest wall ecchymosis and paraplegia may be present. Hypotension and loss of consciousness are late findings. Chest x-ray (CXR) may show a widening mediastinum.
- *Interventions:* Place the patient on a stretcher, apply continuous cardiac monitoring, obtain vital signs and measure pulse oximetry, and perform EKG. Check blood pressure in all extremities. Notify provider of patient signs and symptoms immediately. Prepare for STAT CT angiogram or vascular or cardiovascular surgery consult. Anticipate blood pressure management to systolic blood pressure (SBP) <120, which may need antihypertensive infusions of esmolol, labetalol, and/or Cardene. Start two large-bore IV lines. Send type and cross for 4 units of packed red blood cells (PRBCs).

FAST FACTS

Question: Which type of trauma most commonly causes a descending thoracic aortic laceration?
Answer: Deceleration trauma that causes shearing.

ARRHYTHMIAS

Symptomatic Bradycardia

In symptomatic bradycardia, heart rate is <60 beats per minute, resulting in inadequate circulation. The patient is symptomatic, displaying signs of poor cardiac perfusion such as weak peripheral pulses and delayed capillary refill.

- *Causes:* The cause is not always known, but underlying conditions such as coronary artery disease, heart disease, second- or third-degree heart blocks, hypertension, thyroid disease, medication overdose, Lyme disease, and lung disease can contribute to bradycardia.
- *Signs and symptoms:* Heart rate <60 beats per minute with hypotension. The patient looks and feels unwell (i.e., altered loss of consciousness, chest pain, diaphoretic, and pale).

- *Interventions:* Assess airway, breathing, and circulation (ABCs); provide oxygen as appropriate; start continuous cardiac monitoring and frequent blood pressure readings for the patient; perform EKG; anticipate orders to intravenously push 1 mg of atropine at 3- to 5-minute intervals to a maximum of 3 mg; attach pacing pads; administer medications (dopamine or epinephrine); and prepare for transcutaneous (external) or internal pacer. Anticipate anxiolytics and analgesics if transcutaneous pacing is performed.

Supraventricular Tachycardia

In supraventricular tachycardia (SVT), the heart rate is regular with narrow complexes, but it beats at >150 beats per minute. SVT can be divided into symptomatic/unstable (patient looks unwell) and asymptomatic/stable.

- *Causes:* The cause is not always known. However, some habits and conditions can contribute to it, such as stress, caffeine, smoking, cocaine or other stimulant use, alcohol use, thyroid disease, heart failure, pulmonary embolism, chronic obstructive pulmonary disease, and pneumonia. Some medications for asthma, cold medications, and digoxin can also contribute to SVT (Patocka et al., 2020).
- *Signs and symptoms:* Palpitations, chest pain, diaphoresis, anxiety, and pulse rate >150 beats per minute.
- *Interventions:*
  - *If patient is symptomatic and unstable*, anticipate order to prepare for immediate synchronized cardioversion 50 to 100 J. Be sure to check clearance of the patient and stretcher so no one else receives the jolt. "I'm clear, you're clear, we're ALL CLEAR."
  - *If patient is asymptomatic and stable*, anticipate orders to attempt vasovagal maneuvers, initiate continuous cardiac monitoring, establish at least one IV, provide oxygen, check vital signs, measure pulse oxygen, and perform EKG. Medications that may be prescribed include beta-blockers/calcium channel blockers, amiodarone, or adenosine. Adenosine can be given to treat the SVT or slow conduction to identify the underlying rhythm.
    - Administer adenosine rapidly by IV push. Use a stopcock for rapid administration of adenosine. If possible, place the IV in the right arm and, after pushing the medication, rapidly push a bolus of fluid and have a coworker quickly lift the patient's arm with the hand pointed to the ceiling to facilitate flow of the medication to the heart (Figure 6.3). Remember: The half-life of adenosine is 0.6 to 10 seconds, so anything to facilitate it getting to the cardiac muscle is beneficial.
    - Anticipate that the patient may become bradycardic and asystolic for several seconds—this is expected. During this period, the patient may experience a feeling of doom or significant distress.

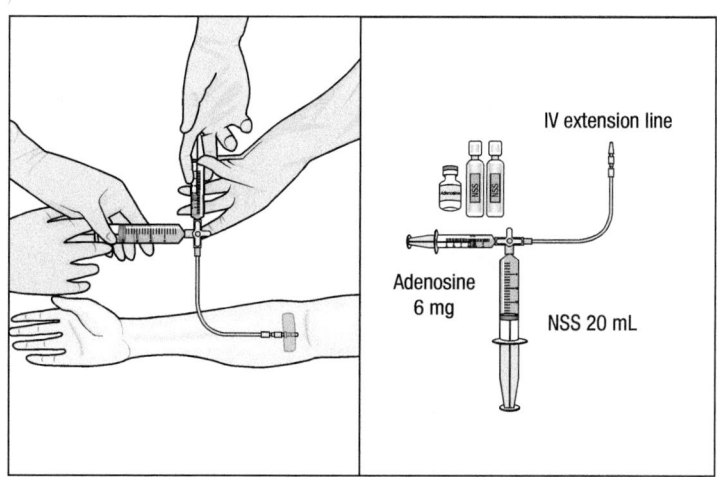

Figure 6.3 Stop-cock method for adenosine administration.

Source: Kotruchin, P., Chaiyakhan, I., Kamonsri, P., Chantapoh, W., Serewiwattana, N., Kaweenattayanon, N., Narangsiya, N., Lorcharassriwong, P., Korsakul, K., Thawepornpuriphong, P., Tirapuritorn, T., & Mitsungnern, T. (2022). Comparison between the double-syringe and the single-syringe techniques of adenosine administration for terminating supraventricular tachycardia: A pilot, randomized controlled trial. *Clinical Cardiology*, 45(5), 583–589. https://doi.org/10.1002/clc.23820. Used under CC BY 4.0 (https://creativecommons.org/licenses/by/4.0/).

As the bedside nurse, in addition to monitoring the patient's vital signs, it is very important to support the patient through this time. Remind the patient that the patient should breathe, that the team is with them, that they are "doing great," and that the feeling will be passing soon. Psychological support can be just as important as physiological support.

- Give the patient a 10-mL syringe and ask them to blow through it to assist vagal maneuvers.

Ventricular Fibrillation or Pulseless Ventricular Tachycardia

Ventricular fibrillation (VF) is always pulseless, and ventricular tachycardia (VT) can be asymptomatic, symptomatic, or pulseless (see Figure 6.4 and Table 6.2).

- *Causes:* Poor cardiac perfusion due to coronary artery disease, shock, hypokalemia, MI, or electrocution.
- *Signs and symptoms:* Palpitations, decreased level of consciousness, no pulse, VF or VT on cardiac monitor.
- *Interventions:* Assess for a pulse within 10 seconds; if no pulse is present, call for help while initiating CPR, starting with chest compressions. Do not interrupt chest compressions while applying

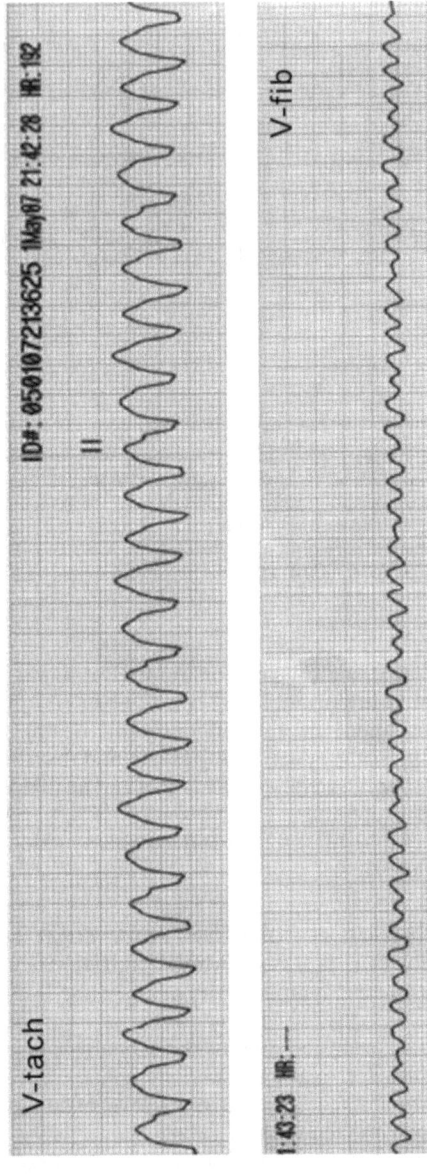

Figure 6.4 Ventricular fibrillation.

TABLE 6.2

Pulseless Ventricular Tachycardia or Ventricular Fibrillation Treatment

Shock at 120 to 200 J biphasic	■ Continuous CPR with ventilation every 6 seconds for 2 minutes ■ Establish IV or IO access and administer epinephrine 1 mg IV/IO during CPR every 3 to 5 minutes
Shock at 200 J biphasic (if still pulseless VT or VF after 2 minutes of CPR)	■ Continuous CPR with ventilation every 6 seconds for 2 minutes ■ Amiodarone 300 mg, 150 mg second dose, or lidocaine during CPR
Shock at 200 J biphasic (if still pulseless VT or VF after 2 minutes of CPR)	■ Continuous CPR with ventilation every 6 seconds for 2 minutes ■ Consider magnesium 1 to 2 g IV/IO for torsades de pointes.

IO, interosseous; VF, ventricular fibrillation; VT, ventricular tachycardia.

cardiac monitor/defibrillation pads. Pulseless VT and VF are shockable rhythms (see Figure 6.4 and Table 6.2). Be sure you know how to set your machine to defibrillation mode, and always make sure your team is all clear before pressing the shock button. Anticipate early defibrillation, early epinephrine, and amiodarone or lidocaine per ACLS protocols. Just remember **DEAL**: **D**efibrillation, **E**pinephrine, and **A**miodarone or **L**idocaine.

PULSELESS ELECTRICAL ACTIVITY

Pulseless electrical activity occurs when a rhythm shows on the monitor but the patient does not have a pulse. Again, you cannot always believe what you see on the monitor. If the monitor shows asystole, ensure all leads are attached and check the rhythm in two leads to confirm.
- *Causes:* Can be attributed to the five "**H**s or five **T**s.":
  - **H**ypovolemia, **H**ypoxia, **H**ydrogen ion (acidosis), **H**yper-/hypokalemia, or **H**ypothermia.
  - **T**oxin (drug overdose), **T**amponade/cardiac, **T**ension pneumothorax, **T**hrombosis, and **T**rauma.
- *Signs and symptoms:* The patient has no pulse, but there is a rhythm on the monitor. Remember that just because there is electrical activity in the heart does not mean the heart is actually pumping.
- *Interventions:* Check for a pulse; if no pulse, perform CPR starting with chest compressions; per order, insert an IV line, monitor oxygen, and administer epinephrine. Consider naloxone (Narcan) for opioid overdose, and treat the underlying causes. Once return of spontaneous circulation (ROSC) is achieved, intubate the patient if this wasn't completed during code.

POST CARDIAC ARREST

The patient has survived a cardiac arrest; now is the time to focus on preserving brain and other vital organ function. The battle is over, but the war has just begun. The patient may still be unstable; thus, achieving stability will require a great team effort.

- *Causes:* ROSC after cardiopulmonary arrest.
- *Signs and symptoms:* The first sign of resuscitation is an increase in end-tidal CO_2 (carbon dixoide). The patient will have regained a pulse after CPR. In most cases, the patient will remain unresponsive, hypotensive, and in need of respiratory and/or circulatory support. This patient is at increased risk for rearrest as epinephrine wears off, so maintain vigilance and frequently confirm a pulse.
- *Interventions:* Document a full primary assessment (ABCs + neurological). Treat any known underlying causes of cardiopulmonary arrest. Assist ED provider with establishing a definitive airway (intubation and ventilator) as needed. Maintain pulse oxygenation between 92% and 98% and continue to monitor capnography. Document Glasgow Coma Scale (GCS), pupillary response, and complete neurological assessment. Anticipate provider insertion of a central IV line with central venous pressure (CVP) monitoring if available. Anticipate diagnostic tests such as arterial blood gas (ABG), CBC, CMP, magnesium, phosphorus, calcium, prothrombin time/international normalized ratio (PT/INR), partial thromboplastin time (PTT), lactate, creatine kinase MB (CK-MB), troponin, amylase, lipase, beta–human chorionic gonadotropin (hCG) on childbearing women without prior hysterectomy, blood glucose, 12-lead EKG, portable CXR, and head CT scan. To preserve organs and prevent fever, consider targeted temperature management (TTM). Evaluate the patient for possible exclusion criteria for TTM such as:
  - Hemorrhagic stroke
  - GCS >8
  - Uncontrolled bleeding or cardiac arrest due to trauma (aka traumatic arrest)
  - Prolonged cardiac arrest >60 minutes
  - Refractory hypotension despite pressor support and adequate fluid resuscitation

(Omairi, 2023)

If the patient meets TTM criteria, consult with the provider to determine if CT imaging is required before initiating cooling measures. Insert core temperature monitoring device (esophageal and/or Foley temperature-sensing probes are more effective than rectal). Attach the cooling unit to the patient according to the manufacturer guidelines. Goal-targeted core temperature will be 33°C to 36°C per order. Goal time for initiation of TTM is within 4 hours per policy. Anticipate orders to administer sedatives and possibly continuous paralytics to prevent shivering. Monitor for anticipated bradycardia, hypotension, hypokalemia, and hypoglycemia during TTM. Prepare for ICU admission where the rewarming phase will occur very gradually over about 24 to 36 hours.

> **FAST FACTS**
>
> Monitor the patient's level of paralysis by using a train-of-four meter. If you turn up the voltage on a train-of-four device high enough, you will elicit a tremor, despite the patient being adequately paralyzed. This is due to interaction with the muscle fibers by surpassing the local nerve fibers.

SUMMARY

Although cardiovascular diseases threaten lives every day, they can often be resolved with quick treatment. Make EKG a priority for all patients with chest pain. From arrival to EKG should be <10 minutes. Study and understand the various dysrhythmias and their treatments. Print out a rhythm strip on your monitored patients and add it to the patient's chart per shift and as needed. An ED nurse needs to understand the basics of cardiovascular assessments and treatments and be certified in ACLS.

REVIEW QUESTIONS

1) A patient with a past medical history (PMH) of CHF presents to the ED with a concern for septic shock. They are hypotensive despite having bilateral lower extremity edema. The provider orders a complete fluid volume resuscitation of 20 mL/kg. What is the appropriate action to take as a bedside nurse?
   a. Prepare the fluid boluses as the provider ordered them.
   b. Refuse to administer this medication.
   c. Clarify the order with the provider.
   d. Wait until the provider comes to you.
2) A patient presents to triage with complaints of chest pain. The patient is pale, diaphoretic, and visibly uncomfortable. What is the next appropriate step?
   a. Obtain an EKG.
   b. Place the patient on oxygen.
   c. Mark the patient an emergency severity index (ESI) 2 and move them to the waiting room until a room in the ED is available.
   d. Obtain a full home medication list.

REFERENCES

American Heart Association. (2023, October 19). *Heart valves and infective endocarditis.* https://www.heart.org/en/health-topics/heart-valve-problems-and-disease/heart-valve-problems-and-causes/heart-valves-and-infective-endocarditis

Chatterjee, K., & Massie, B. (2007, September). Systolic and diastolic heart failure: Differences and similarities. *Journal of Cardiac Failure, 13*(7), 569–576. https://doi.org/10.1016/j.cardfail.2007.04.006

Colucci, W. (2023, October 19). Treatment of acute decompensated heart failure: Specific therapies. *UpToDate.* https://www.uptodate.com/contents/treatment-of-acute-decompensated-heart-failure-specific-therapies

de Alencar Neto, J. N. (2018, January 25). Morphine, oxygen, nitrates, and mortality reducing pharmacological treatment for acute coronary syndrome: An evidence-based review. *Cureus, 10*(1), e2114. https://doi.org/10.7759/cureus.2114

Ferguson, J. J., Diver, D. J., Boldt, M., & Pasternak, R. C. (1989). Significance of nitroglycerin-induced hypotension with inferior wall acute myocardial infarction. *The American Journal of Cardiology, 64*(5), 311–314. https://doi.org/10.1016/0002-9149(89)90525-0

Miller, J., McNaughton, C., Joyce, K., Binz, S., & Levy, P. (2020, April). Hypertension management in emergency departments. *American Journal of Hypertension, 33*(10), 927–934. https://doi.org/10.1093/ajh/hpaa068

Omairi, A. (2023, June 25). *Targeted temperature management.* In StatPearls [Internet]. StatPearls Publishing. Retrieved August 26, 2025, from www.ncbi.nlm.nih.gov/books/NBK556124/

Patocka, J., Nepovimova, E., Wu, W., & Kuca, K. (2020, October 1). Digoxin: Pharmacology and toxicology—A review. *Environmental Toxicology and Pharmacology, 79,* 103400. https://doi.org/10.1016/j.etap.2020.103400

Schranz, A., & Barocas, J. A. (2020). Infective endocarditis in persons who use drugs. *Infectious Disease Clinics of North America, 34*(3), 479–493. https://doi.org/10.1016/j.idc.2020.06.004

Stashko, E. (2023, August 7). *Cardiac tamponade.* In StatPearls [Internet]. StatPearls Publishing. Retrieved August 26, 2025, from https://www.ncbi.nlm.nih.gov/books/NBK431090/

Yiadom, M. Y., Baugh, C. W., McWade, C. M., Liu, X., Song, K. J., Patterson, B. W., Jenkins, C. A., Tanski, M., Mills, A. M., Salazar, G., Wang, T. J., Dittus, R. S., Liu, D., & Storrow, A. B. (2017). Performance of emergency department screening criteria for an early ECG to identify ST-segment elevation myocardial infarction. *Journal of the American Heart Association, 6*(3), e003528. https://doi.org/10.1161/jaha.116.003528

Respiratory Emergencies

Sarah Berry

> Airway, Breathing, Circulation—the ABCs. Of all the acronyms and mnemonics that are used in healthcare, ABC (or any variation thereof) is one of the most important. If the patient's airway loses patency, their risk for decompensation increases exponentially as the seconds pass.

In this chapter, the nurse will learn to:
1. Review the oxygen delivery devices and their flow rates
2. Determine the difference between respiratory distress and respiratory failure
3. Understand the different respiratory and pulmonary diseases and their role in the ED
4. Review the rapid sequence intubation (RSI) checklist and medications

RESPIRATORY EMERGENCIES

Of all emergencies, respiratory problems must be treated first. **Without a patent airway and breathing, patients will die—and nothing else matters.** Therefore, the ED nurse must be able to recognize and rapidly respond to any respiratory emergency. This chapter talks about the most common respiratory conditions seen in the ED. Reviewing this chapter will allow the ED nurse to become familiar with respiratory emergencies and anticipate treatment and care for those emergencies.

It is important to recognize when a patient is in respiratory distress or respiratory failure; however, these terms are often misused.
- *Respiratory distress:* results in *decreased* oxygenation and/or ventilation.
- *Respiratory failure:* results in *inadequate* oxygenation and/or ventilation
  Figure 7.1 details the escalation of oxygen delivery.

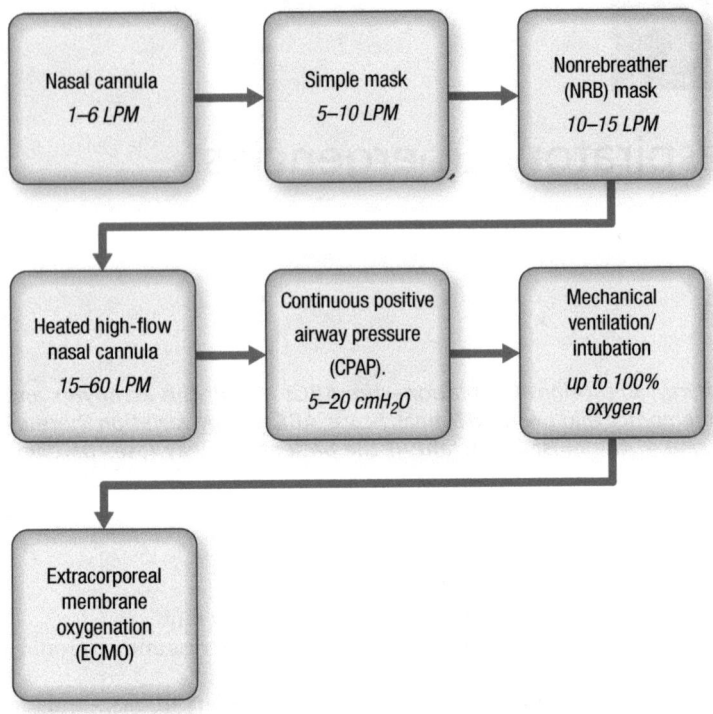

Figure 7.1 Escalation of oxygen delivery.

FAST FACTS

Assess the airway first, then breathing, then circulation. There are cases where the order is rearranged, but in most cases, it is ABC.

ACUTE RESPIRATORY DISTRESS SYNDROME

Acute respiratory distress syndrome (ARDS) can happen to a patient of any age. It can be triggered by either infectious or noninfectious causes. Sepsis is the most common infectious cause of ARDS. Noninfectious causes include pancreatitis, aspiration, traumatic injuries, transfusions, e-cigarette usage, and sometimes drug-induced causes. The result of the damage caused by these sources include decreased lung compliance, ventilation-perfusion (V/P), mismatch, impaired gas exchange, hyaline membrane and alveolar hemorrhage, alveolar collapse, increased dead space and pulmonary hypertension, and ultimately a systemic inflammatory response. Poor oxygen and carbon dioxide exchange is evident, as well as pulmonary edema and decreased oxygen saturation (Bos & Ware, 2022).

- *Causes:* Near drowning, aspiration, trauma, infection or sepsis, toxic inhalation such as e-cigarettes and smoke inhalation, traumatic pulmonary contusions, ischemia related to lung transplantation or endarterectomy, transfusion-related injuries, fat embolism, and other sources of sepsis (Bos & Ware, 2022).
- *Signs and symptoms:* Although there are some signs and symptoms, it is primarily diagnosed based on the Berlin Criteria. Preliminary symptoms include but are not limited to acute hypoxemic respiratory failure with bilateral infiltrates on chest x-ray, shortness of breath, tachypnea, tachycardia, productive cough, cyanosis, extreme fatigue, fever, hypotension, and crackles in the lungs (National Heart Lung and Blood Institute, 2022).
- *Interventions:* Monitor pulse oximetry/waveform capnography; apply continuous cardiac monitoring; establish IV access and obtain ordered lab tests and imaging; advocate for escalation of oxygen therapy as appropriate on the basis of the patient's oxygen saturation; anticipate RSI and ventilation; consider proning (having the patient on their abdomen), either independently if the patient is able or mechanically with coworkers (Gorman et al., 2022).

AIRWAY OBSTRUCTIONS

These can be divided into partial, complete, and upper or lower airway obstructions. A recent study showed abdominal thrusts (previously known as the Heimlich maneuver) and back blows were approximately 48% effective in the choking patient, while only approximately 24% of those survivors had a favorable neurological outcome (Norii et al., 2024). This is not to discourage bystanders from participating in attempting to clear a patient's airway through these measures.

- *Causes:* There are three categories of obstructive causes based on the location of the obstruction: supraglottic, glottic, and subglottic/tracheal (see Table 7.1).
- *Signs and symptoms:* Respiratory distress; tripod position; dyspnea; choking sensation; drooling; wheezing; decreased or no air movement; aphasia; tachycardia; tachypnea; cough; chest retractions; pallor or cyanosis; decreased oxygen saturation; and cardiopulmonary arrest.
- *Interventions:* Clear the airway by performing abdominal thrusts or back blows; initiate basic life support techniques for foreign object obstruction; anticipate foreign body removal with Magill forceps by the provider and orders to administer oxygen; measure pulse oximetry; if alert and coughing, place in high Fowler position for comfort; prepare for intubation and possible cricothyrotomy or tracheostomy; document airway patency changes; and document respiration rate and effort (Norii et al., 2024).

TABLE 7.1

Anatomical Categories of Obstruction

Supraglottic	Glottic	Subglottic/Tracheal
■ Croup ■ Epiglottitis ■ Ludwig angina ■ Angioedema ■ Tumor/abscess ■ Foreign body	■ Vocal cord paralysis ■ Tumor ■ Foreign body	■ Foreign body ■ Subglottic stenosis ■ Tumor

Source: Adapted from Eskander, A., de Almeida, J. R., & Irish, J. C. (2019). Acute upper airway obstruction. *New England Journal of Medicine, 381*(20), 1940–1949. https://doi.org/10.1056/nejmra1811697.

CROUP

Croup is a respiratory disease of the upper airway. It is often secondary to another respiratory illness, with about 75% of croup cases being related to the parainfluenza virus. Croup mostly affects children between the ages of 6 months and 3 years old. Symptoms usually resolve in about 48 hours, but severe obstruction could lead to respiratory distress, failure, and respiratory arrest (Johnson, 2014).

- *Signs and symptoms:* Fever, barking cough that worsens at night, inspiratory stridor, hoarseness, respiratory distress, and retractions or use of accessory muscles while breathing (Johnson, 2014).
- *Interventions:* Prepare for the need for oxygen therapy—this could be either by nasal cannula if the patient can tolerate it or blow-by (oxygen delivered by a mask such as a nonrebreather [NRB] at a rate of 10–15 liters per minute [LPM]; Barends et al., 2018). Dexamethasone is used to decrease inflammation in the airways, allowing for easier air flow and decreasing stridor. A single dose of oral dexamethasone can improve symptoms in mild croup; intramuscular (IM) dexamethasone can be used with patients who are not tolerating the dose by mouth (PO) and nebulized epinephrine (racemic epinephrine) has been shown to reduce symptoms in moderate to severe croup. Patients who require supplemental oxygen to maintain adequate oxygen saturation should be considered for hospitalization. Imaging is not necessary for diagnosis but could be used to exhibit the "steeple sign," visible in the anteroposterior view (Dowdy & Cornelius, 2020).

EPIGLOTTITIS

Epiglottitis is generally caused by a bacterial infection, leading to inflammation and edema. Historically, epiglottitis was predominantly occurring in children between the ages of 2 and 6 years. With the development of the *Haemophilus influenzae* B (Hib) vaccine, the condition became far more common in adults and less common in children (Dowdy & Cornelius, 2020). Other causes include *Streptococcus pyogenes, Streptococcus pneumoniae*, and *Staphylococcus aureus*. Additionally, trauma and foreign body ingestion could potentially lead to epiglottitis (Guerra & Waseem, 2022).

- *Signs and symptoms:* Fever and sore throat; more serious cases with impending airway compromise may exhibit dysphagia, use of the tripod position to facilitate air movement, stridor, and muffled voice. The most prominent and distinguished sign is drooling. A "cherry red edematous epiglottis" is a definitive diagnosis for epiglottitis and can be visualized through either nasolaryngoscopy or laryngoscopy (Dowdy & Cornelius, 2020).
- *Interventions:* If the patient is exhibiting drooling or stridor, *do not* interact with the patient's airway to examine the possibility of swelling. This attempt at visualizing their uvula could cause agitation, leading to rapid decompensation in patient status and ability to maintain their airway (Dowdy & Cornelius, 2020). Initiate continuous cardiac monitoring and pulse oximetry. Have airway supplies readily available near the patient's room, including endotracheal (ET) tubes, stylets, bougies, and direct laryngoscopy and video laryngoscopy blades depending on physician preference. Because the patient's airway is already inflamed and irritated, traditional intubation could be difficult or impossible. It is important to anticipate the need for a potential surgical airway like cricothyrotomy. Initiate IV access. If the patient can tolerate imaging, x-rays could be diagnostic with a lateral neck x-ray. The "thumb sign" is a classic finding that represents epiglottitis (Dowdy & Cornelius, 2020). Much like croup, humidified supplemental oxygen administration may be appropriate if the patient's oxygen saturation indicates the need. Administration of racemic epinephrine may help to improve upper airway edema. Because epiglottitis is generally caused by a bacterial infection, antibiotics are recommended based on culture findings and should be administered as prescribed (Dowdy & Cornelius, 2020). The patient should be admitted to the ICU for close monitoring and transported on a cardiac monitor by an RN whenever they leave the ED.

LUDWIG ANGINA

Ludwig angina is a potentially dangerous phenomenon that could lead to airway compromise. It is characterized by rapidly spreading swelling in the submandibular region that usually has an infectious cause. Because it is bacterial in nature, the most common suspects are *Streptococcus viridans*, *Bacteroides*, and *Staphylococcus*, and treatment is variable (Romero et al., 2022). The occurrence is more common in patients who have poor dentition or who are immunocompromised.

- *Signs and symptoms:* Fever, fatigue, chills, generalized weakness, trismus (spasming of mastication muscles), and meningismus (headache, neck stiffness). With cases of progressing airway compromise, symptoms like drooling, dysphagia, and tripod positioning to facilitate air movement

may be evident. As the airway becomes more compromised, the patient may experience difficulty breathing, new or worsening stridor, and anxiety (Bridwell et al., 2021).
- *Interventions:* ABCs! Because the patient is at risk for rapid decompensation and airway compromise, the nurse should have various oxygen delivery devices and airway management options available at the bedside. This could be as simple as a nasal cannula or NRB or as advanced as intubation or cricothyrotomy equipment. Attach the patient to the cardiac monitor and continuous pulse oximetry. Obtain IV access and anticipate lab work and blood culture collection. The patient may need to get a CT with contrast; use clinical judgment to decide if the nurse should escort the patient to imaging and if cardiac monitoring should be continuously used. Frequently assess the patient's airway and work of breathing. Administer antibiotics and additional medication if written. Anticipate admission to the ICU for close airway and vital sign monitoring (Bridwell et al., 2021).

ANGIOEDEMA AND ANAPHYLAXIS

Currently, four types of angioedema have been identified. Two primary forms are histamine-mediated and bradykinin-mediated angioedema. They present differently, depending on the cause. Histamine-mediated angioedema presents similarly to anaphylaxis, whereas bradykinin-mediated angioedema presents with more face and oropharyngeal involvement. Both types of edema are classically defined as nondependent and nonpitting, which differentiates them from cardiac- or pulmonary-related edema (Long et al., 2019).

In the ED, the most common bradykinin-mediated angioedema is angiotensin-converting enzyme inhibitor (ACE inhibitor)–mediated angioedema. It accounts for approximately 30% of angioedema cases that are seen in the ED. An estimated 11% of the 18% of patients who are admitted to the hospital require ICU-level care because of the high risk of potential airway involvement. African Americans, those who are immunosuppressed, those who take ACE inhibitors, and those who take dipeptidyl peptidase IV inhibitors such as sitagliptin, saxagliptin, linagliptin, and alogliptin are at the highest risk for developing bradykinin-mediated angioedema (Long et al., 2019).
- *Signs and symptoms:* Signs and symptoms are not always obvious and may require some prompting if they are not causing immediate discomfort or distress. Inquire about various types of swelling, but primarily lip or tongue swelling. Patients may also experience nausea, vomiting, or diarrhea depending on the type of anaphylaxis they are experiencing. They may also be experiencing pruritus, syncope, dyspnea, or feelings of lightheadedness. The patient may also experience wheezing, stridor, or changes in their voice (Long et al., 2019).
- *Interventions:* Assess the patient's ABC. Connect the patient to the cardiac monitor, pulse oximeter, and blood pressure cuff. Establish at least one IV site. Establish the patient's baseline mentation so reassessment can be compared as their case evolves. Anticipate administering ordered

medications to treat anaphylaxis such as IM epinephrine, H1 antagonists such as diphenhydramine, H2 antagonists like famotidine, and a corticosteroid. If the patient requires multiple rounds of medication to manage symptoms, the physician may consider a continuous infusion of epinephrine. In cases of presumed ACE inhibitor–mediated angioedema, fresh frozen plasma (FFP) has been recommended for treatment. Prepare for imminent airway compromise and have emergency airway equipment ready at the bedside. Patients with angioedema are at higher risk for difficult airway management and may require fiberoptic intubation. If video, direct, and fiberoptic intubation fail, the patient will require cricothyrotomy to manage their airway. According to Long et al. (2019), 50% of patients who needed a definitive airway required either a cricothyrotomy or tracheostomy. Depending on the level of airway management and assessment required, the patient could be admitted to the ICU (Long et al., 2019).

DRUG-ASSISTED INTUBATION OR RAPID SEQUENCE INTUBATION

Drug-assisted intubation (DAI)/RSI is a technique used to paralyze and sedate a patient just prior to performing ET intubation. This process is usually performed by a team including an ED provider, respiratory therapist, and an RN. In some facilities, a pharmacist may be available for assistance in medication preparation. The RN may consider requesting an additional RN in the room to facilitate bedside care or documentation.

See Table 7.2 for a listing of intubation medication classifications.

RAPID SEQUENCE INTUBATION PREPARATION CHECKLIST

Prepare the Environment and the Patient

1. Attach the cardiac monitor, pulse oximeter, blood pressure monitor, and continuous waveform capnography device to the patient.
2. Obtain the patient's weight for medication dosing.
3. Establish IV or intraosseous access.
4. Preoxygenate the patient with an NRB, a nasal cannula using at least 10 LPM, or a bag valve mask (BVM).
5. Make sure suction equipment and an Ambu bag are available and working properly.
6. Make sure nasal or oral pharyngeal airways are available in appropriate sizes.
7. Make sure ET tubes with stylets and bougies are available in appropriate sizes.

(continued)

8. Make sure nasogastric (NG) or orogastric (OG) tubes are available in the appropriate size. Avoid NG tube usage in patients with nondefinitive head or facial trauma.
9. Make sure a laryngoscope with the physician-preferred size and type of blade is available.
    a. Prepare the video and direct laryngoscope, rescue airway adjuncts such as an iGel or King airway, and cricothyrotomy tray.
10. Make sure a 10-mL syringe to inflate the ET balloon is available.
11. Make sure the ET securement device or cloth tape is available.
12. Ensure a crash cart and ventilator are in the room.
13. Attach the cardiac monitor, pulse oximeter, blood pressure, and continuous waveform capnography device to patient.
14. Obtain the patient's weight for medication dosing.
15. Establish IV or intraosseous access.
16. Preoxygenate the patient with either an NRB, a nasal cannula using at least 10 LPM, or a BVM.
17. Suction equipment and ambu bag is available and working properly.
18. Nasal or oral pharyngeal airways are available in appropriate sizes.
19. ET tubes with stylets and bougies are available in appropriate sizes.
20. NG or OG tube are available in the appropriate size. Avoid NG tube usage in patients with nondefinitive head or facial trauma.
21. Laryngoscope with physician preferred size and type of blade
    a. Prepare the video and direct laryngoscope, rescue airway adjuncts such as iGel or King airway, and cricothyrotomy tray
22. 10-mL syringe to inflate ET balloon is available.
23. ET securement device or cloth tape is available.
24. Crash cart and ventilator is in room.

RAPID SEQUENCE INTUBATION: STEP BY STEP

1. Prepare equipment (see the previous checklist).
2. Pretreat the patient to ensure optimized hemodynamics. If normal vital signs are not possible because of instability but a definitive airway is required, optimize the patient as much as possible without delaying care. Anticipate the need for swift treatment of postintubation consequences such as bradycardia, hypotension, acid–base balance shifts, or even cardiac arrest.
3. Prepare medications for intubation.
    a. Be sure to label all syringes of medications with the name, dose, and concentration of medication; see Table 7.2 for medications.

(continued)

4. Open the airway, maintaining C-spine immobilization if an injury is present.
5. Continue to preoxygenate the patient with 100% oxygen via NRB or BVM.
6. Determine the provider's plan of medication—RSI versus delayed sequence intubation (DSI). Administer medication as ordered by the ED provider; **remember to administer the sedative prior to the paralytic**. The provider will assess whether the patient is relaxed enough to undergo intubation. Look for jaw relaxation and apnea.
    a. RSI is the method of giving the induction agent closely followed by the paralytic medication. DSI is when there is a lapse of time between administering the induction agent and administering the paralytic. This time lapse allows for proper dissociation of the patient, decreasing the chances of delirium or adverse effects of induction medication administration. It also allows for proper preoxygenation of the patient prior to an intubation attempt. DSI is ideal for patients who are not tolerating preoxygenation measures such as bilevel positive airway pressure (BiPAP), continuous positive airway pressure (CPAP), or NRB. With this intolerance of oxygen delivery devices, the team is not able to optimize oxygenation prior to intubation. After administering the induction agent, wait approximately 10 to 15 seconds for the patient to properly dissociate. This allows the patient's airway to relax, and the team can preoxygenate the patient. Once preoxygenation begins, the provider will determine the length of time and hemodynamic indicators required to reach optimization. These indicators may include an ideal blood oxygen saturation or changes in heart rate or blood pressure to show improved stability. After those milestones have been met, the paralytic will be delivered, and the intubation attempt would be completed after the patient shows signs of paralysis (Weingart et al., 2015).
7. Have suction within reach of the provider to evacuate emesis, saliva, or blood from the airway.
8. Monitor the continuous pulse oximeter, waveform capnography, and vital signs while the provider attempts ET intubation.
9. If intubation is successful, assist in removing the stylet and inflate the balloon.
10. If the provider is unsuccessful, be ready to assist ventilations with BVM (one breath every 6 seconds). Assess for chest rise; if chest rise is not witnessed, reposition the patient's head and jaw to open the airway. If an additional person is available, one person would perform a jaw thrust maneuver and secure the BVM over the patient's mouth and nose, while the second person squeezes the

(continued)

ambu bag. Assist with preparation for another pass attempt, and anticipate the need for backup airway adjuncts such as an iGel, a King airway, or a cricothyrotomy.
11. Confirm placement by attaching the BVM to the ET tube; listen over the stomach first for gastric sounds for one breath to ensure an esophageal intubation **did not** take place, **then** assess for bilateral breath sounds; attach the CO_2 detection device; and monitor the waveform capnography.
12. Secure the ET tube with cloth tape or a commercial securement device.
13. Place either the NG or OG tube and obtain an x-ray to confirm placement of both the ET tube and gastric tube. Be mindful that an x-ray confirms depth of the ET tube. To the untrained eye or to even those with experience, the ET tube can be mistaken as in the trachea when in reality it is in the esophagus. That is why additional placement verification processes are used. These include auscultating for air over the stomach, then auscultating the lungs, as well as waveform capnography.
14. Document the time, confirmed placement methods, ET tube size, and tube placement at the teeth or gum. A respiratory therapist will usually attach a ventilator to the ET tube at this time.
15. *Continue sedation, pain management,* and frequent vital sign monitoring.

TABLE 7.2

Intubation Medications

Premedications	Induction	Paralytics
■ Fentanyl ■ Atropine	■ Etomidate ■ Ketamine ■ Propofol ■ Thiopental	■ Rocuronium ■ Succinylcholine ■ Vecuronium

Premedications
- *Fentanyl:* Adults: 1 to 3 mcg/kg
  - *Pediatrics:* 1 mcg/kg
    - An opioid that is used to decrease the sympathetic response and can help to decrease the cough reflex. Monitor for decreases in level of consciousness and blood pressure. Be sure to give this medication over approximately 1 minute to decrease the possibility of thoracic muscle rigidity, also known as rigid chest wall syndrome (Zoorob et al., 2023).

- *Atropine (Atropen):* Adults: 1 mg (max 3 mg)
  - *Pediatrics:* 0.01 to 0.02 mg/kg (max 0.5 mg)
    - Use of atropine helps to decrease rebound bradycardia from medications used to intubate

Induction Medications
- *Etomidate:* 0.3 mg/kg
  - This medication does not alter hemodynamics or change intracranial pressure, making this ideal for trauma patients or those who are hemodynamically unstable.
- *Ketamine (Ketalar):* 1 to 2 mg/kg
  - Ketamine is advantageous for patients with lung disease such as chronic obstructive pulmonary disease (COPD), emphysema, or asthma because of its bronchodilatory effects. It also does not have a significant effect on the patient's hemodynamics like bradycardia or hypotension. Possible adverse effects include increases in intracranial pressure, cardiovascular stimulation, hallucinations, significant muscle rigidity (Vien & Chhabra, 2017), and emergence delirium. Muscle rigidity is sometimes caused when ketamine is administered too quickly when given by IV push. In turn, this can lead to an inability to open the patient's mouth in order to attempt intubation. Emergence delirium is more common in patients who are not going to be sedated continuously following administration.
- *Propofol (Diprivan):* 1 to 2 mg/kg. Check state law for RN administration conditions.
  - This medication does not affect intracranial pressure and provides some amnestic effects for patients. Patients may experience bradycardia or hypotension while on this medication. They may require even closer monitoring and tight titration to achieve a level of comfort for the patient, while not causing hemodynamic instability.
  - Verify the RN's role by the state board of nursing to clarify their administration permissions. Some states do not allow RNs to bolus this medication, and therefore it should be administered by an advanced practice provider (APP) or the physician.

Paralytics
- *Rocuronium (Zemuron):* 1 mg/kg
  - This medication has very little effect on the hemodynamics of patients. Because of its long duration of action, be sure to have contingency plans in place in the event that intubation is unsuccessful.
- *Succinylcholine (Anectine):* 1 to 1.5 mg/kg
  - Succinylcholine is contraindicated in patients who have burns, crush injuries, and renal disease; who are hyperkalemic; or who are bradycardic. In rare cases, genetic disposition may cause **malignant hyperthermia** after receiving succinylcholine. Monitor for severe high fever, muscle spasms/rigidity, tachycardia, sweating, tachypnea, ventricular

tachycardia/ventricular fibrillation, and acidosis. Follow the facility's malignant hyperthermia treatment protocol for cooling measures and administration of the antidote dantrolene (Ryanodex; Watt, 2023).
- *Vecuronium:* 0.1 to 0.2 mg/kg
  - This medication is not routinely used unless a nondepolarizing agent is required and rocuronium is not readily available. Because of this medication's long duration of action, be sure to have a contingency plan in place in the event that intubation is unsuccessful (RSI: medications, dosages, and recommendations).

(Lafferty, 2024)

FAST FACTS

To troubleshoot deterioration or hypoxia after intubation, use the mnemonic **DOPE**: **D**isplacement, **O**bstruction, **P**neumothorax, **E**quipment failure.

TROUBLESHOOTING INTUBATED PATIENTS

When patients are intubated, troubleshooting deterioration in status or hypoxia is not just for respiratory therapists. Remembering the mnemonic DOPE could be beneficial in situations where patients are intubated. **DOPE** stands for **D**isplacement, **O**bstruction, **P**neumothorax, and **E**quipment failure (Piccione, 2021).
- *Displacement:* Check the ventilator circuit. Start at the patient and work backward until the vent is reached. Be sure that the tubing is connected correctly and has not popped off anywhere. Verify that the ET tube has not moved from where it was confirmed after placement. Check that the measurement is 22 cm at the teeth. Additionally, make sure that the ventilator settings are appropriate for the patient's height, ideal body weight, and sex (Piccione, 2021).
- *Obstruction:* Secretions are often thick. Consider suctioning the patient if in-line suction is available to clear secretions from the tube and respiratory tract. Also check that the tube is not kinked anywhere (Piccione, 2021). Again, start at the patient's ET tube and work toward the vent, checking all the connections and intersections of equipment to verify patency.
- *Pneumothorax:* When the ventilator gives a "high pressure" alarm, consider a pneumothorax (Piccione, 2021). Assess the patient's breath sounds. If there is a concern for absence of breath sounds on one side versus the other, alert the provider. A chest x-ray should be obtained to rule out a "right mainstem," which is when the ET tube is either inserted or migrates to the right branch of the trachea. This does not allow for adequate oxygenation and ventilation of the left lung. There would be an

absence of breath sounds on the left side if this is the case. After a right mainstem has been ruled out, evaluate the chest for a pneumothorax. The patient may have other symptoms present such as agitation, pain, tracheal deviation in the event of a tension pneumothorax, dyspnea, decreased oxygen saturation, tachycardia, hypotension, and possible subcutaneous emphysema (Piccione, 2021).
- *Equipment failure:* Ventilators are not perfect. The operators are also not perfect. The environment is certainly not perfect. In the real world, equipment failure can be a daily occurrence. Be sure that the oxygen is hooked up appropriately to the ventilator and whatever oxygen supply is being used. If oxygen delivery is not the problem, consider recalibrating the machine to reestablish a baseline to work from (Piccione, 2021).

CHRONIC OBSTRUCTIVE PULMONARY DISEASE

COPD is an inflammatory process that changes the functionality and structure of the airways. Emphysema, another respiratory disease, falls under the COPD umbrella. Emphysema is characterized by destruction of the alveolar air sacs in the lungs, leading to obstructive damage. In COPD, the alveolar sacs also become less elastic, which does not allow them to rebound to their baseline shape, leading to air trapping in the lungs.

In addition to these structural changes, chronic hyperinflation leads to limited airflow and impaired gas exchange. Because of this impaired exchange, patients with COPD will have elevated carbon dioxide (CO_2) levels and retention. As the disease progresses, the elevated CO_2 levels will make the patient dependent on lower blood oxygen saturation (PAO_2) to regulate ventilations, leading to chronic hypoxia. The dead space is taken up by CO_2, decreasing the surface area to exchange and store oxygen. In doing so, the body begins to compensate for this change and requires less oxygen over time. Patients who have COPD or emphysema have a decreased oxygen saturation, targeted around 88% to 92% (Echevarria et al., 2021).

If patients are given large volumes or concentrations of oxygen, they blow off their CO_2 and could lose their compensatory mechanism. Their hypoxic respiratory drive decreases and can lead to respiratory distress or failure. If patients are in a COPD exacerbation, where something has triggered their lung disease to acutely worsen, the patient may retain even more CO_2 than previously. This could cause changes in mentation, altered blood gas levels, agitation, or lethargy. Consider CPAP or BiPAP in these patients to decrease the compounded CO_2 until the patient returns to their compensatory baseline. After doing so and the patient stabilizes, exchange their oxygen delivery device to something more appropriate (Echevarria et al., 2021).
- *Causes:* Enlargement of the alveoli, loss of lung tissue elasticity, and destruction of the alveolar wall. This chronic lung damage is associated with emphysema, chronic bronchitis, substance inhalation, and cigarette smoking (Agarwal, 2023).

- *Signs and symptoms:* Dyspnea either with exertion or at rest; fatigue; tachypnea; pursed-lip breathing; wheezing; tripod position; use of accessory muscles; barrel chest; tachycardia; hypertension; confusion; cyanosis; premature ventricular contractions; and acute respiratory failure.
- *Interventions:* Administer continuous cardiac monitoring, pulse oximetry, and end-tidal capnography for the patient and have oxygen delivery device options nearby. Anticipate orders to establish an IV and draw blood for lab tests, including either a venous or an arterial blood gas. Monitor for changes in the patient's level of consciousness, work of breathing, and vital signs. Medication orders could consist of inhaled bronchodilators such as albuterol or a nebulizer, corticosteroids by IV such as methylprednisolone that may later be transitioned to a burst pack of prednisone, and possible antibiotics for patients who have cause for infectious concern. If the patient has an abnormal blood gas value, the results may determine if oxygen therapy is needed. If the patient has a concerning level of CO_2 or increased work of breathing, the provider may order CPAP or BiPAP (Sagana, 2022). If the patient fails these interventions, anticipate orders for RSI/DSI and intubation.

ASTHMA

Asthma is a chronic reactive airway disease. It is a complex inflammatory response characterized by large airway inflammation, hyperresponsiveness, and intermittent airflow obstruction. Asthma can be triggered by exposure to allergens or environmental irritants, viruses, cold weather, and exercise.

- *Causes:* Many factors contribute to asthma, including environmental allergens or factors such as pollutants or cold weather, viral respiratory infections, exercise, gastroesophageal reflux disease (GERD), sinusitis or rhinitis, aspirin or nonsteroidal anti-inflammatory drug (NSAID) hypersensitivity, use of beta-blockers, obesity, tobacco smoke, household sprays or perfumes, and emotional factors (Morris, 2024).
- *Signs and symptoms:* Wheezing, coughing, shortness of breath, accessory muscle usage, increased work of breathing, chest/chest wall/rib pain.
- *Interventions:* Apply continuous cardiac monitoring, pulse oximetry, and end-tidal capnography if the patient is disoriented or lethargic. Consider oxygen delivery devices if needed on the basis of patient presentation, vital signs, or provider orders. Medication management depends on the level of severity. Anticipate doses for a short-acting beta$_2$ agonist (i.e., albuterol) through a nebulizer or metered-dose inhaler. Systemic corticosteroids may be ordered, either PO or IV. In addition to the breathing treatments, ipratropium may be added to boost the response of albuterol. If the patient fails treatments and requires high levels of oxygen delivery, the patient may require intubation to manage their symptoms (Pollart et al., 2011). When administered IV, magnesium can have bronchodilating properties. Although this is seen more in children, adults may benefit as well (Cunha et al., 2024). See Table 7.3 for information on asthma severity.

TABLE 7.3
Asthma Severity

Mild	• Dyspnea with exertion • Able to be treated at home with short-acting beta2 agonist • Possible short course of steroids
Moderate	• Dyspnea that interferes with or limits activity • Relief with increased use of short-acting $beta_2$ agonists • Oral steroids
Severe	• ED visit and possible hospitalization • Some relief with short-acting $beta_2$ agonists • PO steroids
Life-threatening	• Requires ED care and possible ICU stay • Minimal to no relief with short-acting $beta_2$ agonists • IV steroids

PO, by mouth.
Source: Adapted from Pollart, S. M., Compton, R. M., & Elward, K. S. (2011, July 1). *Management of acute asthma exacerbations*. American Family Physician. https://www.aafp.org/pubs/afp/issues/2011/0701/p40.html.

STATUS ASTHMATICUS

Status asthmaticus is a rare severe asthma exacerbation that does not respond to therapy. The mortality rate is significantly high.

- *Causes:* Untreated asthma or rapid, severe onset of asthma. History may reveal previous intubations.
- *Signs and symptoms:* Absent breath sounds (silent lung), inability to speak in full sentences or lie flat, pulse oxygen level <90% with supplemental oxygen, altered level of consciousness, fatigue, long expiratory phase, tachypnea with accessory muscle use, and cyanosis (Chakraborty et al., 2024). Waveform capnography may reveal "shark fin"–shaped waveform with elevated CO_2 levels due to air trapping.
- *Interventions:* Treat immediately and aggressively with high-flow oxygen, IV magnesium, BiPAP, or intubation. Ketamine is recommended for sedation with asthmatic intubation. Apply pulse oximetry and end-tidal capnography device. Consider IM or IV epinephrine and extracorporeal membrane oxygenation (ECMO; Chakraborty et al., 2024).

FAST FACTS

Patients who were once wheezing and are no longer making sounds should have their breath sounds evaluated. If they are quiet, it could be that they are improving (no wheezing) or they are worsening (impending respiratory failure due to closed airways).

SPONTANEOUS PNEUMOTHORAX/TENSION PNEUMOTHORAX

Spontaneous pneumothorax is an air leak in the pleural space between the lungs and the chest wall that results in partial or total collapse of the lung. In the event of a tension pneumothorax, intervention is critical for patient survival. As tension pneumothoraxes worsen, the patient's chances of survival dwindle.

- *Causes:* Primary spontaneous pneumothoraxes are not generally caused by something but are more *spontaneous (hence the term)*. Secondary spontaneous pneumothoraxes (SSPs) are associated with underlying disease such as COPD, asthma, cystic fibrosis, pneumonia, and malignancy or lung disease such as sarcoidosis or pulmonary fibrosis. Additionally, connective tissue diseases such as Marfan syndrome, Ehlers–Danlos syndrome, or arthritis are causes of SSP (Costumbrado & Ghassemzadeh, 2023).
- *Signs and symptoms:* Patients may experience sharp, pleuritic chest pain. This is often partnered with dyspnea, increased work of breathing, and tachycardia. Decreased or absent breath sounds may be appreciated on physical exam, as well as jugular venous distention, pulsus paradoxus, hyperresonance on percussion, and decreased tactile fremitus (vibration of the chest wall while the patient speaks; Costumbrado & Ghassemzadeh, 2023). Patients experiencing a tension pneumothorax may exhibit a lot of the same symptoms, but tracheal deviation is the differentiating sign. If not treated immediately, the patient could rapidly decompensate to cardiac arrest (Sahota & Sayad, 2024).
- *Interventions:* Connect the patient to continuous cardiac monitoring and pulse oximetry. Obtain a STAT chest x-ray. Obtain an IV and EKG, and apply oxygen as appropriate. Assess breath sounds, the patient's work of breathing, and any changes in mentation. Prepare the patient for a chest tube or needle thoracostomy in emergency situations. Administer medications as prescribed.

PNEUMONIA

Pneumonia is an infection that encompasses several syndromes caused by various organisms. Three classifications of pneumonia currently exist: community-acquired pneumonia (CAP), hospital-acquired pneumonia (HAP), and ventilator-acquired pneumonia (VAP). CAP is any pneumonia that was obtained outside of the hospital. HAP is pneumonia acquired within 48 hours of being admitted to the inpatient setting that was not already percolating prior to admission. VAP is the type that is acquired within 48 hours of being intubated.

There are several subtypes for each of the pneumonia acquisition types. Each has certain organisms specific to them. This research has made treatment more specific based on the organism found.

- *Causes:* Bacterial infections can develop on their own or from upper respiratory infections such as the flu or a cold. Viral pneumonia can also develop from influenza, rhinovirus, and respiratory syncytial virus. Fungal pneumonia is generally associated with patients who are immunocompromised from chemotherapy or HIV. Aspiration can also lead to pneumonia (U.S. Department of Health and Human Services, 2022).
- *Signs and symptoms:* The patient may experience tachypnea, tachycardia, fever, decreased breath sounds, rhonchi or crackles, and dullness on percussion. The patient may also have increased white blood cell count, decreased oxygen saturation if consolidation is large, and a productive cough (Jain et al., 2023).
- *Interventions:* Attach the patient to continuous cardiac monitoring, the blood pressure cuff, and pulse oximetry. If the team is concerned about possible sepsis with pneumonia being the source, obtain an IV and lab work. Obtain blood cultures and a sputum culture if the patient has a productive cough. Provide medications as prescribed such as antipyretics, analgesia, fluids, and antibiotics. Pneumonia can be painful, so a pain assessment is important. Administer oxygen therapy as appropriate.

SUMMARY

ABC: If the patient does not have an airway and they are not breathing, circulation will quickly follow in failing. Be sure to thoroughly document respiratory assessments. This should include rate, depth, breath sounds, symmetry, skin color, use of accessory muscles (if labored or unlabored), and ability to speak in full sentences before and after each intervention. Recognizing life-threatening respiratory emergencies can make or break a patient's outcome. Confidence comes with practice. Becoming familiar with a facility's products and resources allows one to be prepared with different airway adjuncts or treatments for certain respiratory processes. Use the help and knowledge of the hospital's respiratory therapists for questions and concerns.

REVIEW QUESTIONS

1) What is a common pulmonary cause of septic shock?
    a. Tension pneumothorax
    b. Inhalation burn
    c. Foreign object aspiration
    d. Bacterial pneumonia
2) What is the ideal oxygen saturation for a patient with COPD?
    a. 88% to 92%
    b. 84% to 88%
    c. >95%
    d. 100%

REFERENCES

Agarwal, A. K. (2023, August 7). *Chronic obstructive pulmonary disease.* StatPearls [Internet]. Retrieved August 26, 2025, from https://www.ncbi.nlm.nih.gov/books/NBK559281/

Barends, C. R., Yavuz, P., Molenbuur, B., & Absalom, A. R. (2018). Performance of blow-by methods in delivering oxygen to pediatric patients during transport: A laboratory study. *Pediatric Anesthesia, 28*(12), 1142–1147. https://doi.org/10.1111/pan.13515

Bos, L. D., & Ware, L. B. (2022, October 1). Acute respiratory distress syndrome: Causes, pathophysiology, and phenotypes. *The Lancet, 400*(10358), 1145–1156. https://doi.org/10.1016/s0140-6736(22)01485-4

Bridwell, R., Gottlieb, M., Koyfman, A., & Long, B. (2021). Diagnosis and management of Ludwig's angina: An evidence-based review. *The American Journal of Emergency Medicine, 41,* 1–5. https://doi.org/10.1016/j.ajem.2020.12.030

Chakraborty, R. K., Chen, R., & Basnet, S. (2024, February 9). *Status asthmaticus.* StatPearls [Internet]. Retrieved August 26, 2025, from https://www.ncbi.nlm.nih.gov/books/NBK526070/

Costumbrado, J., & Ghassemzadeh, S. (2023, July 24). *Spontaneous pneumothorax.* StatPearls [Internet]. Retrieved August 26, 2025, from https://www.ncbi.nlm.nih.gov/books/NBK459302/

Cunha, L., Mora, M. R., Afzal, F., Cesar, G. M., Guimaraes, C. R., Pontes, J. P. M., Alves, G. G., & Silveira, A. C. F. (2024, March 16). Standard medical therapy with vs. without nebulised magnesium for children with asthma decompensation. *European Journal of Pediatrics, 183,* 2637–2644. https://doi.org/10.1007/s00431-024-05517-3

Dowdy, R. A., & Cornelius, B. W. (2020). Medical management of epiglottitis. *Anesthesia Progress, 67*(2), 90–97. https://doi.org/10.2344/anpr-66-04-08

Echevarria, C., Steer, J., Wason, J., & Bourke, S. (2021, March 1). Oxygen therapy and inpatient mortality in COPD exacerbation. *Emergency Medicine Journal, 38*(3), 170–177. https://doi.org/10.1136/emermed-2019-209257

Gorman, E. A., Kane, C. M. O., & McAuley, D. F. (2022, October 1). Acute respiratory distress syndrome in adults: Diagnosis, outcomes, long-term sequelae, and management. *The Lancet, 400*(10358), 1157–1170. https://doi.org/10.1016/s0140-6736(22)01439-8

Guerra, A. M., & Waseem, M. (2022, October 17). *Epiglottitis.* StatPearls [Internet]. Retrieved August 26, 2025, from https://www.ncbi.nlm.nih.gov/books/NBK430960/

Jain, V., Vashisht, R., Yilmaz, G., & Bhardwaj, A. (2023, July 31). *Pneumonia pathology.* StatPearls [Internet]. Retrieved August 26, 2025, from https://www.ncbi.nlm.nih.gov/books/NBK526116/

Johnson, D. W. (2014, September 29). Croup. *BMJ Clinical Evidence, 2014,* 0321. PMID: 25263284; PMCID: PMC4178284.

Lafferty, K. (2024, March 22). *Medications used in tracheal intubation.* Medscape. https://emedicine.medscape.com/article/109739-overview

Long, B., Koyfman, A., & Gottlieb, M. (2019). Evaluation and management of angioedema in the emergency department. *Western Journal of Emergency Medicine, 20*(4), 587–600. https://doi.org/10.5811/westjem.2019.5.42650

Morris, M. (2024, August 26). *Asthma.* Medscape. https://emedicine.medscape.com/article/296301-overview#a5

National Heart Lung and Blood Institute. (2022, March 24). *Acute respiratory distress syndrome symptoms*. U.S. Department of Health and Human Services. www.nhlbi.nih.gov/health/ards/symptoms

Norii, T., Igarashi, Y., Yoshino, Y., Nakao, S., Yang, M., Albright, D., Sklar, D. P., & Crandall, C. (2024, June 1). The effects of bystander interventions for foreign body airway obstruction on survival and neurological outcomes: Findings of the MOCHI registry. *Resuscitation*, *199*, 110198. https://doi.org/10.1016/j.resuscitation.2024.110198

Piccione, C. (2021). "DOPES": Acronym to help critical care nurses in the intensive care unit during the COVID age. *Dimensions of Critical Care Nursing*, *40*(2), 129–130. https://doi.org/10.1097/DCC.0000000000000466

Pollart, S. M., Compton, R. M., & Elward, K. S. (2011, July 1). *Management of acute asthma exacerbations*. American Family Physician. https://www.aafp.org/pubs/afp/issues/2011/0701/p40.html

Romero, J., Elkattaway, S., Romero, A., Latif, A., Al-Fiky, E., Al-Nasseri, A., Noori, M. A., & Al-Alwani, K. (2022). Ludwig's angina. *European Journal of Case Reports in Internal Medicine*, *9*(6), e003321. https://doi.org/10.12890/2022_003321

Sagana, R. L. (2022, April). *Care of the hospitalized patient with acute exacerbation of COPD*. National Center for Biotechnology Information. https://www.ncbi.nlm.nih.gov/books/NBK582288/

Sahota, R. J., & Sayad, E. (2024, January 30). *Tension pneumothorax*. StatPearls [Internet]. Retrieved August 26, 2025, from https://www.ncbi.nlm.nih.gov/books/NBK559090/

U.S. Department of Health and Human Services. (2022, March 24). *Causes and risk factors*. National Heart Lung and Blood Institute. https://www.nhlbi.nih.gov/health/pneumonia/causes

Vien, A., & Chhabra, N. (2017). Ketamine-induced muscle rigidity during procedural sedation mitigated by intravenous midazolam. *The American Journal of Emergency Medicine*, *35*(1), 200.e3–200.e4. https://doi.org/10.1016/j.ajem.2016.07.046

Watt, S. (2023, August 17). *Malignant hyperthermia*. StatPearls [Internet]. Retrieved August 26, 2025, from https://www.ncbi.nlm.nih.gov/books/NBK430828/

Weingart, S. D., Trueger, N. S., Wong, N., Scofi, J., Singh, N., & Rudolph, S. S. (2015). Delayed sequence intubation: A prospective observational study. *Annals of Emergency Medicine*, *65*(4), 349–355. https://doi.org/10.1016/j.annemergmed.2014.09.025

Zoorob, R., Uptegrove, L., & Park, B. L. (2023). Case report of very-low-dose fentanyl causing fentanyl-induced chest wall rigidity. *Cureus*, *15*(8), e43788. https://doi.org/10.7759/cureus.43788

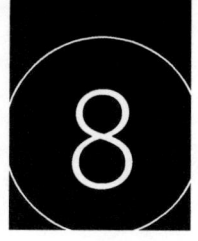

Gastrointestinal Emergencies

Alexander Menard

> The gastrointestinal (GI) system is made up of several organs, including the stomach, liver, pancreas, gallbladder, and intestines. GI emergencies can be a very messy everyday ED occurrence. Ruptured bowels, vomiting, diarrhea, constipation, enemas—you name it; you will see all types of GI problems in the ED. After reviewing this chapter, you will be able to differentiate the types of GI emergencies and their causes, manifestations, and treatments.

In this chapter, you will learn to:
1. Discuss the common GI problems presenting to the ED
2. Identify the signs and symptoms of GI emergencies
3. Review the interventions to address GI emergencies

GASTROINTESTINAL EMERGENCIES

Abdominal emergencies can present with a wide range of symptoms. These can range from severe abdominal pain, to nausea and vomiting, to extensive belching. Careful history taking and physical assessment will help to narrow down the suspected GI issues and inform interventions.

Abdominal Assessment

A thorough abdominal assessment is required when evaluating a patient suspected of having a GI emergency. Provocation, quality, radiation, severity, time (PQRST) is an efficient manner by which to assess a patient's abdominal pain (see Table 8.1).

When evaluating for a GI emergency, you will need to look beyond the abdomen and consider that the GI tract spans from the mouth to the anus. An emergency can occur anywhere along that tract.

TABLE 8.1

PQRST Abdominal Pain Assessment

Component	Description
Provocation	What makes pain better or worse? Position?
Quality or character	Can you describe the pain: burning, aching, sharp, dull, cramping, and stabbing?
Radiation, referral location	Where does pain radiate? Where does it start?
Severity	How severe is pain on a scale of 0–10?
Time	When did it start and end? How long did it last?

PQRST, provocation, quality, radiation, severity, time.

Gastritis
Gastritis is an inflammation of the stomach lining that can be an acute or chronic condition. Chronic gastritis can lead to ulcers and GI bleeding. The most common cause of acute gastritis is secondary to infection. Gastritis can occur in immunocompromised patients as well; examples of this could be herpes simplex or cytomegalovirus gastritis (Valle, 2022).

- *Causes:* Infection; stress; acute illness; gastroesophageal reflux disease (GERD); aspirin; nonsteroidal anti-inflammatory drugs (NSAIDs); alcohol; or food poisoning.
- *Signs and symptoms:* Nausea and vomiting; diarrhea; gastric mucosal bleeding; epigastric pain; malaise; anorexia; and loss of appetite.
- *Interventions:* Anticipate orders to administer fluids IV; arrange for abdominal x-ray; provide blood if blood loss is severe; prepare to collect a complete blood count, *Helicobacter pylori* testing, amylase level, and lipase and basic metabolic panel; and administer medications (e.g., antacids, GI cocktail, histamine receptor antagonists, and antiemetics). Discharge teaching should include lifestyle modifications of six small meals daily, smoking cessation, and prescribed use of antacids.

Gastroenteritis
Gastroenteritis is an inflammation of the stomach or small intestine.

- *Causes:* Viruses, bacteria, parasites, toxins, or allergens. The most common viruses that cause gastroenteritis are *Norovirus* and *Rotavirus* (McAninch & Smithson, 2017).
- *Signs and symptoms:* Nausea, vomiting, and diarrhea; hyperactive bowel sounds; abdominal pain or cramps; fever; dehydration; and hypovolemia in very young or very old people.
- *Interventions:* Educate the patient and family on strict handwashing and contact precautions. Anticipate orders to provide fluids IV,

prepare a basic metabolic panel and complete blood count, administer medications (antibiotics and antiparasitic agents), and provide patient education on a clear liquid and bananas, rice, applesauce, and toast (BRAT) diet.

Discharge teaching should include avoiding meat and dairy products, spicy foods, alcohol, greasy foods, and acidic foods.
- Infants should not stop formula feeding for more than 24 hours.
- Recovering from nausea and vomiting is a gradual process. The patient should have nothing by mouth (NPO) for an hour or so after vomiting. Then clear liquids should be introduced in small increments. Afterwards, the patient can advance to full liquids, avoiding dairy. The next step is the BRAT diet; finally, advancing diet as tolerated.

FAST FACTS

Viral gastroenteritis often produces a secretory diarrhea in the small intestines resulting in a nonbloody diarrhea.

Gastroesophageal Reflux Disease

GERD is commonly called "acid reflux." It occurs when stomach contents cause troublesome symptoms (sore throat or noncardiac chest pain) or complications (esophagitis). Most patients have mild disease, but serious complications can develop in some patients (Papadakis et al., 2025).
- *Causes:* The malfunction of the esophageal sphincter and/or a hiatal hernia are the major causes. Contributing factors are cigarette smoking, lying down after meals, stress, pregnancy, medications, consuming alcohol, large meals, spicy or acidic food, and caffeine. Complications such as scar tissue, dysphagia, and esophageal strictures may result from repeated exposure to gastric contents.
- *Signs and symptoms:* Upper midsternal burning pain and indigestion that worsens with lying down. Most often it occurs 30 to 60 minutes after a meal. Belching, noncardiac chest pain, cough, and hoarseness.
- *Interventions:* Anticipate orders for medications to relieve symptoms like antacids. Educate the patient on avoiding stress, fatty or fried foods, chocolate, alcohol consumption, tobacco products, and overeating. The patient should ensure hydration with water and avoid lying down for 3 hours after eating.

Bowel Obstruction

This is a potentially life-threatening condition resulting in the inability to move GI contents through the large or small bowel. There are two types of obstructions: large bowel and small bowel.

- *Causes:* Previous abdominal surgery, adhesions; hernia; strictures; foreign bodies; volvulus (twisting of bowel); intussusception; tumor; paralytic ileus; mesenteric infarction; and abdominal angina.
- *Signs and symptoms:* Fever; abdominal distention; nausea and vomiting; rapid onset of severe, cramping abdominal pain; diffuse abdominal tenderness and rigidity; dehydration; weight loss or weight gain (due to fluid retention); high-pitched or absent bowel sounds; diaphoresis; weakness; restlessness; and constipation or recent diarrhea.
- *Interventions:* Anticipate orders to arrange for abdominal CT scan, ultrasound, or x-rays; monitor vital signs; designate the patient as NPO; obtain complete blood count, amylase, alkaline phosphatase, lactic acid, and metabolic panel; administer fluids IV, antiemetics, and analgesics; insert nasogastric tube for gastric decompression as ordered; administer antibiotic medications as ordered; and prepare for possible operating room (OR) or admission.

Diverticulitis

Diverticulitis occurs when one or more diverticula become inflamed. This can result in perforation of the thin diverticular wall. If diverticulum perforates, a local abscess or peritonitis may result.
- *Causes:* Inflammation of the diverticula of the colon.
- *Signs and symptoms:* Can vary based on severity. Left lower quadrant pain, fever, nausea, and diarrhea or constipation.
- *Interventions:* Anticipate orders for lab work, including a complete blood count and imaging, which may include an abdominal x-ray, abdominal ultrasound, and abdominal CT scan.

Appendicitis

Appendicitis is an inflammation and obstruction of the appendix. It typically occurs in males ages 10 to 19 but can happen to anyone. If untreated, it can become necrotic or perforate. If it ruptures, it could lead to peritonitis, sepsis, and then septic shock.
- *Causes:* Unknown, but may be attributed to infection, twisting, or obstruction of the appendix.
- *Signs and symptoms:* Constant dull right lower quadrant abdominal pain (McBurney point; see Figure 8.1); rebound tenderness; elevated white blood cell (WBC) count; nausea and vomiting; low-grade fever (usually after first 24 hours); and manifestations of peritonitis (fever, guarding, abdominal pain and distention, hypoactive bowel sounds, and diffuse rigidity). With appendicitis, the pain typically precedes the vomiting. The patient is generally in so much pain that they vomit as a result.
- *Interventions:* Anticipate orders to give the patient analgesics, antibiotics, antiemetics, and fluids IV as well as make them NPO. Arrange for a complete blood count, metabolic panel, type and screen, an abdominal CT scan or ultrasound, and possible surgery.

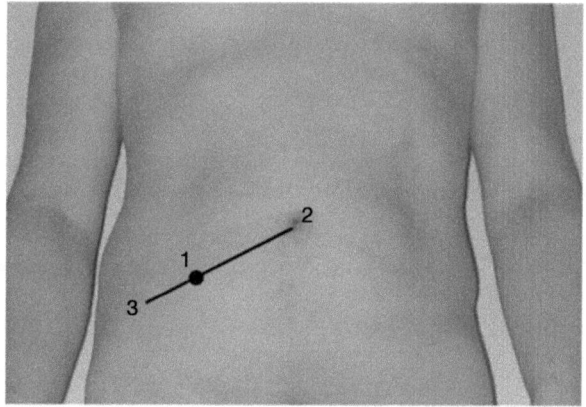

Figure 8.1 McBurney point.

FAST FACTS

A patient sent to surgery should have a completed preoperative checklist and be wearing only a gown. There should be no body jewelry in unusual places, no hearing aids, no dentures, no hairpins, no socks, no underwear—just a patient gown.

FAST FACTS

Manifestations of peritonitis include fever, guarding, abdominal pain and distention, hypoactive bowel sounds, and a diffuse, rigid abdomen.

Acute Cholecystitis
Acute cholecystitis is an acute inflammation of the gallbladder.
- *Causes:* Gallstones (most common), obstruction, or acute inflammation.
- *Signs and symptoms:* Right upper quadrant abdominal pain radiating to the back or right shoulder that becomes worse after eating fatty foods; low-grade fever; tachycardia; clay-colored stool; nausea and vomiting; anorexia; flatulence; possible jaundice; fat intolerance; and positive Murphy sign.
- *Interventions:* Anticipate orders to obtain right upper quadrant ultrasound, complete blood count, liver enzymes, serum amylase, hepatobiliary iminodiacetic acid (HIDA) scan, and abdominal CT;

designate the patient NPO; administer fluids IV; give medications (analgesics, antibiotics, sedatives for smooth muscle relaxation, and antiemetics for nausea and vomiting) as prescribed; and use nasogastric tube for gastric decompression. Arrange for possible surgical intervention.

FAST FACTS

A positive **Murphy sign** is an increased, sharp right upper quadrant abdominal pain that occurs during inspiration when palpating the patient's gallbladder and asking them to take a deep breath.

Mesenteric Ischemia

Mesenteric ischemia is a group of diseases that are characterized by the interruption of blood flow to the intestines. This cessation or decrease in blood flow can result in ischemia. As a result, the ischemia can lead to tissue dysfunction and inflammatory changes. This can result in tissue death or necrosis (Bala et al., 2022).

- *Causes:* Arterial embolism or thrombosis or other low-flow state.
- *Signs and symptoms:* Sudden and severe onset of abdominal pain. The pain may be out of proportion compared to the physical exam findings.
- *Interventions:* Anticipate the patient will need a CT of the abdomen and pelvis with IV contrast. Expect orders for laboratory draws that will include a complete metabolic panel, lactic acid, and complete blood count. Appropriate IV access will be required for resuscitation as well as for the contrast that will be needed for the CT scan. Prepare the patient for potential surgical admission.

FAST FACTS

Pain secondary to mesenteric ischemia may be out of proportion when compared with exam findings.

Esophageal Obstruction

Esophageal obstruction, or food bolus, is a term for food or foreign bodies that get stuck or lodged in the esophagus. Meats such as steak, pork, and poultry can easily become lodged in the esophagus. This may be why some refer to esophageal obstruction as the "steakhouse syndrome."

- *Causes:* Ingestion of a foreign object or simply not chewing well before swallowing. Other conditions pose an increased risk for esophageal obstruction, such as esophageal cancer, eosinophilic esophagitis, nutcracker esophagus, peptic strictures, and Schatzki rings.

- *Signs and symptoms:* Foreign body sensation: "I have something stuck in my throat." The patient may also have acute dysphagia, chest pain, neck pain, pain with swallowing, regurgitation of food, and drooling.
- *Interventions:* Treat any airway concerns first. Anticipate orders to obtain x-rays of the chest and soft tissue films of the neck, administer IV glucagon to relax esophageal smooth muscles, or prepare for endoscopy to retrieve the object. Patient discharge teaching should include chewing food.

Gastrointestinal Bleeding

GI bleeding can be classified as upper or lower.

Upper Gastrointestinal Bleeding

- *Causes:* Peptic ulcer, stomach cancer, infection, esophageal varices, and trauma.
- *Signs and symptoms:* Weakness, hypotension, hypovolemic shock, nausea, and vomiting; bright red to coffee ground color emesis; and black tarry stools (melena) or dark red rectal bleeding.
- *Interventions:* Anticipate orders to apply pulse oximetry; give oxygen; begin cardiac monitoring; start an 18- or 16-gauge IV access; prepare a complete blood count—hemoglobin and hematocrit, metabolic panel, and coagulation studies; arrange for abdominal CT scan; insert nasogastric tube as ordered; document gastric content findings; administer fluids IV; give proton pump inhibitor (PPI) or H2 blocker as ordered; send type and crossmatch; and prepare for possible blood transfusion or endoscopy.

Esophageal Varices

Esophageal varices are enlarged or varicosed veins located in the lower part of the esophagus. It is most concerning when these vessels rupture, resulting in an upper GI bleed.

- *Causes:* Liver damage can lead to poor circulation through the portal vein, causing blood to back up into surrounding smaller vessels, such as esophageal veins. These fragile thin veins in the esophagus can then burst or rupture and bleed out into the esophagus. Other causes include thrombus, infection, and damage from liver cirrhosis.
- *Signs and symptoms:* Vomiting bright red blood or dark and tarry stools. In severe cases, the patient may go into hemorrhagic or hypovolemic shock.
- *Interventions:* Don necessary personal protective equipment (PPE) and treat any airway emergencies first. Anticipate orders to administer oxygen, beta-blockers such as propranolol, and medications to decrease portal vein pressure (octreotide, somatostatin, or vasopressin and nitroglycerin); insert large-bore IV access; monitor vital signs; assess and treat patient for any signs of hypovolemic shock; obtain type and crossmatch for possible blood transfusion; be prepared for potential insertion of balloon tamponade tube per hospital protocol; and prepare for endoscopy.

Lower Gastrointestinal Bleeding
- *Causes:* Internal or external hemorrhoids, constipation, polyps, colitis, diverticulitis, colon cancer, and irritable bowel syndrome.
- *Signs and symptoms:* Bright red rectal bleeding (hematochezia).
- *Interventions:* Anticipate orders to obtain large-bore IV access, prepare a complete blood count and coagulation studies, arrange for abdominal CT scan, assess guaiac gastric contents and stool, administer fluids IV, test blood for type and crossmatch, reverse coagulopathies, and prepare for possible blood transfusion.

SUMMARY

Abdominal pain is a common presenting symptom to the ED. Careful assessment will aid in providing the appropriate nursing interventions. GI emergencies are daily events in the ED. Differentiating between the various types will be a skill developed throughout your time as an ED nurse.

REVIEW QUESTIONS

1) A 72-year-old patient arrives at the ED with sudden, severe abdominal pain that is disproportionate to physical exam findings. The patient has a history of atrial fibrillation and hypertension. The nurse suspects acute mesenteric ischemia. Which of the following interventions is the priority in managing this patient?
   a. Administer PPIs to prevent stress ulcers.
   b. Encourage oral fluid intake to improve perfusion.
   c. Prepare the patient for emergent imaging and notify the provider immediately.
   d. Administer antiemetics and discharge if symptoms improve.
2) A 65-year-old patient with a history of peptic ulcer disease presents to the ED with hematemesis and melena. The patient is hypotensive and tachycardic. Which of the following nursing interventions is the priority?
   a. Administer an oral PPI to reduce gastric acid secretion.
   b. Obtain large-bore IV access and initiate fluid resuscitation.
   c. Place the patient in the Trendelenburg position to improve circulation.
   d. Encourage the patient to drink clear fluids to maintain hydration.

REFERENCES

Bala, M., Catena, F., Kashuk, J., De Simone, B., Gomes, C. A., Weber, D., Sartelli, M., Coccolini, F., Kluger, Y., Abu-Zidan, F. M., Picetti, E., Ansaloni, L., Augustin, G., Biffl, W. L., Ceresoli, M., Chiara, O., Chiarugi, M., Coimbra, R., Cui, Y. ... Moore, E. E. (2022, October 19). Acute mesenteric ischemia: Updated guidelines of the world society of emergency surgery. *World Journal of Emergency Surgery, 17*(1), 54. https://doi.org/10.1186/s13017-022-00443-x. PMID: 36261857; PMCID: PMC9580452.

McAninch, S., & Smithson III, C. C. (2017). Gastrointestinal emergencies. In C. Stone, & R. L. Humphries (Eds.), *Current diagnosis & treatment: Emergency medicine* (8th ed.). McGraw-Hill Education. https://accessmedicine-mhmedical-com.umassmed.idm.oclc.org/content.aspx?bookid=2172&sectionid=165065027

Papadakis, M. A., Rabow, M. W., & McQuaid, K. R. (Eds.). (2025). *Gastroesophageal reflux disease (GERD): Quick medical diagnosis & treatment 2025*. McGraw Hill. https://accessmedicine-mhmedical-com.umassmed.idm.oclc.org/content.aspx?bookid=3516&sectionid=289631890

Valle, J. (2022). Peptic ulcer disease and related disorders. In J. Loscalzo, A. Fauci, D. Kasper, S. Hauser, D. Longo, & J. Jameson (Eds.), *Harrison's principles of internal medicine* (21st ed.). McGraw-Hill Education. https://accessmedicine-mhmedical-com.umassmed.idm.oclc.org/content.aspx?bookid=3095&sectionid=265427594

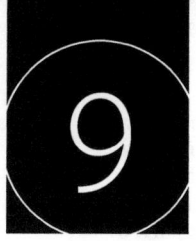

Dental and Ear, Nose, and Throat Emergencies

Sarah Berry

> Dental and ear, nose, and throat (ENT) emergencies are a daily occurrence in the ED. They can vary in severity, depending on the findings of the patient. Consults for these conditions are possible, making interdisciplinary relationships important.

In this chapter, you will learn to:
1. Identify the nonurgent and emergent dental and ENT diagnoses
2. Recognize and treat the dental and ENT conditions in the ED

DENTAL EMERGENCIES

Most of the time, dental problems, and ENT problems are not life threatening. From foreign objects to trauma or infection, this chapter walks through the most common dental and ENT emergencies seen. Be sure to practice using the otoscope and ophthalmic scope and document assessment findings. Upon completing this chapter, nonurgent and emergent dental and ENT emergencies will have been reviewed. For each emergency, causes, manifestations, and interventions will also be covered.

Dental Abscess
A dental abscess is a pocket of infection or pus located in the gums near the base of a tooth.
- *Causes:* They typically are secondary to previous dental problems such as dental caries (cavities), trauma, or failed dental procedures. These are the most common causes, but others include partially erupted teeth (such as budding wisdom teeth), genetic syndromes, bruxism, dry mouth, methamphetamine use, or immunosuppression from chemotherapy or HIV/AIDS (Sanders & Houck, 2023).

- *Periodontal abscess:* An infection from an accumulation of bacteria or foreign body impaction. The type of abscess is generally related to "periodontitis" versus "nonperiodontitis" origins. Periodontitis appears from untreated periodontal disease, and nonperiodontitis is related to foreign body impaction such as food or floss remnants (Yousefi et al., 2023).
- *Periapical abscess:* An infection of the supporting bone around the root structure caused by damage to the pulp (nerve and blood supply) of the tooth. If left untreated, the abscess can spread into the surrounding structures, causing potentially life-threatening infection (Laudenbach & Kumar, 2020).
- *Signs and symptoms:* Manifestation may vary depending on location but usually includes pain (especially with chewing), swelling, toothache, tenderness, fever, and foul breath. Infection may be localized but may also spread into areas of the face and neck, and pain may radiate to the neck, jaw, and ear (Laudenbach & Kumar, 2020).
- *Interventions:* Assess and treat any airway obstructions first. Anticipate orders to set up oral anesthetics and incision and drainage tray or supplies. Administer any IV fluids, pain medication, and antibiotics as ordered. Anticipate diagnostic study orders such as a complete blood count (CBC), erythrocyte sedimentation rate (ESR or sed rate), wound cultures of the abscess, and CT or soft tissue x-ray of the head and neck. Instruct the patient to take prescriptions as ordered until they are completed and rinse with warm salt water when appropriate. It is most important that the patient understands that treatment in the ED is temporary and that their tooth ultimately needs to be treated definitively by a dentist or oral surgeon. They may have to pursue a root canal or extraction of the tooth (Laudenbach & Kumar, 2020).

Fractured Tooth

A tooth fracture is a broken or chipped tooth. This commonly occurs to the "two front teeth," or anterior maxillary teeth, related to facial trauma (Arias et al., 2023).

- *Causes:* Oral, facial, or head trauma.
- *Signs and symptoms:* Vary according to type and location of trauma and may include broken or chipped tooth, bleeding at site of injury, pain, swelling, and embedded tooth fragments.
- *Interventions:* If facial trauma is present, stabilize any airway, breathing, or circulation concerns first. If the patient was able to retrieve the piece(s) of the tooth/teeth, the provider may attempt to reinsert the tooth into the socket. Rinse the tooth off in either milk or water but avoid scrubbing it. Handle the tooth by the crown, and not by the root. This is not always a viable option but is the standard of care if possible. If replacing the tooth into the socket is not possible, place the tooth in a glass of milk. If milk is unavailable, place the tooth in the patient's cheek pouch because saliva is better than storing the tooth in water (McIntosh, 2023). If the patient presents within 30 minutes of the trauma, the chances of viability

are at their best. After 30 minutes, the survival of the tooth diminishes significantly (Alotaibi et al., 2023). Administer oral analgesics and tetanus vaccine as ordered. Referral to a dentist within 24 to 48 hours of injury is critical for proper tooth repair. Set up an emergency dental repair kit for provider administration.

> **FAST FACTS**
>
> If a patient loses a tooth, attempt to replace it in the socket. If replacement is not an option because of remaining fragmentation, bleeding control issues, or pain, place the tooth in milk.

Caries

Dental caries, also known as cavities, is "reported to be one of the oldest and most common diseases found in humans" (Rathee & Sapra, 2023). Commonly, patients show up to the ED for the severe pain associated with caries, known as odontalgia. Patients can have various stages of caries, and they are determined to be either active or inactive based on physical findings.

- *Causes:* Poor oral hygiene and a diet that has frequent consumption of sugar. Snacking or frequent sipping causes continuous acid production in the oral cavity and changes the pH in the mouth. This leads to an area more conducive for bacteria to manifest. In addition to changes in pH, having dry mouth can lead to caries. Saliva has protective properties that help fight caries, and with dry mouth, these properties are scarce. Patients who have areas of dental plaque are at higher risk of developing caries beneath the plaque. Molars and premolars are the areas most affected by caries because they are sometimes difficult to reach while brushing and flossing. Patients who are afflicted with other health issues such as gastroesophageal reflux disease (GERD) or eating disorders such as anorexia and bulimia are susceptible to caries as well. Also, infants and children can acquire cavities if given a bottle to drink at bedtime. Whichever fluid is inside the bottle stays in the infant's mouth for hours, allowing for similar damage to those who sip throughout the day (Mayo Foundation, 2023).
- *Signs and symptoms:* Pain, gray or blackened area noted on affected tooth, toothache, and neck or facial swelling.
- *Interventions:* ED providers may be able to prescribe medication to manage pain, but this is temporary. For definitive treatment, the patient must see a dentist. Discharge instructions should emphasize the importance of good oral hygiene and avoidance of possible causes of caries related to lifestyle.

Tooth Avulsion

Tooth avulsion occurs when the whole tooth is dislocated from its socket. This is a time-sensitive emergency. The best chance of saving the tooth is reimplantation *within 20 to 30 minutes.*

- *Causes:* The most common causes of tooth avulsion are falls. Following falls, cycling accidents, full-contact sports, and physical assaults account for the majority of avulsions. Helmets have not decreased the incidence of trauma to teeth, but the use of mouth guards has helped (Alotaibi et al., 2023).
- *Signs and symptoms:* A gap where the tooth has pain and bleeding (Cleveland Clinic, 2024).
- *Interventions:* Assess for airway, breathing, and circulation concerns due to facial trauma. Offer suction for saliva and bleeding control to maintain the patient's airway. Reimplantation is the choice treatment—within 30 minutes of trauma to increase the likelihood of viability (Alotaibi et al., 2023)—and appropriate storage of a tooth that is not reimplantable is crucial. Anatomical realignment is vital to decrease chances of complications later on from reimplantation growth (Alotaibi et al., 2023). Much like fractured teeth, storing the tooth in milk or in the patient's buccal pocket to use saliva is best. Antibiotics and corticosteroids may be administered to decrease inflammation, known as antiresorption therapy. After the tooth has been reimplanted, radiographic confirmation should be obtained to ensure anatomical alignment (Susarla & Sheller, 2023). Following up with dentistry or oral surgery is vital to track root resorption and likelihood of viability (Alotaibi et al., 2023).

Ludwig Angina

Please refer to Chapter 7 for an extensive review of Ludwig angina.

EAR EMERGENCIES

Foreign Objects

Foreign objects in the ear can sometimes pose a real danger. Because the eustachian tube is continuously narrowing until it reaches the inner ear, foreign objects can easily get jammed farther in until they are next to impossible to remove. If the object goes undetected (like in a small child) and it damages the tissue of the walls of the eustachian tube, it could lead to an ear infection. If the object itself does not lead to an ear infection, attempts to retrieve the object at home could lead to damage to the ear as well, leading to infection. Advise people, especially young children, to not attempt to retrieve foreign objects themselves and bring them to a healthcare professional.

- *Causes:* Foreign object in the ear, such as food, small toys, and other small items found in the home, such as beads—the most common foreign object in the pediatric population (Lotterman, 2022). Adult patients

may have pieces of cotton-tipped applicators, hearing aids, earbud tips, piercings, or insects lodged in their ears.
- *Signs and symptoms:* Visible foreign object; purulent or bloody discharge; discomfort or pain; swelling; redness; foul odor; and foreign body sensation.
- *Interventions:*
  - Assist the ED provider in removing the foreign body with suction, irrigation, alligator forceps, ear curette, or even the pacer magnet for metal objects. Caution should be taken to avoid further lodging it deeper into the nose or ear. Take precautions to avoid possible aspiration with nasal foreign bodies. Provide ear antibiotics or nasal decongestants as ordered. Instruct the patient or caretaker to avoid putting anything in the various orifices.
  - If the patient is not tolerating removal of the object because of discomfort or developmental age, consider conscious sedation for safe retrieval of the object (Brown et al., 2004).
  - If unable to remove a foreign body, the provider may refer the patient to an ENT specialist.

Cerumen Impaction
- *Causes:* Buildup of earwax that blocks the ear drum. Cerumen production is normal because it moisturizes the ear canal and protects it from damage or infection. In those with recurrent impaction, consider fungal or bacterial causes. When tested, the most common fungus found was *Aspergillus terreus*, and bacterial infections consisted of *Staphylococcus aureus* (Sevy et al., 2023). Use of cotton swabs, ear buds, ear plugs, or other foreign bodies can increase cerumen production and sometimes change the composition of the wax (Sevy et al., 2023). Using cotton swabs can also push wax deeper into the ear canal, leading to further wax impaction.
- *Signs and symptoms:* Impaction is generally asymptomatic but can include muffled/decreased hearing, fullness, pruritus, otalgia, tinnitus, and dizziness (Sevy et al., 2023). It is important to explain to patients that simply because an impaction is present, it does not always necessitate removal. If the patient is asymptomatic, cerumen can be beneficial because of its protective properties. Removal could prove to be more detrimental if done unnecessarily.
- *Interventions:* Prior to irrigation or manual removal, it is important to advocate for risk versus benefit in certain populations. Patients who are immunocompromised for various reasons such as HIV, diabetes, transplant, or chemotherapy or those who are anticoagulated are at higher risk of adverse effects from removal. This could lead to superimposed bacterial infections or significant bleeding or development of hematomas. Exercise caution when working with these populations, and advocate for less invasive management for those who are asymptomatic (Sevy et al., 2023).

- When preparing for irrigation, educate the patient on the importance of remaining as still as possible. This decreases risk of injury and allows for communication so that the patient can ask questions and voice understanding of the procedure.
- Three recommended methods of removal:
  - Cerumenolytics help to soften, thin, and break down the ear wax. The most effective ingredient in these products is docusate sodium, which is most beneficial in pretreatment prior to irrigation or manual removal (Sevy et al., 2023).
    - Patients can use these products at home as directed on the box, 1 to 2 times daily, for 3 to 7 days.
  - Irrigation is another effective method of removal, but this should only be performed if the tympanic membrane (TM) can be visualized and is intact. A perforated TM is a strict contraindication of irrigation (Sevy et al., 2023). Mix warm water and hydrogen peroxide at a 50:50 ratio, then slowly express it into the canal, with a basin at the bottom to catch the fluid and cerumen. Try to have the water be close to the patient's body temperature because excessively warm or cold water could cause the patient to experience vertigo (Sevy et al., 2023).
  - Manual removal frequently requires specific equipment to better visualize and remove cerumen. The advantage of this method is decreased risk of infection because the provider does not expose the ear to moisture during irrigation (Sevy et al., 2023).

Acute Otitis Externa (Swimmer's Ear)

Acute otitis externa is an infection of the outer ear that could be infectious or noninfectious. The most common cause is bacterial infection. *Pseudomonas aeruginosa* and *S aureus* are the most common bacteria responsible for infection. If it is noninfectious, it may be fungal: *Candida* or *Aspergillus*. Depending on the length of time the patient has been infected, it can be classified as either acute or chronic, whether it has been less than 6 weeks or more than 3 months, respectively (Medina-Blasini & Sharman, 2023).

- *Causes:* Outer ear infections commonly occur because of frequent swimming or foreign objects in the ear. Bacteria or fungus enters with the water or the foreign object, thereby causing an infection. The inflammatory process is believed to be related to a disruption in the pH of the canal, preceded by a cascading process of damage to the canal, loss of cerumen, and moisture accumulation (Medina-Blasini & Sharman, 2023).
- *Signs and symptoms:* Clinical presentation can vary depending on the chronicity and severity of the infection. Most cases have symptoms consistent with otorrhea, a feeling of fullness, and mild hearing loss (Medina-Blasini & Sharman, 2023). Mild cases can consist of itching, discomfort, and edema. Moderate symptoms include those noted earlier and also possible partial occlusion. Severe cases involve the outer

ear being completely obstructed with edema, causing intense pain, lymphadenopathy to surrounding structures, and fever (Medina-Blasini & Sharman, 2023).
- *Interventions:* Treatment for uncomplicated otitis externa includes antibiotic ear drops and pain management suggestions. For mild to moderate pain management, Tylenol and nonsteroidal anti-inflammatory drugs (NSAIDs) are generally sufficient. For more severe cases, some providers may prescribe a short course of opioids. Within 48 to 72 hours, the patient should have noticeable improvement to their symptoms. In uncomplicated cases, common antibiotic choices consist of ofloxacin or ciprofloxacin. Polymyxin B and neomycin are also common choices that may be combined with a steroid at the provider's discretion (Medina-Blasini & Sharman, 2023). Oral antibiotics are not proven to have significant benefit, but in certain cases they may be warranted. As mentioned earlier, in cases of those with HIV or diabetes, oral antibiotics may be warranted.

FAST FACTS

When examining the ear in an adult, pull *up* and back; in a child younger than 3 years, pull the ear *down* and back.

Acute Otitis Media

Acute otitis media is a middle ear bacterial or viral infection. It is most common in children between the ages of 6 and 24 months and is the second most common diagnosis in the ED after upper respiratory infections (URIs). Ear infections can sometimes coinfect or follow a URI when a virus is the cause of the ear infection (Danishyar & Ashurst, 2023).
- *Causes:* The most common bacterial infections are *Streptococcus pneumoniae, Moraxella catarrhalis,* and *Haemophilus influenzae.* Viral infections consist of "respiratory syncytial virus (RSV), various coronaviruses, influenzas, adenoviruses, human metapneumovirus, and picornaviruses" (Danishyar & Ashurst, 2023).
- *Signs and symptoms:* Recent URI, otalgia, pulling at the ears, fussiness or irritability, headache or sinus pressure, sleeplessness or disturbed sleep patterns, poor appetite and decreased by mouth (PO) intake, vomiting, diarrhea, and sometimes low-grade fevers (Danishyar & Ashurst, 2023).
- *Interventions:* Administer pain management and antipyretics (NSAIDs and acetaminophen [Tylenol] can achieve these goals) and await orders for antibiotics. Anticipate treatment that is based on clinical findings such as a perforated TM; ofloxacin is usually prescribed because it is instilled directly into the eustachian tube via ear drops rather than given as systemic antibiotics. Systemic antibiotics are indicated to treat bacterial infections, with amoxicillin or a second-generation

cephalosporin being most commonly prescribed (Danishyar & Ashurst, 2023). Warm compresses to the area may soothe discomfort. Encourage increased fluid intake and rest while under treatment.

Acute Otitis Interna (Labyrinthitis)

An inflammation to the labyrinth part of the inner ear, which controls balance and hearing, typically affects adults.

- *Causes:* The most common cause is secondary to viral URIs. Congenital deafness is caused by maternal rubella and cytomegalovirus. Mumps and measles lead to viral hearing loss secondary to labyrinthitis. Bacterial meningitis can lead to labyrinthitis, as well as syphilis and HIV (Barkwill & Arora, 2023).
- *Signs and symptoms:* Loss of hearing, nausea, vomiting, tinnitus, imbalance, nystagmus, and severe vertigo (Barkwill & Arora, 2023).
- *Interventions:* Treatment is tailored to the cause. Viral labyrinthitis is typically treated with increased hydration and bed rest. Patients should be advised to seek further treatment if their symptoms evolve into weakness, slurred speech, or gait abnormalities because strokelike symptoms can sometimes be overlooked as labyrinthitis. Oral antibiotics are first-line treatment for bacterial labyrinthitis, depending on the source of the infection. Benzodiazepines, antihistamines, and steroids may be prescribed in the initial 72 hours on symptom onset to treat vertigo. Resting with the patient's eyes closed may be the preferred method to decrease visual stimuli and control the spinning sensation (Barkwill & Arora, 2023).

Ruptured Tympanic Membrane

This is a tear or rupture of the TM (eardrum).

- *Causes:* TMs can be ruptured by infection, trauma, or rapid changes in atmospheric pressure such as on airplanes or scuba diving (Dolhi & Weimer, 2023).
- *Signs and symptoms:* Otalgia, otorrhea, tinnitus, hearing loss, bleeding, and vertigo.
- *Interventions:* TMs usually heal spontaneously and with minimal to no intervention. Advise the patient to keep the ear clean and dry and to not introduce anything potentially traumatizing such as cotton-tipped applicators or other objects. Some providers may prescribe ofloxacin drops to speed up healing time, although this did not support improvement in hearing after healing. Patients should also follow up with an ENT specialist and audiologist to monitor progress (Dolhi & Weimer, 2023).

Ménière Disease

Ménière disease (MD) is a progressive disease with exacerbations. It is a midlife disease process that is diagnosed on average in patients in their 40s, although it can happen at any age. Two classifications of the disease exist: (1) when related to head trauma or an infection and (2) when related to an idiopathic cause that leads to symptoms. It is diagnosed as "definite MD" versus "probable MD." Definite MD consists of "two or more vertigo attacks lasting between 20 minutes and 12 hours, fluctuating low to middle frequency hearing loss while other vestibular diagnoses have been ruled out. Probable MD is defined as two or more vertigo attacks lasting 20 minutes to 24 hours, fluctuating aural symptoms such as tinnitus, hearing loss, or fullness while other vestibular diagnoses have been ruled out" (Mohseni-Dargah et al., 2023).

- *Causes:* The cause is not entirely understood, but there are some genetic variables, as well as environmental factors. Exposure to prolonged loud noise damaging the inner structures of the ears, pathogens (either viral or bacterial), allergens, head trauma, significant changes in atmospheric pressure, and some types of particulate exposures are thought to be leading risk factors (Mohseni-Dargah et al., 2023).
- *Signs and symptoms:* Episodic vertigo, fluctuating progressive hearing loss at different decibels, tinnitus, balance problems, nausea, and a feeling of fullness or pressure (Mohseni-Dargah et al., 2023).
- *Interventions:* Initiate fall precautions and educate patients on changing positions slowly when moving from lying down to sitting, then sitting to standing. Educate on lifestyle modifications including a low-salt diet and decreased alcohol and caffeine consumption. Patients may also benefit from vestibular/balance rehabilitation and hearing aids for hearing loss. Medication options for acute exacerbations could consist of antihistamines, anticholinergic drugs, benzodiazepines, and antiemetics. These are used to treat inflammatory processes and nausea, while helping the patient to relax. More aggressive options include corticosteroids or intratympanic gentamicin. Ultimately, if the disease progresses with significance, surgery may be appropriate, but this is usually far after the ED visit (Mohseni-Dargah et al., 2023).

FAST FACTS

Patients with Ménière disease may experience emotional distress or withdraw from their lifestyle because of the unpredictability of the disease and its attacks.

NASAL EMERGENCIES

Epistaxis

Epistaxis is a nosebleed. It accounts for 1 in 200 ED visits per year (Seikaly, 2021). Generally, treatment is uncomplicated but can be difficult if the patient has underlying conditions that affect their cardiovascular system, they have impaired coagulation from disease or medication, or they have platelet dysfunction (Seikaly, 2021). There are two types: anterior bleeds and posterior bleeds. *Anterior bleeds* are more common and easier to control (Seikaly, 2021).

- *Causes:* There are local, systemic, and idiopathic causes. Local causes consist of those that interact directly with the nares: dry air, trauma to the nose, use of inhaled medications or illicit drugs, infections, inflammation from allergens, or tumors. Systemic issues are diseases or medications that can lead to nosebleeds such as blood dyscrasias, leukemias, hypertension, congestive heart failure, and anticoagulant or antiplatelet medications (Seikaly, 2021).
- *Signs and symptoms:* Nasal bleeding.
- *Interventions:* Position the patient in high Fowler position to decrease risk of aspiration. If the patient is alert and oriented, educate the patient on the use of a suction catheter in their oral cavity to remove blood so that they do not swallow it. Anticipate applying direct pressure to the lower third of the nose for 15 to 20 minutes while leaning forward (Seikaly, 2021). If bleeding continues, anticipate possible topical vasoconstrictors to be utilized. These consist of phenylephrine, epinephrine, or medical cocaine. Although these are topical in the nares, there is an increased risk of effects on the cardiovascular system, and the patient should be monitored closely via telemetry. Tranexamic acid (TXA) may be used topically to control bleeding (Seikaly, 2021). Delivery is provider dependent, but some may choose to soak Rhino Rockets in TXA before placing them in the patient's nares, allowing for the blood vessels to absorb the medication directly. Nasal packing is contraindicated until nasal bone fractures or basilar skull fractures have been ruled out because of possible worsening of fractures (Seikaly, 2021). If a specific area of bleeding can be identified through physical examination, cauterization is another form of treatment. In addition to cautery, if arterial epistaxis is identified, embolization may be warranted (Seikaly, 2021).

FAST FACTS

A reported 80% to 90% of epistaxis episodes are anterior (Seikaly, 2021).

Nasal Fracture

This is a fracture of the nasal bones. They are the most common fracture type of the facial skeleton (Reyad et al., 2024).
- *Causes:* Direct trauma to the nose.
- *Signs and symptoms:* Nasal bleeding, nasal ecchymosis or edema, nasal airway obstruction, and deformity or tenderness over the nasal bridge.
- *Interventions:* Control bleeding and administer analgesia as prescribed. Offer the patient an ice pack. The provider may want to obtain imaging to determine the severity of the fracture or to rule out nearby structures that could also be damaged. Studies show that early surgical intervention for nasal fractures increases patient satisfaction because of improved cosmetic outcomes and improved olfactory function (Reyad et al., 2024). Corrective rhinoplasty can prove to be more expensive and

have less desirable cosmetic results when compared with early surgical intervention (Reyad et al., 2024). Avoid intense or excessive nose blowing to decrease risk of worsening fracture.

Periorbital Cellulitis

Periorbital cellulitis is an infection of the eyelid and surrounding structures. It is most common in children. It is also sometimes referred to as preseptal cellulitis because of its affecting the structures in front of the septum like an eyelid or the skin around the orbital socket. The infection is usually caused by bacteria that are naturally found on the skin or by other bacteria that are introduced to the area (Shih et al., 2022).

- *Causes:* The most common causes consist of insect/animal bites, URIs, facial injuries, dental abscesses, conjunctivitis, and hordeolums. Bacterial infections largely consist of streptococcal and staphylococcal species (Shih et al., 2022).
- *Signs and symptoms:* Swelling, redness, fever, pain in the surrounding structures but no pain with movement, and maintenance of baseline vision (Baiu & Melendez, 2020).
- *Interventions:* Anticipate orders for antibiotics. It is important when triaging to differentiate between periorbital cellulitis symptoms and symptoms similar to sinusitis or allergic rhinitis. Because the symptoms are similar, it can be difficult to differentiate. If left untreated, patients are at risk for vision loss or other life-threatening complications (Shih et al., 2022). Medications consist of vancomycin, amoxicillin/clavulanic acid, or first-generation cephalosporins, depending on the infecting species. Piperacillin/tazobactam may be chosen as well (Shih et al., 2022).

THROAT EMERGENCIES

Pharyngitis/Tonsillitis

This is inflammation of the throat or tonsils. Before developing tonsillitis, the patient may have a recent history of a URI (Singh et al., 2023).

- *Causes:* Bacterial or viral infection.
- *Signs and symptoms:* Sore throat; fever; cervical lymphadenopathy. It may be associated with sinusitis. Strawberry tongue, palatal petechiae, and a red and enlarged uvula (Singh et al., 2023).
- *Interventions:* Arrange a test for streptococcal infection; administer antibiotics such as penicillin or amoxicillin PO or intramuscular (IM) injection as ordered; and monitor airway patency. Educate the patient or their caregiver on the importance of completing the course of antibiotics in order to eliminate the pathogen. If it is left untreated, acute rheumatic fever could develop in the patient (Singh et al., 2023).

Peritonsillar Abscess

This is an abscess of the tonsil. It may be a respiratory emergency if the airway is obstructed.

- *Causes:* Commonly caused by *Streptococcus* bacteria.
- *Signs and symptoms:* Sore throat; unilateral swollen tonsil; swollen cervical lymph nodes; dysphagia; fever; difficulty in opening the mouth; swollen palate; laterally displaced uvula; drooling; and muffled speech (Singh et al., 2023).
- *Interventions:* Prepare for incision and drainage of the abscess with ENT consultant; administer antibiotics; and monitor the airway and pulse oximetry.

SUMMARY

ED nurses see many afflictions of the mouth and ENT. It is important to understand what is abnormal in this anatomical region to spot dangers. Do not be afraid to take an otoscope and assess the patient's mouth, gums, and teeth and ENT. Document preintervention and postintervention findings. Most providers appreciate a good assessment, especially one that is well documented before and after treatment.

REVIEW QUESTIONS

1) When a patient presents with a broken or dislocated tooth, what is the best substance to put the tooth in to maintain its integrity?
   a. Water
   b. Milk
   c. Gatorade
   d. Nothing
2) What is an important assessment to perform prior to irrigating an ear canal?
   a. Determine if the patient is diabetic.
   b. Perform a hearing evaluation.
   c. Visualize the TM to ensure it is intact and not perforated.
   d. Give the patient an ice pack to numb the area.

REFERENCES

Alotaibi, S., Haftel, A., & Wagner, N. (2023, March 6). *Avulsed tooth*. In StatPearls [Internet]. StatPearls Publishing. Retrieved August 26, 2025, from https://www.ncbi.nlm.nih.gov/books/NBK539876/

Arias, Z., Falú Hinojosa Ledezma, H., Patricia Osorio Terán, C., Omori, K., Yamamoto, T., Zahedul Islam Nizami, M., & Takashiba, S. (2023). Reattachment of fractured tooth fragment by multidisciplinary treatment approach. *The Bulletin of Tokyo Dental College*, *64*(1), 13–22. https://doi.org/10.2209/tdcpublication.2022-0019

Baiu, I., & Melendez, E. (2020). Periorbital and orbital cellulitis. *JAMA*, *323*(2), 196. https://doi.org/10.1001/jama.2019.18211

Barkwill, D., Winters, R., & Arora, R. (Updated 2025, July 23). *Labyrinthitis*. In: StatPearls. StatPearls Publishing. Retrieved August 26, 2025, from https://www.ncbi.nlm.nih.gov/books/NBK560506/

Brown, L., Denmark, T. K., Wittlake, W. A., Vargas, E. J., Watson, T., & Crabb, J. W. (2004). Procedural sedation use in the ED: Management of pediatric ear and nose foreign bodies. *The American Journal of Emergency Medicine, 22*(4), 310–314. https://doi.org/10.1016/j.ajem.2004.04.013

Cleveland Clinic. (2024, June 25). *My tooth was knocked out: What to do?* https://my.clevelandclinic.org/health/diseases/21579-avulsed-tooth#symptoms-and-causes

Danishyar, A., & Ashurst, J. (2023, April 15). *Acute otitis media*. In StatPearls [Internet]. StatPearls Publishing. Retrieved August 26, 2025, from https://www.ncbi.nlm.nih.gov/books/NBK470332/

Dolhi, N., & Weimer, A. (2023, August 14). *Tympanic membrane perforation*. In StatPearls [Internet]. StatPearls Publishing. Retrieved August 26, 2025, from https://www.ncbi.nlm.nih.gov/books/NBK557887/

Laudenbach, J. M., & Kumar, S. S. (2020). Common dental and periodontal diseases. *Dermatologic Clinics, 38*(4), 413–420. https://doi.org/10.1016/j.det.2020.05.002

Lotterman, S. (2022, November 28). *Ear foreign body removal*. In StatPearls [Internet]. StatPearls Publishing. Retrieved August 26, 2025, from https://www.ncbi.nlm.nih.gov/books/NBK459136/

Mayo Foundation for Medical Education and Research. (2023, November 30). *Cavities and tooth decay*. Mayo Clinic. https://www.mayoclinic.org/diseases-conditions/cavities/symptoms-causes/syc-20352892

McIntosh, S. (2023, November 8). *Knocked-out tooth in a glass of milk? Ask an emergency dentist*. Distinguished Dental Blog. https://www.distinguished-dental.com/blog/2019/11/14/emergency-dentist-putting-a-tooth-in-milk/

Medina-Blasini, Y., & Sharman, T. (Updated 2023, July 31). *Otitis externa*. In StatPearls. StatPearls Publishing. Retrieved August 26, 2025, from https://www.ncbi.nlm.nih.gov/books/NBK556055/

Mohseni-Dargah, M., Falahati, Z., Pastras, C., Khajeh, K., Mukherjee, P., Razmjou, A., Stefani, S., & Asadnia, M. (2023). Meniere's disease: Pathogenesis, treatments, and emerging approaches for an idiopathic bioenvironmental disorder. *Environmental Research, 238*(1), 116972. https://doi.org/10.1016/j.envres.2023.116972

Rathee, M., & Sapra, A. (2023, June 21). *Dental caries*. In StatPearls [Internet]. StatPearls Publishing. Retrieved August 26, 2025, from https://www.ncbi.nlm.nih.gov/books/NBK551699/#:%E2%88%BC:text=Dental%20caries%20is%20reported%20to,over%20time%2C%20demineralizes%20tooth%20structure

Reyad, K., Elbarbary, A., Naguib, M., & Eldin, M. (2024). Management of acute nasal bone fractures in adults: Systematic review and meta-analysis. *The Egyptian Journal of Plastic and Reconstructive Surgery, 48*(4), 297–308. https://doi.org/10.21608/ejprs.2024.268786.1338

Sanders, J. L., & Houck, R. (2023, February 20). *Dental abscess*. In StatPearls [Internet]. StatPearls Publishing. Retrieved August 26, 2025, from https://www.ncbi.nlm.nih.gov/books/NBK493149/

Seikaly, H. (2021). Epistaxis. *New England Journal of Medicine, 384*(10), 944–951. https://doi.org/10.1056/nejmcp2019344

Sevy, J. O., Hohman, M., & Singh, A. (2023, March 1). *Cerumen impaction removal.* In StatPearls [Internet]. StatPearls Publishing. Retrieved August 26, 2025, from https://www.ncbi.nlm.nih.gov/books/NBK448155/

Shih, E.-J., Chen, J.-K., Tsai, P.-J., Lin, M.-C., & Bee, Y.-S. (2022). Antibiotic choices for pediatric periorbital cellulitis—A 20-year retrospective study from Taiwan. *Antibiotics, 11*(10), 1288. https://doi.org/10.3390/antibiotics11101288

Susarla, H. K., & Sheller, B. (2023). Dental and dentoalveolar injuries in the pediatric patient. *Oral and Maxillofacial Surgery Clinics of North America, 35*(4), 543–554. https://doi.org/10.1016/j.coms.2023.06.002

Yousefi, Y., Meldrum, J., & Jan, A. (2023, June 12). *Periodontal abscess.* In StatPearls [Internet]. StatPearls Publishing. Retrieved August 26, 2025, from https://www.ncbi.nlm.nih.gov/books/NBK560625/

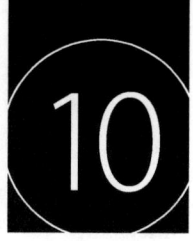

Ocular Emergencies

Alexander Menard

> A variety of eye emergencies will present to the ED. Some are as simple as pink eye, whereas others require emergency ophthalmic surgery. As a nurse, you must be able to differentiate between nonurgent and emergent eye complaints. This chapter guides you through the various types of eye emergencies and reviews the manifestations and interventions for each.

In this chapter, you will learn to:
1. Discuss the ocular emergencies most frequently seen in the ED
2. Identify the red flag warnings for ocular emergencies
3. Review the interventions to address ocular emergencies

OCULAR EMERGENCIES

Ocular emergencies require prompt recognition and immediate intervention to prevent permanent vision loss or serious complications. Nurses play a critical role in the early assessment, triage, and management of patients presenting with acute eye conditions. These conditions can range from chemical burns to retinal detachment to acute angle-closure glaucoma and traumatic injuries. Being able to quickly identify red flag symptoms and coordinate urgent care for the patient is a needed skill.

Central Retinal Artery Occlusion
This is a thrombus- or embolus-associated central retinal artery occlusion (Tripathy et al., 2025). There is a short window of time to restore blood flow. This is a true ocular emergency.
- *Causes:* Thrombi or emboli can occlude the retinal artery, cutting off the blood supply to the eye.
- *Signs and symptoms:* Sudden, painless, unilateral, and complete loss of vision; dilated nonreactive pupil; and pale fundus.

- *Interventions:* Check the patient's visual acuity; obtain eye exam equipment; anticipate orders to obtain IV access, administer vasodilators (e.g., IV nitroglycerin), and anticoagulants as prescribed; arrange STAT ophthalmology consult; and prepare for potential surgical intervention.

Glaucoma

Acute (angle-closure) glaucoma occurs from an obstruction at the access to the trabecular meshwork of the canal of Schlemm. Intraocular pressure is normal when the anterior chamber angle is open. Glaucoma happens when that angle is closed significantly. Chronic (open-angle) glaucoma is characterized by increased intraocular pressure, degeneration of the optic nerve, and visual field loss. Open-angle glaucoma accounts for the vast majority of cases (Kang & Tanna, 2021).

- *Causes:* Open-angle glaucoma is characterized by a disorder of increased intraocular pressure. Angle-closure glaucoma is caused by obstruction.
- *Signs and symptoms:* Diminished vision; deep eye pain; nausea and vomiting; tearing; photophobia; cloudy cornea; rainbow of colors (halos) around lights; semidilated, nonreactive pupils; red conjunctiva; and increased ocular pressure.
- *Interventions:* Perform a visual acuity test; anticipate provider will monitor ocular pressure (tonometry); administer miotic eye drops or topical beta-antagonists as ordered; and obtain ophthalmologist consult.

FAST FACTS

Although open-angle glaucoma makes up the majority of glaucoma cases, angle-closure glaucoma is an acute emergency and often presents with acute eye pain.

Corneal Abrasions

These are scratches or abrasions to the clear surface (cornea) of the eye with or without foreign bodies.

- *Causes:* Anything that can scratch the skin can scratch the cornea. In most cases, the abrasion is caused by some type of foreign body.
- *Signs and symptoms:* Eye pain, corneal irregularity, no corneal luster, photophobia, copious tearing, and foreign body sensation.
- *Interventions:* Assess visual acuity; obtain eye exam equipment (eye kit, Wood's lamp); anticipate orders to administer antibiotic eye drops or ointment, update tetanus/diphtheria shot, administer oral analgesics, and provide ophthalmologist referral. Educate the patient and family on the importance of ophthalmologist follow-up.

Detached Retina

The retina is made of two layers (outer pigmented and inner sensory). A detached retina occurs when these layers separate.
- *Causes:* Vitreous humor leakage, eye trauma, inflammatory disorders, and uncontrolled diabetes.
- *Signs and symptoms:* Painless decreased vision, smoky or cloudy vision, flashing lights, and peripheral floaters (black dots)/"curtain effect."
- *Interventions:* Check visual acuity; position the patient supine; anticipate orders to arrange ophthalmology consult, administer mydriatic drops to dilate pupil as prescribed, and prepare for surgery and admission.

FAST FACTS

Retinal detachment can occur slowly or rapidly, but without pain.

Conjunctivitis/Pink Eye

This is an inflammation of the conjunctiva. Bacterial and viral conjunctivitis are highly contagious.
- *Causes:* Bacteria, viruses, chemicals, or allergies.
- *Signs and symptoms:* Itchy eyes, photophobia, normal visual acuity, purulent or serous eye discharge, reddened conjunctiva, and copious tearing.
- *Interventions:* Assess visual acuity; anticipate orders to instill topical anesthetic, obtain fluorescein staining supplies and Wood's lamp, and instill ophthalmic antibiotic eye drops or ointment as prescribed.

FAST FACTS

Because conjunctivitis is contagious, discharge instructions should include strict handwashing after touching the eye area, no sharing of hand towels, discarding current eye makeup, and disinfecting sunglasses.

Ocular Trauma

Injury to the eye can be devastating and result in vision loss in one or both eyes. Penetrating orbital injuries can result in optic nerve damage and result in immediate vision loss. Corneal injuries can be painful and a result of a foreign body getting into or rubbing against the cornea. Corneal abrasions can be detected by fluorescein staining, penlight, and slit-lamp examination and can aid in revealing foreign material or injury to the eye. Foreign bodies that penetrate the eye should not be removed. They should be secured in place. Penetrating trauma requires immediate ophthalmology consult.

- *Causes:* Vary depending on the situation. Knives, bullets, and nails shot from a nail gun, among many other things. Essentially, anything with enough force behind it can cause penetrating trauma to the eye.
- *Signs and symptoms:* Irregular pupil shape, impaired visual acuity, and decreased intraocular pressure.
- *Interventions:* Prepare for ophthalmology consult; cover injured eye with metal or plastic patch and patch other eye to reduce eye movement; place patient in semi-Fowler position; anticipate orders to administer pain medication or anxiolytic and give tetanus/diphtheria injection as prescribed.

Blunt Ocular Trauma

This is a fracture of the orbital floor.
- *Causes:* Inferior orbital rim trauma.
- *Signs and symptoms:* Change in gaze; diplopia; ecchymosis; subconjunctival hemorrhage; paresthesia; periorbital edema; crepitus; inability to look up due to inferior rectus/inferior oblique muscle entrapment.
- *Interventions:* Apply ice pack; anticipate orders to administer pain medications, arrange for orbital x-rays or CT scan, place patient in semi-Fowler position, and prepare for possible admission or surgery.

Hyphema

Hyphema is a hemorrhage into the anterior chamber of the eye that results in corneal blood staining, secondary glaucoma, visual impairment, or loss of an eye (Gragg et al., 2025).
- *Causes:* Eye trauma.
- *Signs and symptoms:* Blood in anterior chamber of eye, impaired visual acuity, and "seeing red" or floater.
- *Interventions:* Elevate the patient's head of the bed to at least 30 degrees; gently patch both eyes; anticipate orders to arrange immediate ophthalmology consult, monitor intraocular pressure, and administer pain medications as prescribed.

Ocular Burns

Chemical burns are the result of contact with acid or alkali solutions. Alkali chemicals penetrate cells deeper, causing more tissue damage, and can result in loss of vision.
- *Causes:* Foreign chemical contact with the eye. Severity depends on the pH, concentration, and duration of exposure.
- *Signs and symptoms:* Eye pain, visual disturbances, corneal whitening, copious tearing, surrounding skin irritation, and corneal ulceration.
- *Interventions:* Rinse immediately at a sink or eyewash station. Assess visual acuity; check pH with litmus paper; immediately apply copious amounts of normal saline/lactated Ringer's solution; anticipate orders

to maintain continuous irrigation until pH of the eye is 7, administer ophthalmic ointments as prescribed, and arrange ophthalmology referral.

FAST FACTS

Acid burns usually require 30- to 60-minute irrigations. Alkali burns damage tissues more deeply and for longer amounts of time; it may take more than an hour to irrigate. This procedure gets fluid everywhere. You will need to give the patient a gown and a towel and have them lie on the stretcher; place the patient in a slight Trendelenburg position. Then place a basin on the floor at the head of the bed. Finally, place a couple of waterproof bed pads folded like a funnel that drain into a basin on the floor.

SUMMARY

Patients with eye emergencies will present to the ED. It is vital to recognize which ones are emergent and which ones are nonurgent. Be sure to document pupil size, pupil reaction to light, pupil symmetry, and visual acuity. You should now be more confident in recognizing the symptoms and expected treatments for the various types of eye emergencies. However, you need to practice with the current eye supplies at your facility to truly complete your ocular emergency preparation.

REVIEW QUESTIONS

1) A patient presents to the ED with a penetrating eye injury after being struck by a sharp object. The nurse notes a teardrop-shaped pupil and visible foreign material in the eye. What is the nurse's next step?
   a. Instill antibiotic eye drops to prevent infection.
   b. Apply a sterile saline-soaked dressing and patch the affected eye only.
   c. Cover the affected eye with a rigid shield, elevate the head, and designate the patient nothing by mouth (NPO).
   d. Apply direct pressure to the eye to prevent further bleeding.
2) A factory worker presents to the ED after a chemical splash to the eye. The patient reports burning pain, tearing, and blurred vision. What should the nurse do first?
   a. Administer antibiotic eye drops to prevent infection.
   b. Patch the affected eye to reduce irritation and prevent further damage.
   c. Irrigate the eye immediately with copious amounts of normal saline or lactated Ringer's solution.
   d. Instill topical anesthetics before irrigation to minimize pain.

REFERENCES

Gragg, J., Blair, K., & Baker, M. B. (2025, January). *Hyphema* [Updated December 26, 2022]. In StatPearls [Internet]. StatPearls Publishing. Retrieved August 26, 2025, from https://www.ncbi.nlm.nih.gov/books/NBK507802/

Kang, J. M., & Tanna, A. P. (2021, May). Glaucoma. *The Medical Clinics of North America, 105*(3), 493–510. https://doi.org/10.1016/j.mcna.2021.01.004

Tripathy, K., Shah, S. S., & Waymack, J. R. (2025, January). *Central retinal artery occlusion* [Updated May 2, 2024]. In StatPearls [Internet]. StatPearls Publishing. Retrieved August 26, 2025, from https://www.ncbi.nlm.nih.gov/books/NBK470354/

Endocrine Emergencies

Sarah Berry

The endocrine system is a network of glands and organs that produce, secrete, and regulate hormones throughout the body. In the ED, endocrine emergencies can present in different ways and can also sometimes present with neurological symptoms. It is important to recognize and understand these processes and diseases and be able to distinguish between them to anticipate and advocate for appropriate treatment.

In this chapter, you will learn to:
1. Recognize and understand the different endocrine emergencies
2. Anticipate the interventions for patients presenting with different disorders
3. Review the signs and symptoms of endocrine disorders and emergencies that may present in the ED

ENDOCRINE EMERGENCIES

The endocrine system is made up of several complex hormone-secreting glands. These include the pituitary, pineal gland, hypothalamus, parathyroid, thyroid, pancreas, adrenals, testes, and ovaries. When one thinks of the endocrine system, the word that might come to mind is "hormones." While the endocrine system is responsible for hormone production, it also affects metabolism, growth and development, emotions, tissue function, and homeostasis. Although there are many endocrine-related illnesses, this chapter includes only the most common and emergent conditions.

PANCREATIC-RELATED EMERGENCIES

The pancreas is located in the epigastric area and is responsible for production and secretion of insulin and digestive enzymes such as amylase and lipase.

Diabetic Ketoacidosis

Diabetic ketoacidosis (DKA) is a state of metabolic acidosis that is the result of elevated blood sugar (>250 mg/dL). When the blood sugar is this high, the body does not have sufficient insulin to break down sugar for energy. The inability to break down sugar due to a lack of insulin production or ineffective insulin production is generally related to diabetes mellitus. In approximately 25% to 40% of presentations, it is new-onset diabetes mellitus type 1 (DM1; Calimag et al., 2023). To compensate, the body breaks down fat, thereby releasing toxic ketone acids (Gosmanov & Kitabchi, 2023).

- *Causes:* Uncontrolled blood sugar in diabetes mellitus, pancreatitis, illness, dehydration, heat exposure, infection, stress, myocardial infarction, and pregnancy.
- *Signs and symptoms:* Dry, flushed skin; serum glucose level greater than 250 mg/dL; nausea and vomiting; abdominal pain; polyuria; polydipsia; tachycardia; hypotension; weakness; fruity breath; Kussmaul respirations; ketones in urine; change in level of consciousness; and coma (Gosmanov & Kitabchi, 2018).
- *Interventions:*
  - *Initial interventions:* Initiate continuous cardiac monitoring, pulse oximetry, automatic blood pressure readings (frequency is dependent on the stability of the patient), and establish at least two IVs, as multiple infusions and fluid types may be ordered. If the patient has an altered level of consciousness, consider end-tidal waveform capnography for closer monitoring of respiratory changes. Complete ordered bloodwork and plan for frequent redraws and glucose point-of-care testing to monitor the patient throughout treatment. Initial workup should include testing to rule out possible causes inducing DKA, like sending cardiac biomarkers and getting a 12-lead EKG, evaluating for infection with cultures and/or urinalysis, and sending a serum lactic acid sample.
  - *Fluid replacement:* Begin IV fluid replacement per orders (Gosmanov & Kitabchi, 2018). Be cognizant of patients who have a history of congestive heart failure because fluid volume overload needs to be considered in response to rapid infusion.
  - *Correct acidosis:* Check arterial or venous blood gases per policy; address underlying cause of acidosis; administer IV sodium bicarbonate with severe acidosis if ordered (Gosmanov & Kitabchi, 2018).
  - **Balance electrolytes:** Draw blood for lab tests as frequently as ordered to monitor anion gap, glucose level, and potassium (Gosmanov & Kitabchi, 2018). Medicate for nausea and vomiting. Anticipate IV potassium orders for hypokalemia. Insulin administration drives potassium back into the cells, further reducing serum potassium levels. Monitor potassium levels at the ordered frequency. It is also important to be familiar with standing

orders such as "Notify provider if potassium (K) is less than 3.3" or "Hold insulin for potassium (K) less than 3.3." Often the institution will have a protocol for IV fluids, insulin infusions, and electrolyte replacements that the provider will order for the patient with DKA. Continuous communication and documentation on critical patients are key to safe monitoring and treatment.

- *Treat hyperglycemia:* Obtain and monitor hourly blood glucose and a baseline urinalysis; anticipate orders for IV insulin to jump-start treatment. Following this, the provider may order an IV infusion of insulin to continue to lower the patient's blood sugar (Gosmanov & Kitabchi, 2018). Once the patient's blood sugar is <200 to 250 mg/dL, typically a subcutaneous (SQ) insulin dose is ordered to be given 2 hours prior to discontinuing the IV insulin drip (Gosmanov & Kitabchi, 2018). This allows for a smooth transition from IV to SQ insulin. Orders for IV infusion of normal saline with potassium or normal saline with dextrose may be ordered. The dextrose infusion allows for an easier transition to combat insulin infusion and (probable) nothing by mouth (NPO) status until glucose levels reach l≤250 mg/dL. Prepare for ICU admission.

Many orders and procedures are hospital and provider specific. The most important things to monitor in these patients are their mental status, respiratory status, glucose levels, potassium levels, anion gap, telemetry, and IV infusion compatibility. When IV access is potentially limited, IV compatibility is crucial. Check hospital policy or consult with the pharmacy to determine which medications are considered "high alert" or "high risk," such as insulin, and need to be infused alone to tightly control their titration. Best practice also indicates that dual verification by two separate nurses prior to initiating or changing insulin infusion rates decreases error and risk to the patient (Modic et al., 2016).

Hyperosmolar Hyperglycemic Syndrome

This is a severe state of extreme dehydration and hyperglycemia, typically seen in patients with type 2 diabetes. Although hyperglycemia is similar to DKA, the patient with hyperosmolar hyperglycemic syndrome (HHS) has limited acidemia and ketonemia or lacks them altogether, and the glucose level is significantly higher.

- *Causes:* Infection is the leading cause of HHS. Additionally, poor medication management and compliance, cerebrovascular accident, recent myocardial infarction, pancreatitis, trauma, alcohol and drug abuse, and use of corticosteroids or atypical antipsychotics can also lead to HHS (Stoner, 2017).
- *Signs and symptoms:* Profound dehydration with decreased skin turgor; neurological symptoms such as lethargy or coma; dry mucous membranes; sunken eyes; a rapid, thready pulse; low-grade fever; and a marked blood glucose level, generally >600 mg/dL but can be greater than 1,000 mg/dL in some cases (Stoner, 2017).

- *Interventions:*
  - *Fluid replacement:* Anticipate orders for intense fluid resuscitation. Determining volume is based on the patient's body weight in kilograms. Orders for 100 to 200 mL/kg of fluid are recommended (Stoner, 2017). Frequently document vital signs. Use caution if a patient has a history of congestive heart failure or renal failure. Fluid replacement could take several hours to avoid significant shifts in sodium levels or fluid volume overload. As electrolytes and glucose levels change, be aware that orders for different types of fluids may be written (0.9% or 0.45% NaCl). If the patient remains in the ED for a significant portion of the resuscitation, there is a chance the patient may be there once their glucose starts to drop. Although it is dependent on the provider, once the patient's blood glucose decreases to around 300 mg/dL, anticipate orders to change the fluids to one containing dextrose. This will help to smooth the patient's transition out of a state of hyperglycemia with a decreased chance of adverse effects of hypoglycemia (Stoner, 2017). Once fluids have started, be prepared for urinary frequency. Provide urinary solutions such as a urinal, external catheter, or Foley catheter if an order is present. Consider advocating for a Foley catheter for the patient who requires strict intake and output measuring.
  - *Balance electrolytes:* Place the patient on continuous cardiac monitoring and obtain a baseline EKG. As in DKA, serum potassium levels can drop significantly if IV insulin is administered. Once the patient has started to make urine again, anticipate potassium replacement therapy. Also anticipate orders for frequent blood glucose and electrolyte monitoring, either hourly or every 2 hours in the initial phases of the resuscitation (Stoner, 2017). Treatment will be tailored around metabolic panel results, and obtaining those lab tests should be prioritized.
  - *Treat hyperglycemia:* Obtain and monitor blood glucose hourly. Keep in mind that in this state, early insulin administration could be potentially detrimental. The importance of appropriate fluid volume resuscitation prior to insulin administration could save a patient from exacerbated hypotension and subsequent vascular collapse. Treatment with insulin is different depending on adults versus pediatrics. For adults, an insulin bolus followed by an infusion is best practice. The bolus can range from 5 to 10 units of insulin but is generally based on 0.1 unit/kg, followed by a maintenance infusion of 0.1 unit/kg/hr until the patient's blood sugar reaches about 300 mg/dL. It is not recommended that children receive an insulin bolus for initial treatment but instead be started on an insulin infusion. Like adults, children should receive an infusion of 0.1 unit/kg/hr with strict monitoring of blood glucose, electrolytes, and changes in mentation (Stoner, 2017). Although it is more common in children, some adults may experience cerebral edema and worsening alterations in mental status with rapid shifts in glucose or sodium

(Stoner, 2017). IV 5% dextrose 0.45% normal saline (D5½NS) may be ordered as serum sodium returns to normal and glucose levels reach ≤250 mg/dL. This process of stabilization can take several days and often requires an ICU admission.
- *Treatment of precipitating condition(s):* If the patient is hypotensive, febrile, or showing other signs of possible sepsis as being a precipitating cause, anticipate orders for antibiotics after obtaining blood cultures. If it is suspected that the HHS is a side effect from a medication, consider advocating for a change in therapy if the medication is needed for the patient's health and well-being. If necessary, the medication may need to be reduced or discontinued altogether (Stoner, 2017).

Hypoglycemia

Hypoglycemia is defined as low blood sugar (<60–70 mg/dL) and most commonly affects people with type 1 diabetes. There are three classifications of hypoglycemia, delineated into levels: level 1—plasma glucose of <70 mg/dL but >54 mg/dL; level 2—plasma glucose of <54 mg/dL that requires immediate intervention; and level 3—a plasma glucose level that leads to a change in mental status or impairment of the patient's ability to physically function. In this state, the patient is altered to the point that another person would have to intervene on the patient's behalf to correct their glucose (Nakhleh & Shehadeh, 2021).

- *Causes:* Inappropriate use of insulin or antidiabetic medications in relation to dose or timing of administration with regard to a meal, small portions with low carbohydrates, prolonged fasting, excessive alcohol consumption, physical exercise, pregnancy, renal or hepatic failure, or hypothyroidism (Nakhleh & Shehadeh, 2021). Assess if an intentional or unintentional overdose has occurred.
- *Signs and symptoms:* Anxiety, tremor, tachycardia, nausea, diaphoresis, feelings of hunger, vision changes, dizziness, altered mentation, headache, loss of consciousness, and possible seizure (Nakhleh & Shehadeh, 2021).
- *Interventions:* Obtain accurate history, complete neurologic assessment, and assess for cause of hypoglycemia. Anticipate orders to obtain blood glucose, monitor cardiac rhythm and vital signs, provide warm blankets and warming measures if hypothermic, obtain IV access, obtain complete blood count and metabolic panel, and recheck the blood glucose in 1 hour of treatment and as needed. If the patient has an insulin pump, stop it immediately (Nakhleh & Shehadeh, 2021).
  - *If conscious:* Anticipate orders to give simple carbohydrates (20 g) orally in the form of orange juice (150–200 mL), soda, or glucose tabs to quickly raise the blood sugar. If the patient's finger stick glucose level is <70 mg/dL after 30 to 45 minutes, anticipate orders for D10. Once the patient's finger stick glucose is >70 mg/dL and the patient maintains their alertness, give long-acting carbohydrates such as a sandwich or graham crackers (Nakhleh & Shehadeh, 2021).

- *If unconscious:* Have suction available and airway adjuncts prepared. Maintain the patient's airway while treating hypoglycemia. If the patient has an insulin pump, stop it immediately. Anticipate orders to give IV dextrose or intramuscular (IM) glucagon if unable to obtain IV access. Finger stick glucose should be repeated after 10 minutes, and if the concentration is still <70 mg/dL, additional dextrose should be given. IM glucagon is less likely to work with a second administration, so IV access is critical. Once a patient regains consciousness, give simple carbohydrates followed by complex carbohydrates (Nakhleh & Shehadeh, 2021).

Pancreatitis

Acute pancreatitis is an inflammatory process that causes severe abdominal pain. Recurrent pancreatitis could lead to short- and long-term complications that may lead to multiple organ dysfunction, necrosis, or, ultimately, organ failure (Szatmary et al., 2022).

- *Causes:* There are many possible causes for pancreatitis. They range from other organs being inflamed, to poor lifestyle habits, to side effects of procedures. Considerations for pancreatitis consist of cholelithiasis, heavy alcohol consumption, smoking, hyperlipidemia, certain prescription drugs, endoscopic retrograde cholangiopancreatography (ERCP), trauma, viral infections (such as mumps and COVID), scorpion bites, and organophosphate poisoning (Szatmary et al., 2022).
- *Signs and symptoms:* Pancreatitis is hallmarked by epigastric and diffuse abdominal pain, associated distention, and nausea and vomiting. The patient may also experience fever, breathlessness likely related to abdominal distention, irritability, and possible altered mental status. If the patient is experiencing an associated viral infection or sepsis, they may have low oxygen saturation, tachycardia, hypotension, or tachypnea (Szatmary et al., 2022). Some patients may experience foul-smelling, gray stool. Cullen sign (see Figure 11.1) may be present if the patient is experiencing hemorrhagic pancreatitis (Rahbour et al., 2012).
- *Interventions:* Depending on the precipitating cause of the patient's pancreatitis, the treatment may vary. If their oxygen saturation requires support, the clinician should offer the patient supplemental oxygen. The patient should be kept on an NPO diet to allow for rest of the digestive system and to not tax the pancreas by demanding enzyme production from eating. Because the patient is likely being kept NPO, adequate fluid resuscitation, especially in the hypotensive and tachycardic patient, is vital. Early interventions of fluids have been shown to correct third-space volume loss and tissue hypoperfusion. Correcting these complications can help to counteract systemic circulatory impairment and reverse the otherwise subsequent inflammatory cascade (Szatmary et al., 2022). Be sure to have ample IV access for fluids, antibiotics, analgesia, and any additional treatments that may be necessary if further complications

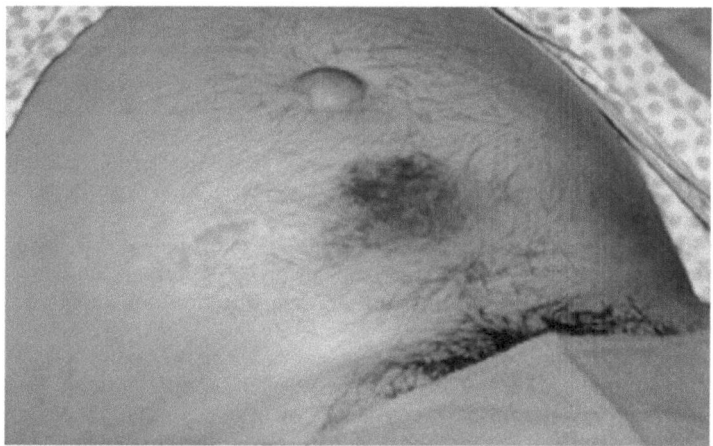

Figure 11.1 Cullen sign.
Source: Herbert L. Fred and Hendrik A. van Dijk. (2008). *Cullen's sign*.

arise. Anticipate orders for antibiotics and pain management. Pancreatitis is a painful disease process, and appropriate analgesia throughout opioid treatment can help manage pain, as well as decrease the need for additional doses throughout admission. If the patient has uncomplicated pancreatitis and their pain does not require the strength of an opioid, nonsteroidal anti-inflammatory drugs (NSAIDs) are an appropriate alternative if their kidney function is adequate (Szatmary et al., 2022). Additionally, in patients with preexisting diabetes mellitus, elevated glucose levels are indicative of a more severe acute pancreatitis. Treatment for hyperglycemia during initial phases is important to decrease the risk of further complications (Szatmary et al., 2022).

THYROID-RELATED EMERGENCIES

The thyroid is a hormone-producing and hormone-regulating organ that is located on the anterior aspect of the throat. The butterfly shape makes it unique to other glands in the endocrine system. It produces hormones throughout the lifespan, controlling growth, metabolism, and development. When certain situations arise and the body calls for more of a specific hormone or function, the thyroid produces what is needed. The three major hormones are triiodothyronine (T_3); tetraiodothyronine, also known as thyroxine (T_4); and calcitonin. Calcitonin is made by C-cells, not the thyroid itself, and is involved in calcium and bone metabolism (Pirahanchi et al., 2023).

Thyroid Storm

"Thyroid storm is a severe manifestation of thyrotoxicosis" and a type of hyperthyroidism (De Almeida et al., 2022). It is most commonly seen as a result of Graves disease but can be caused by other complications of the thyroid, such as cancer, trauma, surgical complications, medication mismanagement, and noncompliance with antithyroid medications (De Almeida et al., 2022). This is a process that can lead to multisystem organ failure and has a high mortality rate if left untreated.

- *Causes:* Uncontrolled hyperthyroidism. Risk factors include history of Graves disease, medication noncompliance, thyroid tumors, certain medications (amiodarone, lithium), trauma, infection, and surgery (De Almeida et al., 2022).
- *Signs and symptoms:* Symptoms are usually exaggerations of hyperthyroidism. Fever, sometimes between 104 and 106°F, with significant diaphoresis, tachycardia of >140 beats per minute (bpm), symptoms of heart failure with peripheral and pulmonary edema, hypotension, agitation, anxiety, nausea, vomiting, diarrhea, abdominal pain, and acute liver failure (Pokhrel et al., 2022).
- *Interventions:* Obtain ordered lab work; maintain the patient's airway, breathing, and circulation. Anticipate orders for aggressive treatment once the diagnosis has been obtained. If there are precipitating factors such as infection, antibiotics will likely be ordered. The majority of treatment is based on supportive measures: administer oxygen if appropriate, administer IV fluids as ordered, apply cooling measures such as blankets or ice packs if the patient is febrile, and start treating hyperthyroidism. To control increased adrenergic tone, a beta-blocker will likely be prescribed. First-line treatment consists of antithyroid drugs such as propylthiouracil, which inhibits thyroid hormone synthesis. After administration, supersaturated potassium iodide (SSKI) may be ordered. Be sure to give propylthiouracil prior to SSKI to offset the sudden increase in thyroid hormone synthesis. Hydrocortisone may be ordered to help with systemic inflammation (Pokhrel et al., 2022). If the patient is critical, an admission to the ICU may be warranted.

FAST FACTS

Patients experiencing thyroid storm may be at risk of hyperthermia, ranging from 104 to 106°F. It is critical to obtain an accurate core temperature and cool the patient steadily to avoid lasting effects.

Myxedema Coma

Myxedema coma is a rare but emergent complication of uncontrolled or undiagnosed hypothyroidism. Even with early recognition and treatment, the mortality rate can be as high as 60% (Elshimy et al., 2023).

- *Causes:* Hashimoto disease (hypothyroidism); infections (both viral and bacterial); burns; trauma; hypothermia or hypoglycemia; congestive heart failure; gastrointestinal (GI) bleeds; and medications including amiodarone, lithium, certain sedatives or tranquilizers, opioids, phenytoin, rifampin, diuretics, and beta-blockers (Elshimy et al., 2023).
- *Signs and symptoms:* Myxedema has effects throughout the body and can lead to multisystem organ dysfunction.
  - *Cardiac:* Hypotension, bradycardia, decreased cardiac output leading to symptoms of congestive heart failure, EKG changes such as bundle branch blocks and complete heart block (Elshimy et al., 2023).
  - *Neurologic:* Lethargy, depression, altered mental status, decreased deep tendon reflexes, paranoia, hypothermia (the lower the core temperature, the worse the prognosis), increased intracranial pressure, and high protein count found on lumbar punctures (Elshimy et al., 2023).
  - *Respiratory:* Patients may experience hypoxia and hypercapnia due to diaphragmatic muscle weakness. Patients who experience congestive heart failure symptoms may have pleural effusions or pulmonary edema, leading to decreased tidal volume (Elshimy et al., 2023).
  - *GI:* Abdominal pain, nausea, vomiting, constipation, decreased appetite, and possible GI bleeding due to increased coagulopathy (Elshimy et al., 2023).
  - *Renal/electrolyte:* Decreased kidney function, hyponatremia, increased secretion of antidiuretic hormone (ADH), and decreased tone of the urinary bladder can lead to urinary retention (Elshimy et al., 2023).
  - *Hematology:* Patients are at risk for having von Willebrand syndrome, leading to decreases in factors V, VII, VIII, IX, and X (Elshimy et al., 2023). This is reversible with T_4 therapy.
- *Interventions:* As always, airway, breathing, and circulation are the highest priorities. Patients may experience airway complications and subsequent breathing abnormalities. Support the patient's airway and breathing through supplemental oxygen. If the patient is altered to the point that they cannot tolerate or do not improve with noninvasive oxygen therapy, anticipate the probability of intubation. Patients often are altered and are at increased risk for aspiration; have suction available and ready for use. Consider advocating for a Foley catheter for accurate intake and output. Anticipate orders for fluid resuscitation and repeat lab work to acutely monitor sodium levels. While rewarming the patient, monitor for hypotension. As the vessels dilate due to warmth, the patient is at increased risk for hypotension and impending cardiovascular collapse. If the patient is not responsive to IV fluid resuscitation, they may require vasopressors until thyroid replacement therapy (levothyroxine) has had time to start working. IV fluids may be changed to dextrose to combat

persistent hypoglycemia. Patients with severe hyponatremia may qualify for 3% hypertonic saline, followed by furosemide to combat fluid volume shifts. With hyponatremia being slowly reversed, the patient's mental status should begin to improve. The ultimate line of treatment is levothyroxine administration to correct hypothyroidism. IV therapy is the initial preference, followed by oral doses as the patient's mental status and stability improve (Elshimy et al., 2023). In addition to the treatment for myxedema, expect treatment of precipitating factors such as possible sepsis or other infections to warrant antibiotic therapy. Because of the complexity of patients with this syndrome, their multisystem dysfunction, and high mortality rate, ICU orders and admission should be anticipated.

Diabetes Insipidus

Diabetes insipidus (DI) is characterized by high volumes of dilute urinary output, significant thirst, and dehydration. It can be further broken down into two subcategories, central and nephrogenic. Central DI is more common.

- *Causes:* Decreases in regulation and release of ADH; this is usually caused by acquired factors such as a traumatic brain injury, infection (tuberculosis, toxoplasmosis, meningitis, and HIV; Christ-Crain & Gaisl, 2021), decreased perfusion to the posterior pituitary gland where ADH is produced, neurosurgery complication, genetic abnormalities, or tumors (Mutter et al., 2021).
- *Signs and symptoms:* Fluid consumption of >3 to 3.5 L in a 24-hour period in adults or urine volume of 50 mL/kg of body weight, significant craving for cold water, and marked dehydration. If left untreated, subsequent complications such as hypotension, acute tubular necrosis due to renal hypoperfusion, and shock could arise. Patients may experience irritability, altered levels of consciousness, seizure, and coma (Christ-Crain & Gaisl, 2021).
- *Interventions:* Advocate for a Foley catheter for accurate intake and output measurement to help with both diagnosis and treatment. Therapy for management consists of replacement of free water deficit with adequate rehydration, replacement of ADH, and treatment of the underlying cause (Christ-Crain & Gaisl, 2021). While participating in fluid replacement, it is important to correct plasma osmolality over approximately 72 hours. Approximately 50% of the initial replacement should be administered in the first 24 hours and the additional 50% over the following 48 hours to avoid cerebral edema secondary to water shifts (Christ-Crain & Gaisl, 2021). Desmopressin (DDAVP) is a synthetic form of ADH and is dosed based on individual patient needs.

SUMMARY

Those little hormones can affect so much more than just our moods. The endocrine system can affect multiple body systems. Document a full primary assessment, all interventions, and any changes in lab results. Be sure to accurately document intake and output hourly in critically ill patients. Early recognition, thorough assessment, and rapid treatment are crucial to the survival of an endocrine-related emergency.

REVIEW QUESTIONS

1) Which of the following symptoms are *not* characteristic of DKA?
   a. Blood glucose >250 mg/dL
   b. Presence of ketones in urine
   c. Fruity breath
   d. Blood glucose <100 mg/dL
2) Which lab value should cause a nurse to pause and contact the provider prior to administering IV insulin?
   a. Serum potassium <3.3 mEq/L
   b. Blood sugar of 520 mg/dL
   c. Carbon dioxide of 40 mmHg
   d. Sodium of 140 mEq/L
3) There are different routes for glucose administration when patients are being treated for hypoglycemia. When choosing the appropriate route, what consideration should be taken as priority?
   a. Urgency of need for correction
   b. The patient's Glasgow Coma Score (GCS) and mentation
   c. The patient's blood pressure
   d. The patient's preferred method of treatment despite their level of mentation

REFERENCES

Calimag, A. P., Chlebek, S., Lerma, E. V., & Chaiban, J. T. (2023). Diabetic ketoacidosis. *Disease-a-Month, 69*(3), 101418. https://doi.org/10.1016/j.disamonth.2022.101418

Christ-Crain, M., & Gaisl, O. (2021). Diabetes insipidus. *Presse medicale, 50*(4), 104093. https://doi.org/10.1016/j.lpm.2021.104093

De Almeida, R., McCalmon, S., & Cabandugama, P. K. (2022). Clinical review and update on the management of thyroid storm. *Missouri Medicine, 119*(4), 366–371. PMID: 36118802; PMCID: PMC9462913

Elshimy, G., Chippa, V., & Correa, R. (2023, August 13). *Myxedema*. In StatPearls [Internet]. StatPearls Publishing. Retrieved August 26, 2025, from https://www.ncbi.nlm.nih.gov/books/NBK545193/

Ghimire, P., & Dhamoon, A. S., (Updated 2023, August 8). *Ketoacidosis*. In StatPearls [Internet]. StatPearls Publishing. Retrieved August 26, 2025, from https://www.ncbi.nlm.nih.gov/books/NBK534848/

Modic, M. B., Albert, N. M., Sun, Z., Bena, J. F., Yager, C., Cary, T., Corniello, A., Kaser, N., Simon, J., Skowronsky, C., & Kissinger, B. (2016). Does an insulin double-checking procedure improve patient safety? *JONA: The Journal of Nursing Administration, 46*(3), 154–160. https://doi.org/10.1097/nna.0000000000000314

Mutter, C. M., Smith, T., Menze, O., Zakharia, M., & Nguyen, H. (2021). Diabetes insipidus: Pathogenesis, diagnosis, and clinical management. *Cureus, 13*(2), e13523. https://doi.org/10.7759/cureus.13523

Nakhleh, A., & Shehadeh, N. (2021). Hypoglycemia in diabetes: An update on pathophysiology, treatment, and prevention. *World Journal of Diabetes, 12*(12), 2036–2049. https://doi.org/10.4239/wjd.v12.i12.2036

Pirahanchi, Y., Tariq, M., & Jialal, I. (2023, February 13). *Physiology, thyroid*. In StatPearls [Internet]. StatPearls Publishing. Retrieved August 26, 2025, from https://www.ncbi.nlm.nih.gov/books/NBK519566/

Pokhrel, B., Aiman, W., & Bhusal, K. (2022, October 6). *Thyroid storm*. In StatPearls [Internet]. StatPearls Publishing. Retrieved August 26, 2025, from https://www.ncbi.nlm.nih.gov/books/NBK448095/

Rahbour, G., Ullah, M. R., Yassin, N., & Thomas, G. P. (2012). Cullen's sign—Case report with a review of the literature. *International Journal of Surgery Case Reports, 3*(5), 143–146. https://doi.org/10.1016/j.ijscr.2012.01.001

Stoner, G. (2017). Hyperosmotic hyperglycemia state. *American Family Physician, 96*(11), 729–736. PMID: 29431405.

Szatmary, P., Grammatikopoulos, T., Cai, W., Huang, W., Mukherjee, R., Halloran, C., Beyer, G., & Sutton, R. (2022). Acute pancreatitis: Diagnosis and treatment. *Drugs, 82*(12), 1251–1276. https://doi.org/10.1007/s40265-022-01766-4

Genitourinary Emergencies

Alexander Menard

> Genitourinary emergencies are routinely seen and treated in the ED. Most of the time, they are minor problems that can be treated with medications. However, genitourinary problems such as testicular torsion can result in loss of the testicle(s) if untreated. This chapter guides you through the genital and urinary problems commonly faced in the ED. After reviewing this chapter, you will understand the causes, manifestations, and interventions for common genitourinary emergencies.

In this chapter, you will learn to:
1. Discuss the common genitourinary problems presenting to the ED
2. Identify the signs and symptoms of genitourinary emergencies
3. Review the interventions to address genitourinary emergencies

GENITOURINARY EMERGENCIES

Genitourinary emergencies encompass a wide range of acute conditions affecting the kidneys, ureters, bladder, and reproductive organs, many of which require immediate intervention to prevent serious complications. From urinary tract infections to urinary retention to testicular torsion and pyelonephritis, these conditions can cause significant pain, hemodynamic instability, and potential loss of organ function if not promptly identified and managed. Nurses play a critical role in the early assessment, triage, and stabilization of patients presenting with genitourinary emergencies.

Urinary Tract Infection
This is a bacterial infection of the bladder and urethra, also known as a lower urinary tract infection.

- *Causes:* Because of their anatomy, urinary tract infections are more common in women than in men. Other contributing factors are holding urine, not drinking enough water, intercourse, kidney stones, and pH imbalances.
- *Signs and symptoms:* Dysuria; hematuria (gross or microscopic); frequency; nocturia; urgency; cloudy urine; foul-smelling urine; fever; urinary retention; and abdominal/suprapubic pain or discomfort.
- *Interventions:* Obtain clean-catch urine or catheterized urine if vaginal bleeding is present, administer antibiotic as ordered, encourage fluids, discourage bubble baths, encourage sitz baths, teach to wipe from front to back after toileting, and teach sexually active females to void and cleanse the perineal area after intercourse. If administering urinary analgesia (phenazopyridine), indicate that it will turn the urine orange and permanently stain underwear.

Pyelonephritis

This is a bacterial infection of the renal pelvis or renal tissue and can involve one or both kidneys (Sommers, 2023a).
- *Causes:* Pyelonephritis usually starts as a urinary tract infection in the urethra or bladder that travels all the way up to the kidneys.
- *Signs and symptoms:* Flank pain; painful urination (dysuria); hematuria (macro or micro); frequency; urgency; cloudy urine; foul-smelling urine; fever; chills; costovertebral tenderness; nausea and vomiting; and anorexia. Urinalysis may reveal elevated white blood cell (WBC) counts, nitrates, elevated red blood cell counts, and bacteria.
- *Interventions:* Obtain clean-catch urine or catheterized urine if vaginal bleeding is present, urinalysis, urine culture, blood cultures, complete blood count (CBC), IV fluids, and antibiotic/antipyretics/antiemetics and pain medications as ordered; encourage intake of fluids, discourage bubble baths, encourage sitz baths and bed rest; teach females to wipe from front to back after toileting; teach sexually active females to void and cleanse the perineal area before and after intercourse; and prepare for possible admission.

Renal Calculi

Renal calculi, or nephrolithiasis, are stones of various sizes along the urinary tract that are commonly known as "kidney stones" (Figure 12.1). Stones form in the kidney from the crystallization of minerals and/or other substances that should normally dissolve in the urine (Sommer, 2023a).
- *Causes:* Kidney stones are usually made of calcium or uric acid salt deposits, possibly resulting from urine that is too alkaline or too acidic. Kidney stones have been associated with dehydration, urinary obstruction, and calcium levels.
- *Signs and symptoms:* Severe flank pain radiating to the groin; restlessness; diaphoresis; nausea and vomiting; urgency; frequency; dysuria; hematuria; oliguria; pallor; low-grade fever; and guarding.

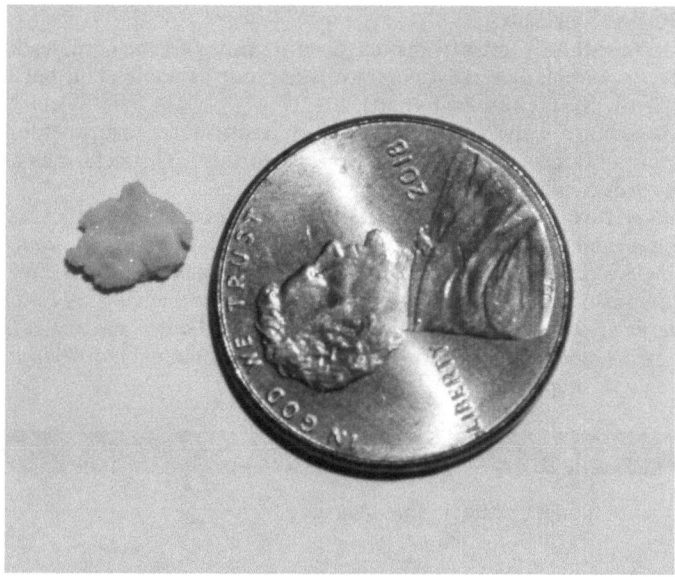

Figure 12.1 Renal calculi.

- *Interventions:* Anticipate orders to obtain clean-catch or catheter urine if vaginal bleeding is present; obtain IV access; administer analgesics as prescribed and document effectiveness; administer antiemetic medications as prescribed; instruct to strain all urine; and prepare for CT scan of abdomen/pelvis without contrast.

Epididymitis

Epididymitis is the inflammation or infection of the epididymis. The epididymis carries sperm from the testicle to the urethra. This is the most common intrascrotal infection and is often unilateral. If left untreated, this can lead to infection of the testicle, which can lead to sterility (Sommers, 2023b).
- *Causes:* Sexually transmitted diseases, urinary tract infections, prostate obstruction, urethral stricture.
- *Signs and symptoms:* Penile discharge, bacteria in urinalysis, gradual scrotum pain that is relieved with elevation, fever, epididymis swelling, and chills.
- *Interventions:* Anticipate orders for ice pack to the scrotum, gonorrhea and chlamydia (G&C) culture, and antibiotics; instruct to abstain from sexual intercourse until repeat urine culture is negative for infection.

FAST FACTS

Untreated epididymitis leading to testicular infection can lead to sterility.

Testicular Torsion

This occurs when a testis twists one or more times on the cord, leading to possible ischemia. The most common age group is adolescent, but it can occur at any age (Schick & Sternard, 2025).

- *Causes:* It is not always known, but it can be attributed to an anatomical abnormality known as the "bell clapper deformity." This deformity allows the cords to twist more easily.
- *Signs and symptoms:* Acute, sudden, severe testicular pain radiating to the groin or abdomen not relieved with testicle elevation; nausea and vomiting; and elevated, swollen, and tender testes. Absence of the cremasteric reflex (elevation of the affected testis when aspect of inner thigh is gently stroked).
- *Interventions:* Anticipate orders for IV crystalloid fluids and analgesics, ice packs, and testicular ultrasound; prepare for manual reduction of the torsion or prepare for surgery as indicated.

FAST FACTS

Testicular torsion is a urologic emergency!

Penile Fracture

Penile fracture is an acute rupture in the membrane (tunica albuginea) that surrounds the corpora cavernosa (Adkins et al., 2017).

- *Causes:* Trauma or abrupt bending of the erect penis commonly associated with aggressive sexual intercourse or masturbation.
- *Signs and symptoms:* The patient may report hearing a cracking or popping sound upon injury, immediately followed by pain, flaccidity, hematoma, swelling, deformity, and dark bruising of the penis. Other symptoms may include hematuria, blood noted at the urethral meatus, and inability to void.
- *Interventions:* Anticipate orders to administer pain medications, insert IV access, obtain urinalysis if possible, contact emergent consulting urologist, and give patient nothing by mouth and no urethral catheterizations. Prepare for retrograde urethrogram and surgical intervention with transfer to the operating room.

Urinary Retention

Urinary retention (ischuria) is the inability to void or to fully empty the bladder.

- *Causes:* Enlarged prostate, constipation, infection, nerve dysfunction, urethral obstruction or strictures, kidney stones, blood clots, and some medications such as opioids, amphetamines, anticholinergics, antidepressants, and cyclooxygenase-2 (COX-2) inhibitor medications.
- *Signs and symptoms:* Unable to void or "only a little comes out"; bladder "feels full" or is distended; lower midabdominal pain; and patient may appear anxious.

- *Interventions:* To properly treat urinary retention, one must first find the cause by obtaining an accurate urologic history and assessment. Anticipate orders to obtain urology consult and insert a urinary catheter. If resistance is met upon urinary catheter insertion, do not force; reattempt with a smaller or specialty urinary catheter per order. Once inserted, the patient typically finds instant relief. To avoid bladder spasms, clamp the urinary catheter after the first 1,000 mL empties. If blood clots are present, a bladder irrigation system may be ordered by the provider.

Genital Warts

Genital warts (condylomata acuminate) is a viral sexually transmitted infection. The virus responsible is the human papilloma virus (HPV). It is estimated that about 50% of sexually active males and females will acquire HPV in their lifetime (Buettner, 2022).
- *Causes:* Sexual contact with an infected partner.
- *Signs and symptoms:* Painless single or multipapular-type rash in various shapes such as plaque or cauliflowerlike appearance on the genital areas. Areas affected may include perianal, vulva, penis, perineum, and cervix. The oral pharynx or larynx may also be affected. Warts may spontaneously increase or decrease without treatment.
- *Interventions:* Because it is a viral infection, there is no cure. Treatments may include laser therapy, surgical excision, and cryotherapy. The treatment goal is to remove symptomatic warts to induce more "wart-free" periods. Although there is no cure, we can educate our patients on prevention. The Gardasil vaccine is now available to prevent cervical cancer and other diseases associated with HPV.

Priapism

Priapism is a prolonged penile erection lasting longer than 4 hours (Silberman, 2025).
- *Causes:* Spinal cord injury, leukemia, sickle cell disease, psychotropic drugs, multiple sclerosis, prolonged sexual stimulation, penile tumor, urethral tumor, anticoagulant therapy, and impotence treatments.
- *Signs and symptoms:* Prolonged painful penile erection for more than 4 hours.
- *Treatments:* Anticipate treatment of underlying causes by provider that may include observation of the patient; ice packs; penile or groin pressure; intracavernous injections (with drugs such as epinephrine, norepinephrine, and ephedrine); needle aspiration; or surgery.

SUMMARY

Although most genitourinary emergencies can be treated with medications, some require immediate interventions. Remember that renal infections, obstructions, or poor perfusion can lead to renal failure; early intervention is key. Document your urine and genital assessments. Maintain and respect patient privacy; provide a chaperone when necessary.

REVIEW QUESTIONS

1) A 45-year-old female presents to the ED with fever, chills, flank pain, nausea, and dysuria. Upon assessment, you find costovertebral angle (CVA) tenderness and a temperature of 102.2°F. What is the next best step?
    a. Administer oral antibiotics and discharge the patient with a follow-up appointment.
    b. Obtain blood and urine cultures, then initiate IV fluids and broad-spectrum antibiotics.
    c. Encourage the patient to drink fluids and monitor urine output before initiating treatment.
    d. Perform a bladder scan and insert a urinary catheter to relieve symptoms.
2) A 28-year-old male presents to the ED with gradual onset of scrotal pain, swelling, and tenderness over the past 2 days. He also reports dysuria and urethral discharge. The nurse performs an assessment and notes that the pain improves with scrotal elevation. What is the most appropriate initial nursing intervention?
    a. Apply ice packs to the scrotum and instruct the patient to limit activity.
    b. Obtain a urine sample for urinalysis and culture, then anticipate administration of antibiotics.
    c. Prepare the patient for emergent surgical intervention to prevent testicular infarction.
    d. Perform manual detorsion of the testicle to relieve pain and restore blood flow.

REFERENCES

Buettner, J. R. (2022). *Fast facts for the ER nurse: Guide to a successful emergency department orientation*. Springer Publishing Company.

Schick, M. A., & Sternard, B. T. (2025, January). *Testicular torsion* [Updated June 12, 2023]. In StatPearls [Internet]. StatPearls Publishing. Retrieved August 26, 2025, from https://www.ncbi.nlm.nih.gov/books/NBK448199/

Silberman, M., Stormont, G., Leslie, S. W., & Hu, E. W. (2025, January). *Priapism* [Updated May 30, 2023]. In StatPearls [Internet]. StatPearls Publishing. Retrieved August 26, 2025, from https://www.ncbi.nlm.nih.gov/books/NBK459178/

Sommers, M. S. (2023a). *Davis's diseases & disorders: A nursing therapeutic manual* (pp. 1043–1046). F.A. Davis Company.

Sommers, M. S. (2023b). *Davis's diseases & disorders: A nursing therapeutic manual* (pp. 227–221). F.A. Davis Company.

Hematologic Emergencies

Sarah Berry

> Among the various types of emergencies seen in the ED, hematologic emergencies are less common but not less important. Various symptoms such as severe pain or fever can seem equivocal but ultimately can make or break a patient visit or diagnosis. A clear medical history and medication list can sometimes reveal the possible diagnosis quickly. These cases can be life threatening and should be taken as seriously as any other type of emergency.

In this chapter, you will learn to:
1. Discuss the possible hematologic emergencies and disorders that present to the ED
2. Identify the signs and symptoms of patients experiencing hematologic emergencies or disorders
3. Review the interventions and treatment options for hematologic emergencies

HEMATOLOGIC EMERGENCIES

Hematologic emergencies have different etiologies. Some may be related to diseases or their sequelae such as hemolytic transfusion reactions due to blood group incompatibility or pain related to a sickle cell crisis. A fever in the setting of neutropenia related to chemotherapy or immunotherapy treatment is just as life threatening and requires similar critical interventions as would a fever in a septic patient. A thorough history from the patient can help the nurse to narrow down and anticipate possible diagnoses and pending interventions.

Anemia
Anemia is a condition that is defined by a reduced number of red blood cells (RBCs), or a lower hemoglobin. Hemoglobin is the oxygen-carrying portion of the cells, and when there is an insufficient oxygen-carrying capacity, it leads

to anemia. Anemia can be classified as acute or chronic and mild or severe. When someone's oxygen-carrying capacity is altered, the body attempts to compensate. When the body is unable to compensate, this results in anemia. Chronicity and severity are determined by the precipitating factors and associated lab values. Anemia is characterized by a low hemoglobin and hematocrit (H&H) level and any associated symptoms. In males, the normal hemoglobin level is l<13.5%, and the hematocrit level is <39 g/dL. In females, the normal hemoglobin level is <12%, and the hematocrit level is <36 g/dL (Newhall et al., 2020).

- *Causes:* There are two main mechanisms for RBC destruction (Turner et al., 2023).
  - *Blood loss*
    - *Acute:* Hemorrhage, surgical blood loss, trauma, and menorrhagia
    - *Chronic:* Heavy menstruation, gastrointestinal (GI) bleeding, and urinary losses
  - *Hemolytic anemia*
    - *Acquired:* Caused by autoimmune diseases, infection, blood transfusion reactions, splenic diseases or injury, snake bites/venom, disseminated intravascular coagulation (DIC)
    - *Hereditary:* Sickle cell disease (SCD) and additional disorders affecting hemoglobin
- *Types of anemia:* There are three main deficiencies (Cascio & DeLoughery, 2017):
  - *Microcytic:* Iron deficiency anemia, thalassemia, inflammatory anemia, and lead poisoning
  - *Normocytic:* Inflammatory anemia, acute hemolysis, renal disease, aplastic anemia, and multiple myeloma
  - *Macrocytic:* Liver disease; aplastic anemia; hypothyroidism; liver, renal, and thyroid disease; reticulocytosis; iron, vitamin B_{12}, and folate deficiency; chemotherapy-related anemia; and myelodysplastic syndrome
- *Signs and symptoms:* Symptoms are generally dependent on the rate at which blood is lost and its chronicity. The patient may report weakness, fatigue, shortness of breath (especially with exertion), and overall exercise intolerance. The nurse may witness signs like hypotension, pallor, jaundice, swelling of the spleen or liver, tachycardia, or melena on rectal exam (Turner et al., 2023).
- *Interventions:* Attach the patient to the cardiac monitor, pulse oximetry, and blood pressure cuff to monitor for acute changes in vital signs that could be related to decreased blood volume or decreased oxygen-carrying capacity. Anticipate orders to establish an IV and obtain lab work. Lab tests will depend on the diagnostic differential. If the patient is hemodynamically unstable due to acute blood loss, anticipate either fluid resuscitation or rapid blood transfusion. It is important to become familiar with the department's rapid infuser. Be aware of how to prime it, operate it, and troubleshoot it. The cause of the anemia will guide

additional treatment after the acute phase and the patient becomes stable. Additional tests or procedures, such as an upper endoscopy or colonoscopy, may need to be performed to find the source of any suspected GI bleeding. The patient may require nutritional supplements that are started in the ED. Additional studies may be indicated later but are not necessarily performed in the ED (Turner et al., 2023).

Sickle Cell Anemia

Sickle cell anemia (also known as SCD) is a blood disorder that is inherited from a gene mutation of the beta-globin gene. The gene mutation affects millions of people but is more common among people of African, Mediterranean, Middle Eastern, and South Asian descent (Elendu et al., 2023). The gene mutation produces abnormal hemoglobin in the shape of a sickle called hemoglobin S (HbS). In a healthy adult, hemoglobin A is the structure that is present. The irregular shape of the HbS encourages the cells to become stiff and sticky, making it difficult for them to pass through the vessels without sticking together (Elendu et al., 2023).

- *Causes:* Genetic mutation that results in an inherited disorder. Sickle cell anemia is a recessive condition because the patient must inherit one copy of the gene from both parents.
- *Signs and symptoms:* Signs and symptoms vary in both presentation and severity. Recurrent episodes of severe pain related to vaso-occlusive crises are one of the tell-tale symptoms. Additional signs and symptoms include fatigue, anemia, and increased susceptibility to infection (Elendu et al., 2023). Newborn screenings in the United States test for SCD upon birth if the disease is not known to the parents prior to conception (Elendu et al., 2023). Additional signs, symptoms, and complications include acute chest syndrome, delayed growth and development, stroke, end-organ damage of the spleen or kidneys, retinopathy, and avascular necrosis (Elendu et al., 2023).
- *Interventions:* Establish cardiac monitoring, pulse oximetry, and blood pressure monitoring. Establish an IV with the anticipation of fluids and pain medication to be ordered. Because pain is one of the leading symptoms, pain management is of great importance. Patients with SCD frequently require nonsteroidal anti-inflammatory drugs (NSAIDs), opioids, and, in some, cases patient-controlled analgesia (PCA). Additionally, the nurse can offer heat therapy if the patient can pinpoint the pain. Hydration can help the patient prevent vaso-occlusive crises by increasing intravascular volume and allowing for sickle-shaped cells to pass through vessels more easily (Elendu et al., 2023). Some patients may require blood transfusions if they are experiencing anemia, acute chest syndrome, or stroke. Transfusions can also increase the patient's oxygen-carrying capacity because sickle-shaped hemoglobin does not have the same capacity as regular hemoglobin cells (Elendu et al., 2023). If the patient's oxygen saturation is insufficient, consider oxygen administration.

> **FAST FACTS**
>
> Patients with pain related to SCD are considered high risk, according to the emergency severity index (ESI). The suggested ESI level is 2, or high-risk priority.

Disseminated Intravascular Coagulation

DIC is often secondary to another disruptive process. The most common cause is sepsis, leading to systemic organ dysfunction and coagulation disruption. DIC is a process that causes both blood clots and bleeding at variable rates that can determine the patient's prognosis.

- *Causes:* DIC is a secondary process that is a result of another illness. Sepsis accounts for the majority of primary causes. Additional causes include but are not limited to various cancers including solid tumors or hematologic cancers, obstetric emergencies such as HELLP syndrome, preeclampsia and amniotic fluid embolisms, cardiac arrest, aortic aneurysm, and head trauma (Adelborg et al., 2021).
- *Signs and symptoms:* Patient history may indicate recent infections, hepatic failure, obstetric complications, or cancer (Costello et al., 2024). Patients may experience bleeding from anywhere such as their gums, areas of recent surgery, or through orifices such as the vagina or rectum. Patients may also have bleeding from areas of medical devices such as arterial or central lines, IV catheters, or urinary catheters. Symptoms such as hematuria, oliguria, and anuria may be indicative of DIC-induced renal injury or failure (Costello et al., 2024). If the patient is experiencing thrombosis related to DIC, they may experience shortness of breath or changes in oxygenation status from pulmonary embolism or chest pain related to developing coronary occlusions (Costello et al., 2024). Skin findings may consist of ecchymosis, hematomas, petechiae, cyanosis, jaundice, or necrosis depending on the end-organ damage that is involved (Costello et al., 2024).
- *Interventions:* Start the patient on continuous cardiac monitoring, pulse oximetry, and blood pressure monitoring. The patient's hemodynamic status dictates the frequency of blood pressure monitoring. The nurse should monitor for new or increased bruising or petechiae, especially where IVs or medical devices are present such as under the blood pressure cuff. Additionally, if the patient has lacerations, abrasions, or skin tears, the nurse should monitor these areas for new oozing and notify the provider if there are changes. Anticipate orders for lab tests to measure coagulants, H&H, platelets, and blood type. If the patient is experiencing excessive bleeding, there may also be an order to use extreme caution or limit the number of venipunctures or invasive medical procedures such as Foley catheters, arterial line insertions, or central line insertion. These procedures may be necessary if the patient requires strict monitoring or several medications with limited IV access.

The nurse must monitor these sites for new or worsening bleeding after completion.
- *Primary management:* Primary management for DIC is treating the underlying cause, then treating any overt symptoms. Treatment for the underlying cause will differ depending on the cause. For infections, prompt antibiotics and fluid resuscitation for hypotension are appropriate. For obstetric emergencies, treatment for postpartum hemorrhage is a priority to mitigate impending DIC. Patients who are experiencing thrombosis should be treated with anticoagulants to impede worsening thrombosis (Adelborg et al., 2021). In cases of bleeding, platelets and coagulation factors should be transfused to replace those that were lost or inactivated. In the setting of septic-induced DIC, antithrombin is inactivated; therefore it would be reasonable to see orders for antithrombin administration (Adelborg et al., 2021). Additionally, fibrinolysis is common, but treatment with antifibrinolytics is not indicated. However, in cases of cancer-induced DIC, use of antifibrinolytics and tranexamic acid (TXA) may be appropriate if the patient is experiencing excessive bleeding or hemorrhage (Adelborg et al., 2021). For patients in the postpartum setting, TXA is widely accepted and an established practice, but if the patient is experiencing obstetric DIC prior to birth, treatment should be more carefully gauged (Adelborg et al., 2021).

Hemophilia

Hemophilia is a rare, X-linked congenital bleeding disorder with as many as 30% to 40% of cases arising from spontaneous genetic mutations with no prior familial history (Page, 2019). The more severe disorders tend to affect males more, while mild symptoms of bleeding are seen in females. Hemophilia A and B are the most common severe disorders; however, numerous other disorders require treatment (Page, 2019). In addition to genetic bleeding disorders, there are also acquired types of hemophilia that have various causes related to several different organ systems, diseases, or medications (Haider & Anwer, 2022).
- *Causes:* Hemophilia A and B are a result of genetic mutations, whereas other disorders such as von Willebrand disease are characterized by a deficiency in factors I, II, V, VII, VIII, X, XI, and XII and inherited platelet disorders (Page, 2019).
- *Signs and symptoms:* Bleeding can occur anywhere in the body; however, bleeding into the joints (particularly ankles, knees, and elbows) and muscles is the most debilitating with pain (Page, 2019). Bleeding that occurs in the brain or GI tract or overt hemorrhaging from a traumatic event can be life threatening (Page, 2019). Assess the patient for areas of swelling, ecchymoses, petechiae, or vital signs consistent with internal bleeding or hemorrhage such as tachycardia, tachypnea, and hypotension.

- *Interventions:* Anticipate orders to obtain IV access and immediate administration of IV clotting factor VIII or IX as indicated. Other orders may include desmopressin acetate (DDAVP) administration for minor bleeding. Although other synthetic clotting factors are available, DDAVP is a viable and well-researched option to treat minor to moderate bleeding in patients with hemophilia A(Loomans et al., 2018). In cases of major bleeding, consider using bypassing agents such as activated prothrombin complex concentrate (aPCC) or recombinant activated factor VII (rFVIIa) (Haider & Anwer, 2022). While immediate bleeding is being controlled and first-line treatment is underway, some patients may benefit from inhibitor eradication. These treatments should happen simultaneously to increase chances of improved patient outcomes (Haider & Anwer, 2022). Anticipate orders for the use of prednisone as it is a first-line treatment and can be used with cyclophosphamide to increase chances of a better patient outcome (Haider & Anwer, 2022). During treatment, assess the patient for bleeding and encourage joint elevation, ice, and immobilization for swelling or pain. Other orders might include hematologist consultation or topical thrombin for nosebleeds. Diagnostic tests may include CTs, x-rays, complete blood count (CBC), prothrombin time (PT), partial thromboplastin time (PTT), and factor levels. It is important that these not delay factor replacement. Avoid unnecessary venipunctures or excessive peripheral blood pressure cuff usage. Be mindful when removing adhesive dressings and observe for pressure injuries. Avoid intramuscular (IM) injections because of increased risk of muscle damage and excessive bleeding. If it is difficult to obtain IV access on the patient, consider using a more experienced nurse or someone who is trained in ultrasound-guided IV insertion to decrease the risk of unnecessary vessel damage.

FAST FACTS

For patients with hemophilia, use caution when using venipuncture, central line, or arterial line cannulation because of increased bleeding risk. Be prepared to control any potential bleeding because it may be excessive (Dolan et al., 2021).

Acute Leukemia

Leukemia is a cancer of the blood, blood-producing organs, and bone marrow. Acute leukemia is a result of mutations that take place during the hematopoiesis process—the making of blood cells (Rose-Inman & Kuehl, 2017). Depending on the hematologic cell lineage with the mutation, the patient could have either acute myeloid leukemia (AML) or acute lymphocytic leukemia (ALL). Myeloid cells mature within the bone marrow, and lymphoid cells mature within lymphoid organs such as lymph nodes, spleen, and thymus (Rose-Inman & Kuehl, 2017).

- *Causes:* Mutations in the production of red and white blood cells cause different types of leukemias. Possible risk factors include exposure to benzene, ionizing radiation, or previous exposure to chemotherapy or radiation (Puckett et al., 2023). Newer studies suggest that despite ALL not being a "familial disease," there are possible genetic predispositions for its development. In addition to exposure and possible genetic predisposition, it also seems to be more common in patients with trisomy 21 (Down syndrome), neurofibromatosis type 1, Bloom syndrome, and ataxia telangiectasia (Puckett et al., 2023).
- *Signs and symptoms:* Symptoms of acute leukemia may include fever, pallor, shortness of breath, fatigue, bleeding, petechiae, excessive bruising, bone pain, lymphadenopathy, splenomegaly, hepatosplenomegaly, gingival hyperplasia, or a dermatologic phenomenon known as leukemia cutis (Rose-Inman & Kuehl, 2017).
- *Interventions:* While in the ED, interventions should be directed around recognition of possible disease through a thorough triage, history, and physical. If the patient already has a diagnosis of leukemia or any type of cancer, ask if they are undergoing chemotherapy, radiation, or any additional type of treatment. If they are undergoing treatment, isolation is important to protect them from secondary infection that could be acquired in the ED because these patients are immunocompromised. Do not give the patient any fresh fruit or vegetables without thoroughly washing them. Perform frequent and thorough hand hygiene, wear gloves, and consider placing the patient on reverse isolation precautions to protect them from the environment (Puckett et al., 2023).
  - Obtain IV access and anticipate orders for potential blood administration if the patient is actively bleeding. Lab orders may include type and screen, CBC with differential, and coagulation studies. Apply supplemental oxygen and continuous pulse oximetry monitoring if the patient appears or states they are short of breath. If a patient presents with lymphadenopathy or organomegaly, anticipate they will be sent for diagnostic imaging, which could include CT scans, ultrasounds, or x-rays.

TUMOR LYSIS SYNDROME

Tumor lysis syndrome (TLS) is a life-threatening oncologic emergency. Patients who experience TLS undergo a large release of potassium, phosphate, and nucleic acids into their circulatory system after tumor cells are destroyed (Barbar & Sathick, 2021). Because of the metabolic derangements and the end-organ failure that often accompany this syndrome, rapid recognition and intervention are necessary. TLS is most common in "bulky" hematologic malignancies such as non-Hodgkin lymphoma (NHL), Burkitt lymphoma, chronic lymphocytic leukemia (CLL), AML, and ALL. Some reports of TLS in small cell carcinoma, breast cancer, and neuroblastomas have been recorded as well (Barbar & Sathick, 2021).

- *Causes:* TLS is the result of ruptured tumor cells, allowing for excessive release of potassium, phosphorus, nucleic acids, and cytokines to be released into the bloodstream. This burden far exceeds the kidneys' ability to metabolize and excrete them (Barbar & Sathick, 2021). Nucleic acids undergo abnormal conversions, resulting in increased uric acid production and crystalizing uric acid, calcium, phosphate, and xanthine oxidase in the renal tubules, leading to inflammation and obstruction (Barbar & Sathick, 2021). This then leads to acute kidney injury (AKI). Risk factors according to Barbar and Sathick (2021) are as follows: large tumor burden, extensive metastases, rapid proliferation, high cell lysis potential, intensity of initial chemotherapy, bone marrow involvement, splenomegaly and hepatomegaly, markedly elevated lactate dehydrogenase (LDH), preexisting renal impairment, kidney infiltration of tumor, obstructive uropathy from tumor, volume depletion, hypotension, nephrotoxic exposures to NSAIDs and iodinated contrast, and acidic urine.
- *Signs and symptoms:* Signs and symptoms of TLS can vary based on the metabolic derangements the patient is experiencing. If a patient is severely hypocalcemic, they may have positive Chvostek or Trousseau signs, or even seizures. Manifestations of AKI or uremia from TLS include weakness, lethargy, malaise, nausea, vomiting, joint pain, and generalized pruritus. Patients may also exhibit signs of fluid overload including rales and rhonchi or muffled heart sounds (Adeyinka & Bashir, 2021). Laboratory values demonstrating hyperkalemia, hyperphosphatemia, hyperuricemia, hypocalcemia, and elevated LDH levels can be indicative of TLS when correlated clinically.
- *Interventions:* Attach the patient to continuous cardiac monitoring, pulse oximetry, and blood pressure cuff. Determine the frequency of blood pressure reading based on the patient's stability. Establish IV access. If the patient has a port for chemotherapy or because of limited venous access, consult hospital policy and the provider about accessing it. Lab work and treatment can usually be completed through the port if there is adequate blood return. Treatment is based on the presenting symptoms and lab values.
    - Anticipate orders for aggressive IV therapy to help with hypovolemia and to increase urine flow. Increased urine output will help to decrease uric acid. Pay special note to orders, especially if they include the administration of rasburicase. Rasburicase rapidly and effectively reduces uric acid levels, ultimately decreasing the risk of acute renal failure (Alakel et al., 2017). Following its administration, uric acid lab tests should be sent on ice to delay further uric acid degradation leading to falsely low levels. IV hydration is vital because it helps to decrease the concentration of electrolytes from dangerous levels. It treats hyperphosphatemia, which exacerbates hypocalcemia. The breakdown of calcium into calcium phosphate is further exacerbated by treatment for hyperkalemia because of

calcium gluconate being part of its mainstay treatment (Barbar & Sathick, 2021). Maintaining a balance between potassium, calcium, and phosphorus poses a significant challenge in the setting of this condition, and close monitoring by the nurse in these critically ill patients is vital. Anticipate orders for treatment for hyperkalemia, which can be life threatening (Barbar & Sathick, 2021). Treatment for hyperkalemia has become more standardized over the years to include a calcium gluconate infusion, insulin, dextrose, beta-adrenergic agonists, and sodium bicarbonate (Palmer & Clegg, 2024). Additional treatments can be added and tailored to specific patients. Ideally, the order of administration is calcium gluconate, dextrose, insulin, and sodium bicarbonate. Calcium gluconate helps to stabilize the cardiac membrane. Although calcium gluconate does not act directly on the potassium level, calcium acts on the sodium-potassium channels. Then dextrose should be administered to offset any possible hypoglycemia when the insulin is administered. Dextrose is given prior to insulin administration as a safeguard. If insulin is given and then IV access is subsequently lost because of an unforeseen reason, the patient now has a bolus of insulin without counter-treatment available. This could lead to life-threatening hypoglycemia while attempting to obtain new access. Insulin is given to reduce extracellular potassium by promoting cellular uptake of potassium (Palmer & Clegg, 2024). Anticipate orders for IV regular insulin to push potassium into the cell. After treatment is complete, anticipate or request orders for blood glucose finger sticks for 4 hours after. Monitoring the patient's blood sugar for 4 hours is done to cover the duration of the insulin action (Palmer & Clegg, 2024). Some providers may order beta-adrenergic agonists such as nebulized albuterol. This treatment is not always used because it can have complications such as tachyarrhythmias or myocardial ischemia in patients who have coronary artery disease. In patients with end-stage renal disease, the effectiveness of this branch of treatment is significantly lower (Palmer & Clegg, 2024). Lastly, sodium bicarbonate should be reserved for those who have severe metabolic acidosis. The potential complications of sodium bicarbonate administration can outweigh the benefits in most patients (Palmer & Clegg, 2024).

SUMMARY

Because of advances in treatment options, patients today are surviving and living longer with hematologic and oncologic diseases. Anemia, sickle cell crisis, and hemophilia are more commonly seen in the ED than other hematologic emergencies. Neutropenic fever and TLS are two of the most common oncologic emergencies. Be familiar with hospital policies regarding typical blood product transfusion (consent, retrieval of blood products, and administration) and how they may differ from emergent mass transfusion. It is also important to be competent in the utilization of the department's rapid infuser in the event of an emergency.

REVIEW QUESTIONS

1) A patient with acute leukemia is receiving chemotherapy and begins to show signs of TLS. Which of the following lab findings would the ED nurse most likely expect?
    a. Increased calcium, decreased phosphate, decreased uric acid, and increased potassium
    b. Decreased calcium, increased phosphate, increased uric acid, and increased potassium
    c. Increased calcium, increased phosphate, increased uric acid, and decreased potassium
    d. Decreased calcium, decreased phosphate, decreased uric acid, and increased potassium
2) Which of the following clinical signs would most likely indicate the development of DIC in a patient?
    a. Bradycardia and hypertension
    b. Petechiae and oozing from IV sites
    c. Jaundice and green-tinged urine
    d. Hyperreflexia and muscle spasms

REFERENCES

Adelborg, K., Larsen, J. B., & Hvas, A. (2021). Disseminated intravascular coagulation: Epidemiology, biomarkers, and management. *British Journal of Haematology*, *192*(5), 803–818. https://doi.org/10.1111/bjh.17172

Adeyinka, A., & Bashir, K. (2021). *Tumor lysis syndrome*. In StatPearls [Internet]. StatPearls Publishing. Retrieved August 26, 2025, from https://www.ncbi.nlm.nih.gov/books/NBK518985/

Alakel, N., Middeke, J. M., Schetelig, J., & Bornhäuser, M. (2017). Prevention and treatment of tumor lysis syndrome, and the efficacy and role of rasburicase. *OncoTargets and Therapy*, *10*, 597–605. https://doi.org/10.2147/ott.s103864

Barbar, T., & Sathick, I. (2021). Tumor lysis syndrome. *Advances in Chronic Kidney Disease*, *28*(5), 438–446. https://doi.org/10.1053/j.ackd.2021.09.007

Cascio, M., & DeLoughery, T. (2017). Anemia: Evaluation and diagnostic tests. *Medical Clinics of North America*, *101*(2), 263–284. https://doi.org/10.1016/j.mcna.2016.09.003

Costello, R., Leslie, S., & Nehring, S. (2024, May 1). *Disseminated intravascular coagulation*. In StatPearls [Internet]. StatPearls Publishing. Retrieved August 26, 2025, from https://www.ncbi.nlm.nih.gov/books/NBK441834/

Dolan, G., Benson, G., Bowyer, A., Eichler, H., Hermans, C., Jiménez-Yuste, V., Ljung, R., Pollard, D., Santagostino, E., & Šalek, S. Z. (2021). Principles of care for acquired hemophilia. *European Journal of Haematology*, *106*(6), 762–773. https://doi.org/10.1111/ejh.13592

Elendu, C., Amaechi, D. C., Alakwe-Ojimba, C. E., Elendu, T. C., Elendu, R. C., Ayabazu, C. P., Aina, T. O., Aborisade, O., & Adenikinju, J. S. (2023). Understanding sickle cell disease: Causes, symptoms, and treatment options. *Medicine, 102*(38), e35237. https://doi.org/10.1097/md.0000000000035237

Haider, M., & Anwer, F. (2022, December 13). *Acquired hemophilia*. In StatPearls [Internet]. StatPearls Publishing. Retrieved August 26, 2025, from https://www.ncbi.nlm.nih.gov/books/NBK560494/

Newhall, D. A., Oliver, R., & Lugthart, S. (2020). Anaemia: A disease or symptom? *The Netherlands Journal of Medicine, 78*(3), 104–110. PMID: 32332184.

Loomans, J. I., Kruip, M. J. H. A., Carcao, M., Jackson, S., van Velzen, A. S., Peters, M., Santagostino, E., Platokouki, H., Beckers, E., Voorberg, J., van der Bom, J. G., Fijnvandraat, K., & RISE consortium (2018). Desmopressin in moderate hemophilia A patients: a treatment worth considering. *Haematologica, 103*(3), 550–557. https://doi.org/10.3324/haematol.2017.180059

Page, D. (2019). Comprehensive care for hemophilia and other inherited bleeding disorders. *Transfusion and Apheresis Science, 58*(5), 565–568. https://doi.org/10.1016/j.transci.2019.08.005

Palmer, B. F., & Clegg, D. J. (2024). Hyperkalemia treatment standard. *Nephrology Dialysis Transplantation, 39*(7), 1097–1104. https://doi.org/10.1093/ndt/gfae056

Puckett, Y., Chan, O., & Doerr, C. (2023, August 26). *Acute lymphocytic leukemia (Nursing)*. In StatPearls [Internet]. StatPearls Publishing. Retrieved August 26, 2025, from https://www.ncbi.nlm.nih.gov/books/NBK568716/

Rose-Inman, H., & Kuehl, D. (2017). Acute leukemia. *Hematology/Oncology Clinics of North America, 31*(6), 1011–1028. https://doi.org/10.1016/j.hoc.2017.08.006

Turner, J., Parsi, M., & Badireddy, M. (2023, August 8). *Anemia*. In StatPearls [Internet]. StatPearls Publishing. Retrieved August 26, 2025, from https://www.ncbi.nlm.nih.gov/books/NBK499994

Musculoskeletal and Wound Care Emergencies

Alexander Menard

> You will see all types of musculoskeletal and wound emergencies in the ED. You need to be familiar with many different pieces of orthopedic equipment. In addition to using the equipment, the ED nurse is also responsible for teaching the patient how to use the orthopedic equipment. Assess and document circulation, motion, and sensation before and after splinting.

In this chapter, you will learn to:
1. Discuss the common musculoskeletal injuries presenting to the ED
2. Identify the signs and symptoms of musculoskeletal and wound care emergencies
3. Review the interventions to address musculoskeletal and wound care emergencies

MUSCULOSKELETAL AND WOUND CARE EMERGENCIES

Musculoskeletal and wound care emergencies are presentations seen in all EDs. These patient presentations range from fractures, dislocations, and crush injuries to lacerations and burns. Prompt assessment, stabilization, and wound management are essential to prevent complications such as neurovascular compromise, infection, and impaired healing.

Systematic inspection assesses obvious signs of musculoskeletal injury such as extremity deformity or bone protruding from skin. Other signs indicating potential for injury include ecchymosis, edema, and visible muscle spasm, all of which can be indications of an underlying musculoskeletal injury and need to be evaluated further. Alterations in extremity color can be an indication of underlying musculoskeletal pathology. A pale-appearing

TABLE 14.1

Findings With Palpation of the Musculoskeletal System

Assess For	Finding	Can Indicate
Deformity	Misshapen, misaligned bone or joint	Fractured bone, joint dislocation Arthritis, previous injury
Pain	Palpation over site of suspected injury	Fractured bone, damaged tissue, joint damage
Crepitus	A crunching or grating sound or sensation	Fractured bone, joint damage
Sensation	Inability to differentiate between sharp and dull or loss of proprioception	Neuronal compression or injury
Pulses and capillary refill	Decreased pulses or capillary filling time <2 seconds	Vascular compromise Compartment syndrome
Movement	Decreased range of motion from baseline*	Fractured bone, bone/joint dislocation, neurovascular injury
Muscle spasm	Presence of spasm Absence of spasm over injury	May represent underlying fracture May indicate neuronal injury

*Bones and joints with obvious injury should not be assessed for range of motion because of the potential for further neurovascular injury.

extremity can indicate inadequate arterial blood flow, where a dusky/blueish appearance can indicate venous congestion. Each extremity must be fully palpated to assess for deformity, pain, crepitus, sensation, pulses, movement, and muscle spasm. Findings must be documented because each evaluation can indicate underlying disease (see Table 14.1).

Strains

A strain is a pull or tear to a tendon or muscle.
- *Causes:* Injury resulting in a pull or tear to a tendon.
- *Signs and symptoms:* Pain, swelling, ecchymosis, edema, point tenderness, spasm, and decreased range of motion.
- *Interventions:* Mnemonic **PRICE** (**P**rotect [splint, cast, sling], **R**est, **I**ce, **C**ompression [ACE wrap], **E**levate); x-ray; instruct patient on use of crutches for light to no weight-bearing status per provider/consultant orders; and arrange orthopedic follow-up.

Sprains

A sprain is a pull or tear to a ligament, commonly in the knees, ankles, and shoulders.

- *Causes:* Injury resulting in a pull or tear to a ligament.
- *Signs and symptoms:* Pain, swelling, ecchymosis, edema, point tenderness, spasm, and decreased range of motion.
- *Interventions:* Mnemonic PRICE; x-ray; instruct patient on light to no weight bearing (crutches) per provider/consultant orders; and arrange orthopedic follow-up.

Fractures

A fracture is a broken bone or disruption in normal continuity of bone, cartilage, or both.

- *Types* (see list and Figure 14.1):
    - *Closed:* Skin intact.
    - *Open:* Broken bone with break in the skin surrounding the fracture. Patient is at high risk for developing an infection in the bone (osteomyelitis).
    - *Avulsion:* Insertion site bone fragment breaks away because of forceful muscle contraction.
    - *Comminuted:* Two or more bone fragments.
    - *Depressed:* Flat bone injury due to blunt trauma.
    - *Greenstick:* Incomplete compression force-type fracture (common in school-age children).
    - *Spiral:* Twisting injury.
    - *Oblique:* Linear oblique fracture.
    - *Transverse:* Horizontal linear fracture.
    - *Segmented:* Broken in two or more places.
    - *Salter–Harris:* Fracture involving the growth plate.
    - *Boxer fracture:* Occurs to the fourth or fifth metacarpals after punching-type injury.
- *Causes:* Injury or disease process resulting in a break in the bone. Consider corresponding injuries to surrounding tissue, nerves, blood vessels, or internal organs.
- *Signs and symptoms:* Pain; tenderness; swelling; redness; ecchymosis; deformity; shortening/rotation in hip fracture; decreased range of motion; inability to bear weight; muscle spasm; crepitus; weak or absent pulses; pallor; and shock.
- *Interventions:* Administer pain medication promptly as ordered and document effectiveness; immobilize; assist in applying traction for femur fracture; remove any rings or jewelry to the fractured extremity; cover open fractures with sterile saline-soaked dressing; mnemonic PRICE; x-ray; instruct patient on light to no weight bearing (crutches); prepare for possible closed reduction; give nothing by mouth; give instructions for possible surgical repair; teach cast care instructions and crutch training; check peripheral pulses; anticipate orders to start IV access; possibly give IV fluids and tetanus immunization if open fracture; and arrange orthopedic follow-up.

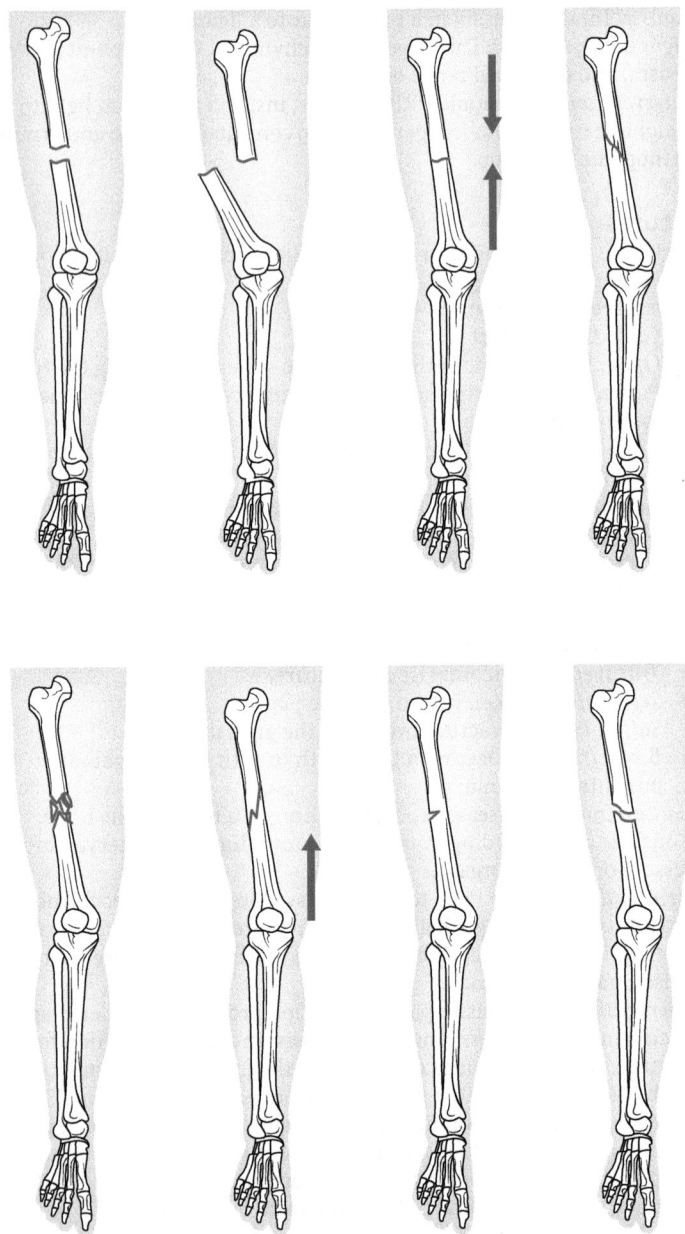

Figure 14.1 Types of fractures.

Source: OpenStax College. (2013). *Types of fractures*.

FAST FACTS

If a patient with a long bone fracture suddenly develops an altered mental status, visual disturbances, respiratory distress, tachycardia, petechial chest rash, or thrombocytopenia, consider fat embolism syndrome.

Dislocations and Subluxations
Dislocations and subluxations occur when a joint is pulled out of place.
- *Causes:* Injury or movement resulting in joint dislocation.
- *Signs and symptoms:* Severe joint pain; joint deformity/asymmetry; decreased or absent range of motion; weak or absent pulse; edema; and shortening of extremity.
- *Interventions:* Anticipate orders to obtain x-ray films, prepare for conscious/moderate sedation for closed reduction, apply ice pack, start IV access, prepare a neurovascular assessment, immobilize joint postreduction, and obtain postreduction x-ray.

FAST FACTS

Dislocation is a complete displacement of bone from the normal position, and subluxation is a partial dislocation.

Amputation
Amputation is a partial or complete separation of a limb.
- *Causes:* Injury/trauma resulting in separation of a limb.
- *Signs and symptoms:* Completely or partially detached extremity.
- *Interventions:* Treat airway, breathing, and circulation (ABC) first. Administer oxygen and initiate two large-bore IV accesses. Wrap the amputated part in sterile saline-soaked gauze and place in a sterile plastic bag or container. Place the bag or container on crushed ice and water. Never put the amputated part directly on ice. Control bleeding (direct pressure, wound packing, and tourniquet); apply sterile saline-soaked dressing to amputation site; anticipate orders to administer pain medications, antibiotics, and tetanus immunization and evaluate effectiveness of medications; and prepare for surgery.

Acute Compartment Syndrome
This occurs when a compartment of the limb becomes full of fluid or blood, thereby hindering circulation to that extremity (Colancecco, 2018). This is a limb- and life-threatening emergency.
- *Causes:* Usually occurs with trauma.
- *Signs and symptoms:* The six **P**s: **P**ain, **P**ressure, **P**aresthesia, **P**ulselessness, **P**aralysis, and **P**allor.

- *Interventions:* Administer anti-inflammatory drugs as ordered, elevate the affected limb to the level of the heart, and reassess neurovascular status. Prepare for intramuscular pressure measurements (normal is 0–8 mmHg) and possible emergency fasciotomy. Ice is contraindicated because it will compromise circulation. Discharge teaching should include instructions to return for any increasing pain, pallor, or decreased circulation below the cast or splint.

FAST FACTS

Assess and document circulation, motion, and sensation before and after splinting.

Lacerations Versus Cuts

Lacerations are breaks or tears in the skin due to blunt trauma. Cuts occur from sharp objects.
- *Causes:* Everything from pieces of glass, knives, and razors to umbrellas, coffee tables, and baseball bats. You name it; almost anything can cause a laceration or cut.
- *Signs and symptoms:* Bleeding, cuts, and open wounds. An arterial laceration will intermittently squirt blood with each pulse. If a vein is cut, it will constantly ooze. Superficial lacerations are easily repaired in the ED. Deep wounds through the muscle fascia or tendons may require a plastic surgeon.
- *Interventions:* Apply pressure to control bleeding; update tetanus shot if more than 5 years since the last one; cleanse wound; prepare patient for wound closure with Dermabond, Steri-Strips, or sutures per provider order; bandage accordingly.

Burns

Most burn injuries are from thermal injury, with less than 10% of burns resulting from electrical or chemical sources. Flame and scald burns are considered thermal burns and are the leading cause of burns in adults. Burn injuries differ from other traumas because of the overwhelming inflammatory response that occurs moments after injury. The first 48 hours of burn care are the most critical, having the greatest influence on morbidity and mortality.
- *Causes:* Chemicals, sun, heat, radiation, fire, electrical, or even cold substances such as dry ice.
- *Signs and symptoms:*
  - *First degree:* Superficial pink color or redness; pain; blanches; area feels warm.
  - *Second degree:* Partial thickness, redness; blistering; break in the first layer of skin down to the second layer of skin; pain.
  - *Third degree:* White, waxy areas or charred, black areas to skin; painless; full thickness: all layers of skin affected; requires skin grafts.

Chapter 14 Musculoskeletal and Wound Care Emergencies 155

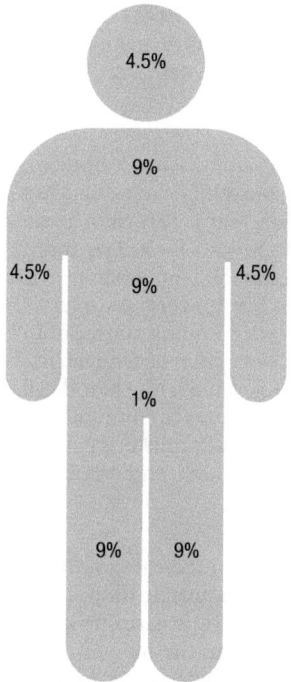

Figure 14.2 "Rule of nines" for adult burn victims.

- *Fourth degree:* Painless, full-thickness burn extending down into muscle layers and bone requiring amputation.
- *Interventions:* Stop burning process. Check ABC first. The patient may have smoke/burn inhalation or carbon monoxide poisoning; consider proactive intubation. For minor burns, give pain medication as ordered; cleanse burns; and apply antibiotic ointment or silver sulfadiazine (Silvadene) cream and nonadherent dressings as ordered. Screen the patient for possible abuse. If it is a major burn, do not apply creams or ointments; instead, cover with dry sterile drape or clean sheet, start IV access, give analgesics, and prepare for admission to a burn center. Use the "rule of nines" (see Figure 14.2) as a fast way to determine a patient's percentage of burned surfaces using multiple of nines, rule of palm, or modified Lund and Browder chart to determine total burn surface area (TBSA).

Burn care and management is nursing intensive. Nurses may be required to perform dressing changes on the burn patient or frequently wet dressings that are in place. Burn dressing changes are performed with aseptic technique. Detailed instructions are provided by the trauma, burn, plastic surgery, and other consulting teams regarding timing and specifics of dressing changes. Burn care requires interdisciplinary collaboration. It is recommended that any burn over 20% TBSA, circumferential burns, burns involving the face or genitals, full-thickness burn, or electrical injury be transferred to a certified burn center (Vrouwe & Shahrokhi, 2023).

Osteomyelitis

Osteomyelitis is an infection of the bone, bone marrow, and soft tissue that surrounds the bone. Osteomyelitis can be acute or chronic. Acute osteomyelitis refers to an infection that is less than 1 month in duration. Chronic refers to an infection that persists for longer than 4 weeks (Sommers, 2023).

- *Causes:* Direct contamination from open fractures, penetrating wounds, or surgical procedures. The longer the surgery, the greater the risk. *Staphylococcus aureus* is a common source of infection.
- *Signs and symptoms:* Fever, pain, or tenderness over infected area; edema; redness; drainage; and elevated white blood cell (WBC) count.
- *Interventions:* Anticipate orders to immobilize the extremity, obtain blood and wound cultures, administer IV antibiotics, perform bone scan, assist with surgical debridement, and monitor for development of sepsis.

Rhabdomyolysis

Rhabdomyolysis is a complex medical condition that results from significant cellular damage or lysis to muscle tissues (breakdown of muscle tissue). Excessive amounts of myoglobin, creatinine kinase, electrolytes, and lactate dehydrogenase are released into the bloodstream and extracellular tissues. Because myoglobin is a large molecule, it gets trapped in the renal tubules resulting in renal failure.

- *Causes:* Most commonly musculoskeletal crush injury trauma. However, infection, toxins, electrolyte imbalances, prolonged immobilization, extreme exercise, third-degree burns, snake venom or spider bites, metabolic disorders, muscle ischemia, and hyperthermia can also lead to rhabdomyolysis.
- *Signs and symptoms:* Classic triad.
  1. Tea or cola-colored (red or brownish) urine (due to myoglobinuria)
  2. Muscular pain (soft tissue damage and bruising)
  3. Muscular weakness or paralysis
- *Interventions:* Anticipate orders for aggressive IV fluid resuscitation, large-bore IV access, urinalysis, creatinine kinase levels, hemoglobin levels, and metabolic panel; monitor and document urine output, use cardiac monitoring, provide pharmacologic and nonpharmacologic pain relief, and prepare for admission and, in severe cases, dialysis.

SUMMARY

You should have a better understanding of musculoskeletal and wound care emergencies, symptoms, and treatments. Be sure to familiarize yourself with the musculoskeletal and wound care supplies at your local facility. Thoroughly document your assessments, being sure to include what the distal pulses, capillary refills, deformities, and symmetry are; whether bleeding is controlled; and when and how the injury occurred. Use personal protective equipment, especially with arterial bleeds. Teach patients the importance of an orthopedic follow-up; the ED visit goal is to stabilize, and small fractures may not be visible until swelling subsides.

REVIEW QUESTIONS

1) A 55-year-old patient presents to the ED with a closed tibial fracture after a fall from a ladder. The patient had a splint placed on arrival to the ED. The affected leg is swollen, deformed, and extremely painful. The nurse notes diminished pedal pulses and increasing pain despite pain medication. What should the nurse do first?
   a. Apply a warm compress to promote circulation and reduce swelling.
   b. Elevate the affected limb above heart level to decrease swelling and pain.
   c. Encourage early ambulation to prevent complications such as deep vein thrombosis.
   d. Loosen any restrictive dressings or splints and notify the provider immediately.
2) A college student presents to the ED after being found on the ground after prolonged physical exertion on a hot day. The patient reports severe muscle pain, weakness, and dark-colored urine. Bloodwork reveals elevated creatine kinase (CK) levels. What is the nurse's next intervention?
   a. Ensure appropriate IV access for expected IV fluid orders.
   b. Encourage ambulation to improve circulation and reduce muscle stiffness.
   c. Restrict fluids to prevent fluid overload and worsening renal function.
   d. Administer diuretics to promote urine output and eliminate myoglobin.

REFERENCES

Colancecco, E. (2018). Management of patients with musculoskeletal trauma. In J. L. Hinkle & K. H. Cheever (Eds.), *Brunner & Suddarth's textbook of medical-surgical nursing* (14th ed., pp. 1194–1221). Wolters Kluwer Health/Lippincott Williams & Wilkins.

Sommers, M. S. (2023). *Davis's diseases & disorders: A nursing therapeutic manual* (pp. 873–877). F. A. Davis Company.

Vrouwe, S. Q., & Shahrokhi, S. (2023). Critical care of the burn patient. In G. A. Schmidt, J. P. Kress, & I. S. Douglas (Eds.), *Hall, Schmidt and Wood's principles of critical care* (5th ed.). McGraw Hill. https://accessmedicine-mhmedical-com.umassmed.idm.oclc.org/content.aspx?bookid=3350&sectionid=279567889

Infectious Disease Emergencies

Sarah Berry

> Infectious diseases are common in the ED, but that does not make them any less troubling. Oftentimes, the infected person is unaware they are infected and contagious, increasing the risk of unknowingly transmitting disease. Proper hand hygiene and application of appropriate isolation precautions are just the beginning when it comes to protecting ourselves and protecting others.

In this chapter, you will learn to:
1. Discuss the common infectious diseases presenting to the ED
2. Identify the signs and symptoms of infectious emergencies
3. Review the interventions to treat infectious emergencies

INFECTIOUS DISEASES EMERGENCIES

Infectious diseases make up about 13.5% of all ED visits among adults older than the age of 65 (Liang & Chin, 2018). Usually, it is the triage nurse who is first exposed to an unknown case of tuberculosis (TB), meningitis, or new viral pandemic. Most patients do not know what is wrong with them when they come to the ED. Most facilities have a travel screening that asks questions about whether the patient has symptoms of common pathogens or whether the patient has been to a high-risk area recently. If the triage or travel screening is positive, nurses must follow the facility's protocol; this usually requires transmission-based precautions. Use the time during the triage period to assess the patient for rashes, respiratory or gastrointestinal (GI) symptoms, or inability to turn their head due to nuchal rigidity. Upon completing screening, initiate precautions, whether it is placing the patient in a negative pressure room, masking, or isolating them from the rest of the department. Always practice standard or universal precautions when caring for any patient, and practice hand hygiene. This chapter investigates different infectious pathogens and how to care for those afflicted.

> **FAST FACTS**
>
> Always practice standard/universal precautions.

INFECTIOUS DISEASES

Infectious Colitis

Colitis is an encompassing term that includes several different bacterial, viral, and parasitic pathogens that cause acute diarrhea. This diarrhea is a result of inflammatory responses in the GI tract and can lead to different symptoms, frequently bringing patients to the ED.

- *Causes:* Bacterial colitis pathogens include *Campylobacter jejuni (C. jejuni), Salmonella, Shigella, Escherichia coli (E. coli), Yersinia enterocolitica, Clostridioides* (formerly *Clostridium*) *difficile (C difficile),* and *Mycobacterium tuberculosis.* Common causes of viral colitis include *Norovirus, Rotavirus, Adenovirus,* and *Cytomegalovirus.* Parasitic infestation, such as *Entamoeba histolytica,* a protozoan parasite, is capable of invading the colonic mucosa and causing colitis (Azer & Tuma, 2022). There are several other pathogens, but these are the most common. Men who participate in sex with men where the rectum is penetrated are at risk for sexually transmitted diseases that could cause diarrhea. Those include *Neisseria gonorrhoeae, Chlamydia trachomatis,* herpes simplex virus (HSV), and *Treponema pallidum,* and these also occur in patients who are positive for HIV (Azer & Tuma, 2022).
- *Signs and symptoms:* Inquire about past medical history; those with a history of advanced age, sickle cell anemia, hemolytic anemia, immunosuppression from steroids, chemotherapy, and HIV/AIDS are at higher risk for contracting *Salmonella* (Azer & Tuma, 2022). Patients who recently underwent antibiotic treatment should be screened for possible *C. difficile.* Symptoms include fever, weakness, excessive diarrhea, vomiting, nausea, and abdominal pain (Azer & Tuma, 2022).
- *Interventions: Apply contact enteric precautions for the patient and implement strict handwashing with soap and water. Have the patient undergo cardiac monitoring to check for potential arrhythmias related to electrolyte changes from profuse diarrhea or vomiting.* Initiate IV access and obtain lab work per orders. Anticipate orders for IV fluids and potential antibiotics. Not all patients with diarrhea will require antibiotic therapy; therefore, it is important to identify the causative infection. A stool sample is necessary to determine which pathogen is making the patient sick (Azer & Tuma, 2022). Once the pathogen has been identified, appropriate treatment can begin. For select populations, such as those with HIV/AIDS, cancer, a history of transplant or prosthetic implants, and valvular heart disease and those of significant age, antibiotic therapy should be given for their infecting organism (Azer & Tuma, 2022). In severe cases of *C difficile*, patients may receive

vancomycin by mouth (PO) along with IV metronidazole for treatment (Azer & Tuma, 2022). In most cases, these pathogens are self-limiting and will improve with time and supportive therapy. Encourage increased hydration, a bland diet, and rest. Hygiene and cleanliness are keys to stopping the spread of infection. Educate the patient and their family on proper hand hygiene and cleansing of high-touch surfaces such as door handles, sinks, and toilet handles. If the patient is able, consider recommending that the patient be confined to the use of a specific bathroom in their household, while the rest of the family uses another bathroom. This could decrease the chances of contamination. After the symptoms have subsided, deeply clean the bathroom with an effective cleanser to decrease reinfection. While in the hospital, if the patient is unable to have a private bathroom or is unable to make it to the bathroom because of the urgency or frequency of defecation, consider a bedside commode for the patient. If the patient is experiencing weakness, having a bedside commode nearby could help with safety risk as well because they are not walking any distance to reach the bathroom. If the patient is undergoing antibiotic treatment that continues in the outpatient setting, it is imperative that the patient understand the importance of finishing the antibiotics. If they do not complete the course, the chance of relapse or worsening condition is significant and should not be overlooked (Azer & Tuma, 2022).

Meningitis

Meningitis, inflammation of the meninges and subarachnoid space, can be caused by viral, bacterial, or fungal pathogens. Infectious meningitis can be caused by several pathogens and has a high morbidity and mortality rate (Poplin et al., 2020).

- *Causes:* The most common bacteria to cause meningitis are *Streptococcus pneumoniae* and *Neisseria meningitidis* with high morbidity and mortality rates (van de Beek et al., 2016). Pathogens, including enterovirus, herpes simplex viruses, and influenza viruses, can lead to viral meningitis. Enterovirus has been found to be the leading cause of most viral cases of meningitis worldwide (Kohil et al., 2021). The most common fungal pathogen is *Cryptococcus neoformans* (Pagliano et al., 2020). Fungal meningitis (FM) is growing in frequency as patients become immunocompromised. These patients are often undergoing chemotherapy or taking other immunosuppressing drugs, or they are living with HIV/AIDS (Pagliano et al., 2020). The use of conjugate vaccinations has greatly decreased certain strains of bacterial and viral infections that could lead to meningitis (McGill et al., 2016). This has improved immensely, especially in the more vulnerable pediatric population, through the administration of *Haemophilus influenzae* type b (Hib) vaccines (McGill et al., 2016).
- *Signs and symptoms:* Bacterial meningitis can be difficult to diagnose clinically because the classic triad of neck stiffness, fever, and an altered

level of consciousness is present in <50% of patients (McGill et al., 2016). Although the triad occurs in <50%, often at least two symptoms are present in up to 95% of patients that include headache, fever, neck stiffness, and an altered level of consciousness.

- *Kernig and Brudzinski signs* are sometimes used to support the diagnosis with up to 95% specificity, depending on the clinician, but their reliability is often questioned (McGill et al., 2016).
  - *Kernig sign:* The patient experiences pain when, in a supine position, the knee is flexed to a 90-degree angle, then the hip is flexed to a 90-degree angle, and the knee is then extended upward toward the examiner. If the patient experiences pain or significant resistance in the hamstring, this is considered positive for meningitis (Mehndiratta et al., 2012).
  - *Brudzinski sign:* The patient is placed in the supine position and the examiner passively flexes the patient's neck such that their chin approaches their chest. When the examiner flexes the patient's chin toward their chest, their legs reflexively draw upward at the knees toward their chest as well (Mehndiratta et al., 2012).
- Symptoms of viral meningitis may include fever, chills, abdominal pain, nausea, and headache. Patients may also experience tachypnea, anorexia, nuchal rigidity and pain, sensitivity to light, double vision, and difficulty concentrating (Kohil et al., 2021). FM is often difficult to diagnose because of its reported nonspecific symptoms and absence of meningeal irritation or inflammation on imaging (Pagliano et al., 2020).
- *Interventions:* Place the patient on droplet precautions as soon as possible to decrease the risk of further transmission (Gottenborg & Barron, 2016). The patient is to remain in droplet precautions until meningitis is ruled out, whether it is the definitive diagnosis or not. Additional orders for treatment may include frequent neurological assessments to observe for seizures or show any changes or deterioration in the patient's mental status. Establish an IV and obtain lab work per provider's orders. In cases of suspected bacterial meningitis, antibiotics should be administered as soon as possible after specimens have been collected. For diagnosis of suspected viral meningitis, the gold-standard tool is a polymerase chain reaction (PCR) that tests for DNA or RNA in the patient's cerebrospinal fluid (CSF; Kohil et al., 2021).
  - The nurse may be asked to assist the provider in a lumbar puncture (LP) to obtain CSF. The results of this test can help determine if the patient is experiencing bacterial or viral meningitis. Assist the patient in getting into position for the procedure, which can either be lateral recumbent or sitting. In either position, the patient should be instructed to bring their chin to their chest and draw their knees upward, arching their back "like a cat" (Jane & Wray, 2023). LPs are an aseptic procedure, so healthcare professionals assisting in the procedure or observers should be masked and wearing a

bonnet to cover their hair. When collecting the CSF, four vials are collected. The order of collection is important and should be followed numerically, based on the numbers printed on the vials (Jane & Wray, 2023). The most common complication of LPs is a post-LP headache. Ensuring that the stylet has been replaced in the needle prior to removal can decrease the incidence of spinal headache (Jane & Wray, 2023). Historically, patients have been advised to increase hydration and maintain a supine position after completing an LP. A recent systematic review showcasing results of 2,996 participants concluded that limiting a patient's activity and advising increased hydration did not show obvious decrease in post-LP headaches (Arevalo-Rodriguez et al., 2016). It later suggested that adequate hydration and encouraging the patient to participate in activity that matches their individual comfort level may be a more appropriate approach to postprocedure treatment (Arevalo-Rodriguez et al., 2016).
- Viral meningitis is generally self-limiting and does not require hospitalization. Treatment consists of symptom alleviation, including antipyretics, antiemetics, and analgesics. Some providers may prescribe antivirals to shorten the course of the virus, but there is not significant evidence to support their use (Kohil et al., 2021). If patients are unable to care for themselves or they require monitoring because of concern for seizurelike activity, they may be admitted to the hospital for observation (Kohil et al., 2021). See Table 15.1 for more information.

Influenza

Influenza A, B, and C are seasonal viruses that typically infect between the months of October through May, with the peak season taking place between December and February (Bigham, 2024). In the 2023 to 2024 flu season, it was estimated that between 35 and 65 million people were affected by the flu, 390,000 to 830,000 people were hospitalized because of influenza, and about 25,000 to 72,000 people died in relation to the flu (Bigham, 2024). Patients in certain subgroups are at increased risk of complications from the flu. These populations include patients who have neuromuscular diseases; cerebral palsy; history of stroke, seizure disorders, or dementia; asthma or other pulmonary diseases; chronic kidney or liver disease; heart disease; conditions or medications that can lead to immunocompromise; diabetes mellitus; obesity; or sickle cell anemia. Addition special groups include adults 65 years and older, children younger than 5 years, patients who live in nursing homes or chronic care facilities, and pregnant and postpartum women (Gaitonde et al., 2019). Although influenza is not generally a complicated respiratory illness, the possible complications with the flu can be detrimental. Complications can affect any system in the body and are extensive, including strokes, ischemic heart disease, myocarditis, hemolytic uremic syndrome, thrombotic thrombocytopenia, myositis, rhabdomyolysis, acute disseminated encephalomyelitis, encephalitis, Guillain–Barré syndrome, encephalopathy, Reye syndrome, transverse myelitis, conjunctivitis, optic neuritis, retinopathy, uveal effusion syndrome, acute respiratory

TABLE 15.1
Lumbar Puncture Findings

	Appearance	Opening Pressure (cm)	White Blood Cells (cells per µL)	Predominant Cell Type	Protein (g/L)	Glucose (mmol)
Normal	Clear	10–20	<5	None	<0.4	2.6–4.5
Bacterial	Turbid, cloudy, purulent	Increased	Increased (>100)	Neutrophils	Increased (>1.0)	Decreased
Viral	Clear	10–20 or mildly increased	Increased (<1,000)	Lymphocytes	Mildly increased (0.5–1)	2.6–4.5 or slightly decreased

Source: McGill, F., Heyderman, R. S., Panagiotou, S., Tunkel, A. R., & Solomon, T. (2016). Acute bacterial meningitis in adults. *The Lancet, 388*(10063), 3036–3047. https://doi.org/10.1016/s0140-6736(16)30654-7.

distress syndrome (ARDS), diffuse alveolar hemorrhage, hypoxic respiratory failure, viral pneumonia, secondary bacterial pneumonia, acute kidney injury, and multisystem organ failure (Gaitonde et al., 2019).
- *Causes:* Influenza is a highly contagious respiratory illness that is transmitted through droplets in the air. Patients who sneeze, cough, or have insufficient hand hygiene while sick risk transmission to others around them.
- *Signs and symptoms:* The patient may experience a sudden onset of fever, sore throat, chills, sweats, cough, myalgias, and fatigue (Gaitonde et al., 2019). GI symptoms are also common and include nausea, vomiting, and diarrhea (Ghebrehewet et al., 2016).
- *Interventions:* Ensure that the patient in the waiting room uses a mask and initiate droplet isolation precautions per hospital protocol. In mild cases, anticipate orders to obtain a flu swab and discharge home with antiviral prescriptions if appropriate for the patient. The antiviral medication is most effective if administration is started within 24 hours of symptom onset (Gaitonde et al., 2019). Anticipate education for patients for at-home supportive care. This includes antipyretics for fever, analgesias for aches and pains, adequate fluid intake, rest, and time taken off from work or school until they are fever free for more than 24 hours (Ghebrehewet et al., 2016). In more severe cases, treatment is based on patient symptoms and presentation. Anticipate orders to obtain imaging such as a chest x-ray to rule out pneumonia or bronchitis. Establish an IV for medications for nausea or vomiting and hydration. Provide the patient with the appropriate oxygen adjunct to meet their requirement and to maintain an oxygen saturation that is appropriate for that patient. Encourage rest and good hand hygiene. Anticipate the possibility of the patient being admitted to the hospital for complicated influenza if the patient is unable to care for themselves at home, cannot maintain adequate hydration and has lab values that indicate dehydration, or has a new oxygen requirement.

HUMAN IMMUNODEFICIENCY VIRUS/ACQUIRED IMMUNODEFICIENCY SYNDROME

HIV is a virus that attacks the immune system, primarily targeting the CD4+ T-lymphocyte helper cells (Swinkels et al., 2024). This leads to complete immune suppression and to increased chances of opportunistic infections. If the patient has not received treatment for their HIV or the diagnosis is discovered late, it eventually evolves into AIDS. At that stage of the infection, the immune system is not able to fight off any type of infection, and the patient usually ultimately succumbs to an opportunistic infection and dies (Swinkels et al., 2024).
- *Causes:* Contamination with HIV-infected blood or bodily fluids. This contamination is usually through transmission of sex, drug paraphernalia sharing, and blood transfusions (Swinkels et al., 2024). When triaging patients, the ED staff should ask about social interactions, including

participation in unprotected sex and use of needle sharing during drug injection (Swinkels et al., 2024).
- *Signs and symptoms:* Most patients with HIV experience symptoms within the first 4 weeks after the primary infection has started to replicate. These symptoms are usually self-limiting and nonspecific. They can include fever, fatigue, myalgias, rash, headache, sore throat, swollen lymph nodes, joint pain, night sweats, and diarrhea (Swinkels et al., 2024). If patients are not investigated and treatment is not started during this period or shortly thereafter, the patient's viral load will increase exponentially, and their prognosis becomes bleaker (Swinkels et al., 2024).
    - AIDS is later diagnosed regardless of CD4+ count if the patient has AIDS-specific conditions such as candidiasis of the digestive tract or pulmonary system, invasive cervical cancer, extrapulmonary or disseminated coccidioidomycosis, histoplasmosis, or cryptococcosis, including cryptococcal meningitis, intestinal cryptosporidiosis, cytomegalovirus retinitis, Kaposi sarcoma, HIV encephalitis, TB, primary lymphoma of the brain, non-Hodgkin lymphoma, Burkitt lymphoma, mycobacterial infections, *Pneumocystis jirovecii* pneumonia, progressive multifocal leukoencephalopathy, *Salmonella* septicemia, and HIV-associated wasting syndrome (Swinkels et al., 2024).
    - These illnesses are generally found concurrently with a low CD4+ count and are indicative of advanced AIDS (Swinkels et al., 2024).
- *Interventions:* Patients should start treatment immediately after diagnosis is confirmed (Swinkels et al., 2024). Treatment may be delayed but generally only when the patient has a current opportunistic infection that requires treatment first (Swinkels et al., 2024). Treatment consists of multimodal medications that require strict adherence. Management is generally built around the patient's ability to obtain medications and adhere to the regimen. The goal with antiretroviral therapy is to maintain viral suppression through serial testing (Swinkels et al., 2024). Education is key. Understanding their medication regimen and the importance of adherence is one of the most important aspects of HIV education for patients. Following care for the patient, education on preventing transmission is also of significant importance. Practicing safe sex, not sharing needles during illicit drug administration, and adhering to the medication regimen to decrease viral load are frontline defenses against transmission. Disclosing their HIV status in the appropriate situations should be encouraged to the patient. These situations may include recent, current, or future sexual partners; illicit drug participation; medical treatment where possible contamination to a healthcare worker is possible; or an increase of their viral load.

FAST FACTS

Standard/universal precautions are sufficient when caring for patients with HIV.

Hepatitis

Hepatitis is an inflammation or infection of the liver.

- *Causes:* There are an abundance of possible causes of hepatitis. There are hepatotropic and nonhepatotropic viruses, including hepatitis A, B, C, D, and E; Epstein–Barr; cytomegalovirus; herpes; coxsackievirus; adenovirus; Dengue virus; and COVID-19. In addition, there are bacterial, fungal, and parasitic possibilities. Toxin- or substance-related causes include significant alcohol ingestion, acetaminophen overdose, and other toxins. Patients who are experiencing other medical conditions can have hepatitis as a side effect or comorbidity (Schaefer & John, 2023).
    - *Hepatitis A:* Contracted via the fecal/oral route.
    - *Hepatitis B:* Contracted via blood or body fluids.
    - *Hepatitis C:* Contracted via blood or body fluid, commonly in IV drug abusers.
    - *Hepatitis D:* Contracted via blood or body fluids and requires coinfection of hepatitis B.
    - *Hepatitis E:* Contracted via the fecal/oral route with a higher mortality rate than hepatitis A.
- *Signs and symptoms:* Patients may or may not have specific symptoms and may also be asymptomatic, with elevated liver function tests being the only indicator. When present, symptoms can consist of fever, malaise, fatigue, altered mental status, decreased appetite, vomiting, diarrhea, and abdominal pain (Schaefer & John, 2023). Patients may also have yellowing of their sclera (icterus), skin (jaundice), dark-colored urine, or light-colored stool (Schaefer & John, 2023). It is important during triage to ask patients about these possible symptoms, and, if the patient has known hepatitis, ask if their level of jaundice has recently worsened.
- *Interventions:* Anticipate orders to obtain lab work consistent with a complete blood count (CBC), complete metabolic panel (CMP) focusing on liver enzymes and bilirubin levels, ammonia level, lactate, hepatitis panel, albumin levels, and coagulation studies (Schaefer & John, 2023). The patient may undergo imaging to rule out other abdominal etiology (Schaefer & John, 2023). If the patient is presenting because of an acute acetaminophen overdose, timely treatment is crucial to salvage liver functionality and deter liver failure. Treatment with N-acetylcysteine can be given either orally or IV, depending on the patient's willingness and ability to participate in treatment. Loading doses are administered, with additional doses being administered that are based on the patient's weight (Schaefer & John, 2023). Other than acetaminophen ingestion, treatment is specific to the etiological factor. Supportive treatment includes treatment of symptoms related to hepatitis, whether it be IV fluids, antiemetics, and avoidance of alcohol or drug abuse (Schaefer & John, 2023).

Coronavirus-19

The COVID-19 pandemic changed the face of medicine and nursing care for many. With the "shutdown" of the world in 2020, social distancing, mandatory wearing of face masks, overrun EDs, high hospital admission rates, and outstanding mortality rates worldwide, healthcare providers and "frontline workers" sustained a life-changing experience. Although there are several, less problematic strains of coronavirus, COVID-19 is caused by the novel severe acute respiratory syndrome coronavirus 2 (SARS-CoV-2; Wiersinga et al., 2020). COVID-19 initially begins with flulike symptoms and can rapidly evolve. After the initiation of flulike symptoms, an inflammatory response begins. The epithelial barrier of the pulmonary capillaries becomes compromised, leading to thickening alveolar walls in the lungs and pulmonary edema (Wiersinga et al., 2020). The pulmonary edema and changes to alveolar walls compromise oxygen exchange and transmission, leading to impaired oxygen saturation and the early stages of ARDS (Wiersinga et al., 2020). Late-stage COVID-19 activates coagulation but also consumes clotting factors. This leads to diffuse intravascular coagulation (DIC), deep venous thrombosis (DVT), pulmonary embolisms, ischemic limbs, strokes, and myocardial infarctions. Respiratory failure, sepsis, and multisystem organ failure are the ultimate detriments of these patients (Wiersinga et al., 2020).

- *Causes:* Coronavirus is a large, single-stranded RNA virus that is transmitted through droplets from the respiratory tract, which is what encouraged the social distancing and mask-wearing. Prolonged exposure (within 6 feet for >15 minutes) without taking precautions showed increased risk of contracting COVID-19 (Wiersinga et al., 2020).
- *Signs and symptoms:* Fever, dry cough, shortness of breath, fatigue, myalgias, nausea and vomiting or diarrhea, headache, weakness, and rhinorrhea. Lab values include increased lymphopenia, increased inflammatory markers (particularly ferritin), and abnormal coagulation results (Wiersinga et al., 2020). Imaging frequently showed bilateral, lower-lobe infiltrates or ground-glass opacities (Wiersinga et al., 2020).
- *Interventions:* When assessing patients, be sure to screen for recent travel or common symptoms they may have experienced in the last 14 days. Initiate cardiac monitoring, pulse oximetry, and blood pressure (BP) monitoring. The frequency of BP measurements should be determined by the stability of the patient. Establish IV access and initiate droplet precautions as soon as possible. Assess the patient and anticipate treatment that is based on supporting their symptoms. Assessing the patient's need for supplemental oxygen is vital for this disease process. According to the *Journal of the American Medical Association (JAMA)*, more than 75% of patients hospitalized required supplemental oxygen. Start with a nasal cannula and escalate treatment as needed on the basis of the patient's response to oxygen therapy. Anticipate the possibility of the patient's needing to undergo intubation and follow the appropriate preintubation preparation steps. After the patient's airway and respiratory status has been stabilized, additional treatments may require proning (laying the patient on their abdomen), which allows for increased

expansion of the pleural space with ventilation (Wiersinga et al., 2020). Additional treatments for medications are determined by patient presentation, lab findings, and symptom support. Antivirals for COVID-19, antibody therapy, and anti-inflammatory agents such as steroids, anticoagulants, and antipyretics are likely to be prescribed (Wiersinga et al., 2020). Hand hygiene and rest are always encouraged. Anticipate the need for an ICU admission if the patient is unstable and needs significant oxygen therapy or vasopressors because of COVID-induced sepsis.

Tick-Borne Illnesses

These are infectious diseases caused by ticks. "Ticks are the most common arthropod vectors of disease in the United States and the second most common vector worldwide" (Choi et al., 2016). People who own dogs are five times more likely to contract Rocky Mountain spotted fever (RMSF; Choi et al., 2016).

Lyme disease: A *Borrelia burgdorferi* bacterial infection (see Figure 15.1). Lyme disease is the most common vector-borne infectious disease in the United States (Choi et al., 2016). It consists of three stages of infection, and if the tick is attached for longer than 48 to 72 hours, the risk of transmission increases significantly (Choi et al., 2016).

- *Causes:* Usually spread by black-legged ticks, also known as deer ticks
- *Signs and symptoms:* See Table 15.2.

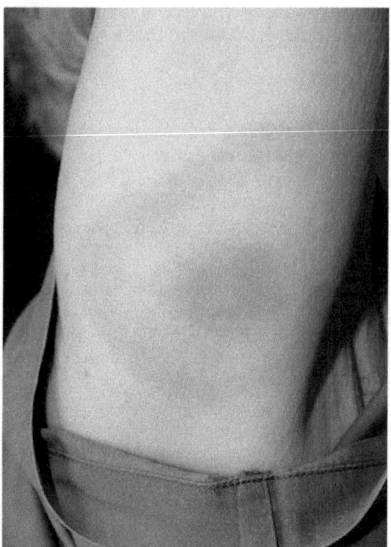

Figure 15.1 Bull's-eye rash of Lyme disease, known as erythema migrans.
Source: Centers for Disease Control and Prevention.

TABLE 15.2

Lyme Disease Symptom Progression

Stage I	Recognition of symptom onset is generally between 7 and 10 days. ■ Fever ■ Malaise ■ Local lymphadenopathy ■ Myalgias ■ Erythema migrans in 75% of patients

Stage II	After days to weeks, the skin rash can disseminate into the bloodstream and/or lymphatic system.
	■ "Bull's-eye" rash evolves into a more widespread rash, sparing the palms and soles of the feet
	■ Up to 60% of patients may experience musculoskeletal symptoms.
	   ■ Monoarticular arthritis
	   ■ Joint swelling of the knees
	■ Up to 40% of patients may experience neurological symptoms.
	   ■ Meningitis
	   ■ Encephalitis
	   ■ Meningoencephalitis
	   ■ Lethargy
	   ■ Forgetfulness
	   ■ Disorientation
	   ■ Somnolence
	   ■ Dizziness
	   ■ Photophobia
	   ■ Lack of coordination
	   ■ Bell palsy (may persist for several months and resolve spontaneously)
	■ 10% of patients may have GI symptoms.
	   ■ Hepatitis
	   ■ Hepatomegaly
	   ■ Generalized abdominal pain
	■ 10% of patients may have cardiac symptoms.
	   ■ They are rarely life-threatening.
	   ■ Conduction delay in the AV node (first-degree heart block and PR interval exceeding 300 ms)
	   ■ Complete heart block—requires temporary pacing and potentially a permanent pacemaker

Stage III	Lyme disease about a year or more after the initial presentation
	■ 50% of patients experience rheumatological symptoms.
	   ■ Degenerative arthritis or joint effusions that are evident on imaging
	■ Neurological symptoms are progressive and persistent.
	   ■ Encephalomyelitis
	      ■ Ataxia
	      ■ Cognitive impairment
	      ■ Spastic paresis
	      ■ Impairment of cranial nerves VII and VIII
	   ■ MRI exhibits changes in white matter consistent with encephalopathy.

AV, atrioventricular; GI, gastrointestinal.
Source: Choi, E., Pyzocha, N. J., & Maurer, D. M. (2016). Tick-borne illnesses. *Current Sports Medicine Reports, 15*(2), 98–104. https://doi.org/10.1249/jsr.0000000000000238.

- *Interventions:* Remove all ticks after a thorough skin assessment. According to the length of symptom presentation, the patient may require additional tests such as bloodwork or imaging. Inflammatory markers such as erythrocyte sedimentation rate (ESR), C-reactive protein (CRP), antinuclear antibodies (ANAs), and rheumatoid factors will typically be negative (Choi et al., 2016). A tick-borne disease panel (enzyme immunoassay) should be drawn to confirm the diagnosis of Lyme disease and rule out additional possibilities of other tick-borne illnesses. The return time for this bloodwork is typically 1 to 4 days, and antibiotics should be started immediately. Without antibiotics, patients are at increased risk for evolving to stages II and III (Choi et al., 2016). If the initial bloodwork comes back positive or equivocal, confirmation should be completed through an immunoblot test immunofluorescence assay (IFA/Western blot; Choi et al., 2016). Antibiotic administration of doxycycline may be offered prophylactically (Choi et al., 2016). Education regarding doxycycline should be given to the patient. In children aged 8 years and younger, the medication may cause permanent yellowing or graying of teeth (Puckey, 2024). If the patient is pregnant or breastfeeding, inform the provider immediately. This may deter them from prescribing this antibiotic because it passes from mother to the baby. It may cause yellowing or graying of the baby's teeth even prior to birth or during breastfeeding because doxycycline passes through breast milk (Puckey, 2024). When taking this medication, the patient may take it with food or milk to help decrease the risk of upset stomach. It is also crucial that the patient wear protective clothing while outside or in sunlight. Patients are at increased risk of sunburn while taking this medication. The most important part of antibiotic therapy is to take the medication until the prescription is complete to avoid further infection (Puckey, 2024).

Rocky Mountain spotted fever: A bacterial infection transmitted by ticks (see Figure 15.2)

- *Causes:* Bite from the wood tick *Dermacentor andersoni* contaminated with *Rickettsia rickettsii* bacteria in the western United States and the dog tick *Dermacentor variabilis* in the eastern and southern regions of the United States (Choi et al., 2016). The most common cases occur between April and September in all states with the exception of Maine, Hawaii, and Alaska. Inoculation can take place as quickly as 6 hours after attachment, and the mortality rate can be as high as 30% without antibiotics (Choi et al., 2016).
- *Signs and symptoms:* Patients frequently recall recent exposure to ticks, and symptoms usually begin around 5 to 7 days after interaction. Patients may experience sudden onset of headache, fever, chills, or rash. Unlike Lyme disease, the rash is present on the soles of the feet. It is also present on the palms, wrists, ankles, and forearms, where it then spreads proximally. The lesions can cause skin necrosis in areas like the fingertips, toes, nose, and genitalia. If left untreated, late stages of disease can lead to hypovolemia and shock, as well as DIC, renal failure, metabolic acidosis, cardiac and respiratory complications, and neurological changes (Choi et al., 2016).

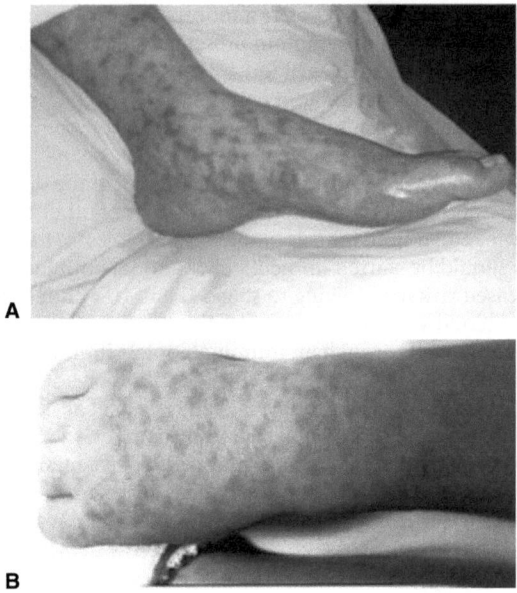

Figure 15.2 Rocky Mountain spotted fever rash of the (A) foot and (B) hand.
Source: Centers for Disease Control and Prevention. www.cdc.gov/rmsf

- *Interventions:* Anticipate orders for a thorough skin assessment and removal of all possible ticks or insects. The provider will likely order antibiotics to be initiated as soon as possible if RMSF is part of the differential diagnosis. Doxycycline is the most common antibiotic and shows the most efficacy in preventing death if started within 5 days of symptom presentation (Choi et al., 2016).

Tuberculosis

In most major cases of TB, the point of entry is the lung. On initial infection, the patient may exhibit little to no signs of illness. It can take approximately 4 to 6 weeks before symptoms begin to develop (Lyon & Rossman, 2017). In most cases, the patient's immune system is able to contain the infection locally, keeping it primarily in the lung. If the disease is not contained by the immune system and undergoes dissemination into the extrapulmonary space through the lymphatic system, the patient then begins to manifest the major clinical manifestations and radiographic findings of TB (Lyon & Rossman, 2017). The first encounter with the infection is frequently clinically inconsequential and goes unrecognized because of its nonspecific symptoms. There, it will lie dormant indefinitely or until a future breakdown in the patient's immune system occurs, leading to secondary occurrence and further manifestation (Lyon & Rossman, 2017).

- *Causes: Mycobacterium tuberculosis* is spread through droplets from the respiratory tract; therefore, patients should be moved to airborne isolation as soon as possible. In its dormant stage, TB is not contagious, and the patient is asymptomatic. Populations who are susceptible to TB are generally those with a compromised immune system due to decreased resistance to the microorganism (Lyon & Rossman, 2017). These populations include but are not limited to adolescents; older adults; pregnant women; patients who have comorbidities such as malnutrition, diabetes mellitus, renal failure, lymphoma, or HIV/AIDS; those undergoing adrenocortical steroid therapy or immunosuppressive therapy; and those with a history of transplant (Lyon & Rossman, 2017).
- *Signs and symptoms:* Symptoms vary and are broken down into two categories. Primary TB infections are generally minimally symptomatic or asymptomatic. Symptoms accompanying primary and reactive TB are similar and include cough, fever, weight loss, and hemoptysis. A pivotal symptom is the classic "night sweats" (Lyon & Rossman, 2017). Fevers that develop late in the afternoon and break during sleep lead to night sweats. Additional symptoms include malaise, unusual fatigue, irritability, weakness, headache, and weight loss. As the disease progresses, tissue in the lung develops caseation necrosis. This is a type of cell death that causes the tissue to crumble, leading to liquefaction of the crumbling area (Lyon & Rossman, 2017). Once this takes place, hemoptysis may become obvious if the patient coughs because of breakdown in the vasculature of the lung tissue.
- *Interventions:* Screen patients for TB in triage and provide a mask to patients suspected of infection. Then place the patient in a room on respiratory isolation. Anticipate orders to obtain IV access, prepare for a chest x-ray or CT scan, and obtain labs, including a sputum culture if the patient is able to produce one. Administer antibiotics (e.g., isoniazid and rifampicin; Tiberi et al., 2018) and prepare for possible admission. Instruct family members and caregivers to get TB testing. Educate the patient on the importance of complying with the medication regimen despite the duration of treatment. "Treatment can last at least 6 months, requiring the patient to take on average ten pills a day during the intensive phase" (Tiberi et al., 2018). Initially, for the first 2 months of treatment, isoniazid, rifampicin, pyrazinamide, and ethambutol are taken daily. After the initial 2 months, an additional 4 months of treatment are completed with isoniazid and rifampicin (Tiberi et al., 2018).

FAST FACTS

Rifampin can turn the patient's urine orange, much like phenazopyridine (Pyridium).

PARASITIC AND INSECT INFESTATIONS

Scabies (*Sarcoptes scabiei* Var. *Hominis*)

Scabies are little contagious mites that affect 100 to 130 million people yearly. They are considered a parasitic infection because they burrow under the skin and can cause both physical and psychosocial complications (Jannic et al., 2018). They are common in tropical regions with low resources. Additionally, in wealthier parts of the world, prevalence is equal between the sexes, all age groups, and all socioeconomic groups (Jannic et al., 2018). Children younger than the age of 2 years and disadvantaged populations are most at risk (Jannic et al., 2018).

- *Causes:* Transmission of a single pregnant mite is sufficient to infest a human host. For common scabies, intense skin-to-skin contact for at least 5 to 10 minutes is required. They can survive outside the body for 24 to 48 hours at room temperature without a host (Sunderkötter et al., 2021).
- *Signs and symptoms:* After approximately 10 to 14 days after contact, patients may experience "intense itching . . . vesicles, or papulonodular erythematous lesions, located on the finger webs, wrists, axillae, breasts, buttocks, and genitalia" (Jannic et al., 2018).
- *Interventions:* Initiate contact precautions and encourage frequent hand hygiene while in the hospital. Treatment consists of both topical and PO medications that have to be repeated 1 to 2 weeks after the initial treatment to wipe out any cyclical survivors of the first round of treatment. Ivermectin is the PO agent of choice. Topical treatments consist of permethrin and benzyl benzoate, which are the standard regimens (Jannic et al., 2018). Discharge instructions should include applying scabicide cream to the entire body from the neck down, including all web spaces and folds, to clean skin (after a shower or bath) daily for the prescribed length of time. For reinfection to be avoided, instructing all partners or persons who had skin-to-skin contact in the past month to be examined and treated at the same time is important. All bed linens and clothing should be laundered in hot water or a hot dryer. Nonwashable items may be sealed in plastic bags for at least 72 hours at 70°F in a dry location (Sunderkötter et al., 2021). Clean all high-touch surfaces; vacuum furniture and its cushions, mattresses, carpets, and floors; and use disposable gloves while doing these tasks (Sunderkötter et al., 2021).

Bedbugs

Cimex lectularius are tiny 1- to 7-mm flat bugs that feed on human and animal blood while they sleep. Although it is not common to treat bedbug bites in the ED, sometimes bedbugs hitch a ride on our patients and their belongings when they come to the ED. If not identified, this can quickly become an infectious disease problem for the entire hospital.

- *Causes:* Bedbugs can be picked up easily when traveling from hotels, buses, trains, luggage, cruise ships, and dorm rooms. They can hide in

the seams of fabric mattresses, box springs, headboards, dressers, seats, wallpaper, and clothes in suitcases.
- *Signs and symptoms:* Painless, itchy bug bites to the face, neck, arms, legs, or other body parts while sleeping. Bedbugs or their exoskeletons may be found in the folds and seams of the mattress and sheets.
- *Interventions:* Initiate contact precautions and contact your hospital infection preventionist. Topical creams may be prescribed to the patient to help with itching and healing. Antibiotics may be ordered if secondary infection occurs. If the patient is to be admitted, special environmental interventions may be implemented, such as sealing all the patient's belongings into plastic bags while having the patient shower. The patient's belongings may be taken home or placed in their car. Decontamination of the room with insecticides may be implemented after the patient leaves the room.

FOOD AND DRINKS AT WORKSTATIONS

It is important to stay hydrated as an ED nurse. However, the ED environment is not the safest place for your food or drinks—not if you are trying to avoid getting sick, that is. Potential contamination may occur if food and drinks are left at workstations; therefore, **do not eat or drink in these areas**. A simple solution may be a designated hydration station. These designated areas have been determined to represent less risk for contaminated food and drinks.

ENVIRONMENT OF CARE

Even if the bed was wiped down and new sheets were applied, many germs may linger on the call button, side rails, cabinet handles, thermometer, monitors, bedside table, otoscope handles, or light switches. It is important to make a habit of wiping down high-touch surfaces when cleaning a room. Any equipment that goes from patient to patient or room to room also needs to be disinfected between patients and rooms. This includes things like BP machines and cuffs, blood glucometers, and wheelchairs. Wipe the equipment thoroughly with the appropriate disinfectant; let it dry completely. Make an effort to wipe work areas as well as the patient rooms, especially the high-touch surfaces.

SUMMARY

Most EDs do not allow new graduate nurses to be involved with triage until proper training and experience are achieved. This is partly because the triage nurses are the front line when it comes to exposure to infectious diseases. Therefore, it is crucial to thoroughly screen all patients who come through triage for infectious diseases. If an infectious disease is suspected, proper isolation must be implemented. Make sure to become familiar with each facility's isolation protocols and equipment and know how to use it. The ED is the doorway to the hospital for patients many times. The importance of infection control is significant. The key is **good handwashing**, universal precautions, triage travel screening, proper isolation, and notification of appropriate personnel.

REVIEW QUESTIONS

1) In addition to contact precautions for *C difficile* what act is crucial to prevent the spread?
    a. Using hand sanitizer dispensers when entering and exiting patient rooms
    b. Wearing a mask to prevent inhalation of contaminated droplets
    c. Washing hands with soap and water prior to exiting the patient's room
    d. Limiting the number of staff members who care for this patient population
2) What is the recommended length of time for nonwashable objects to be sealed in plastic to decrease transmission of scabies?
    a. 72 hours or longer
    b. 24 hours
    c. 12 hours
    d. 30 minutes

REFERENCES

Arevalo-Rodriguez, I., Ciapponi, A., Roqué-Figuls, M., Muñoz, L., & Bonfill Cosp, X. (2016). Posture and fluids for preventing post-dural puncture headache. *Cochrane Database of Systematic Reviews, 2021*(4), CD009199. https://doi.org/10.1002/14651858.cd009199.pub3

Azer, S., & Tuma, F. (2022, September 26). *Infectious colitis.* In StatPearls [Internet]. StatPearls Publishing. Retrieved August 26, 2025, from https://www.ncbi.nlm.nih.gov/books/NBK544325/

Bigham, J. (2024, September 9). Preparing your family medicine practice for the 2024–2025 flu season. *Family Practice Management, 31*(5), 29–34. https://www.aafp.org/pubs/fpm/issues/2024/0900/preparing-for-flu-season.html

Choi, E., Pyzocha, N. J., & Maurer, D. M. (2016). Tick-borne illnesses. *Current Sports Medicine Reports, 15*(2), 98–104. https://doi.org/10.1249/jsr.0000000000000238

Gaitonde, D. Y., Moore, F. C., & Morgan, M. K. (2019, December 15). Influenza: Diagnosis and treatment. *American Family Physician, 100*(12), 751–758. https://www.aafp.org/pubs/afp/issues/2019/1215/p751.html

Ghebrehewet, S., MacPherson, P., & Ho, A. (2016). Influenza. *BMJ, 355*, i6258. https://doi.org/10.1136/bmj.i6258

Gottenborg, E. W., & Barron, M. A. (2016). Isolation precautions in the inpatient setting. *Hospital Medicine Clinics, 5*(1), 30–42. https://doi.org/10.1016/j.ehmc.2015.08.004

Jane, L. A., & Wray, A. A. (2023, July 24). *Lumbar puncture*. StatPearls [Internet]. StatPearls Publishing. Retrieved August 26, 2025, from https://www.ncbi.nlm.nih.gov/books/NBK557553/

Jannic, A., Bernigaud, C., Brenaut, E., & Chosidow, O. (2018). Scabies itch. *Dermatologic Clinics, 36*(3), 301–308. https://doi.org/10.1016/j.det.2018.02.009

Kohil, A., Jemmieh, S., Smatti, M. K., & Yassine, H. M. (2021). Viral meningitis: An overview. *Archives of Virology, 166*(2), 335–345. https://doi.org/10.1007/s00705-020-04891-1

Liang, S. Y., & Chin, R. L. (2018). Here to stay: Infectious diseases in emergency medicine. *Emergency Medicine Clinics of North America, 36*(4), 17–18. https://doi.org/10.1016/j.emc.2018.08.001

Lyon, S. M., & Rossman, M. D. (2017). Pulmonary tuberculosis. *Microbiology spectrum, 5*(1), 10.1128/microbiolspec.tnmi7-0032-2016. https://doi.org/10.1128/microbiolspec.TNMI7-0032-2016

McGill, F., Heyderman, R. S., Panagiotou, S., Tunkel, A. R., & Solomon, T. (2016). Acute bacterial meningitis in adults. *The Lancet, 388*(10063), 3036–3047. https://doi.org/10.1016/s0140-6736(16)30654-7

Mehndiratta, M., Nayak, R., Garg, H., Kumar, M., & Pandey, S. (2012). Appraisal of Kernig's and Brudzinski's sign in meningitis. *Annals of Indian Academy of Neurology, 15*(4), 287–288. https://doi.org/10.4103/0972-2327.104337

Pagliano, P., Esposito, S., Ascione, T., & Spera, A. M. (2020). Burden of fungal meningitis. *Future Microbiology, 15*(7), 469–472. https://doi.org/10.2217/fmb-2020-0006

Poplin, V., Boulware, D. R., & Bahr, N. C. (2020). Methods for rapid diagnosis of meningitis etiology in adults. *Biomarkers in Medicine, 14*(6), 459–479. https://doi.org/10.2217/bmm-2019-0333

Puckey, M. (2024, April 23). *Doxycycline: Uses, dosage, side effects, warnings*. Drugs.com. https://www.drugs.com/doxycycline.html

Schaefer, T. J., & John, S. (2023, July 10). *Acute hepatitis* (Archived). In StatPearls [Internet]. StatPearls Publishing. Retrieved August 26, 2025, from https://www.ncbi.nlm.nih.gov/books/NBK551570/

Sunderkötter, C., Wohlrab, J., & Hamm, H. (2021). Scabies: Epidemiology, diagnosis, and treatment. *Deutsches Ärzteblatt International, 118*(41), 695–704. https://doi.org/10.3238/arztebl.m2021.0296

Swinkels, H. M., Justiz Vaillant, A. A., Nguyen, A. D., & Gulick, P. G. (2024, July 27). *HIV and AIDS*. In StatPearls [Internet]. StatPearls Publishing. Retrieved August 26, 2025, from https://www.ncbi.nlm.nih.gov/books/NBK534860/

Tiberi, S., du Plessis, N., Walzl, G., Vjecha, M. J., Rao, M., Ntoumi, F., Mfinanga, S., Kapata, N., Mwaba, P., McHugh, T. D., Ippolito, G., Migliori, G. B., Maeurer, M. J., & Zumla, A. (2018). Tuberculosis: Progress and advances in development of new drugs, treatment regimens, and host-directed therapies. *The Lancet Infectious Diseases, 18*(7), E183–E198. https://doi.org/10.1016/s1473-3099(18)30110-5

van de Beek, D., Brouwer, M., Hasbun, R., Koedel, U., Whitney, C. G., & Wijdicks, E. (2016). Community-acquired bacterial meningitis. *Nature Reviews Disease Primers, 2*(1), 1–20. https://doi.org/10.1038/nrdp.2016.74

Wiersinga, W., Rhodes, A., Cheng, A., Peacock, S., & Prescott, H. (2020). Pathophysiology, transmission, diagnosis, and treatment of coronavirus disease 2019 (COVID-19). *JAMA, 324*(8), 782–793. https://doi.org/10.1001/jama.2020.12839

Shock Emergencies

Sarah Berry

Patients in shock are on a slippery slope. Without proper, prompt, and definitive recognition, these patients have an exponentially higher risk of morbidity and mortality in relation to other patients. There are various types of shock, and each one is unique in its treatment.

In this chapter, you will learn to:
1. Identify the three stages in any form of shock
2. Identify the signs and symptoms of various forms of shock
3. Review the interventions to treat forms of shock

SHOCK

Shock is a term used to describe "circulatory failure that causes an imbalance between cellular oxygen supply and demand resulting in organ dysfunction" (Patel et al., 2022). Shock is one of the most common causes of admission to the ICU around the world (Khorsand et al., 2023). It is broken down into four categories, generally with a common denominator of hypotension and hypoperfusion: cardiogenic, distributive, obstructive, and hypovolemic (Khorsand et al., 2023).

There are three stages to any form of shock.
- *Compensated:* This is the earliest stage of shock, where the body is still able to compensate for the changes in pathophysiology. These mechanisms decrease tissue perfusion by increasing heart rate, peripheral vascular resistance, and changes in blood pressure (Koya & Paul, 2023).
- *Decompensated or progressive:* This stage is indicated by the more classic signs of shock, resulting from progressive deterioration of compensatory mechanisms (Koya & Paul, 2023).
- *Irreversible or refractory:* The final stage of shock is marked by irreversible organ dysfunction, multiorgan failure, and ultimately death (Koya & Paul, 2023).

Each category of shock can be further broken down into subcategories depending on its precipitating factor.
- *Hypovolemic*—loss of volume
  - Hemorrhagic
  - Nonhemorrhagic (dehydration)
  - Cardiogenic—pump problem
  - Obstructive
  - Cardiac tamponade
  - Tension pneumothorax
  - Massive pulmonary embolism (PE)
  - Ductal-dependent congenital heart lesion (obstructs flow from left side to aorta)
  - Distributive
  - Anaphylactic
  - Septic
  - Neurogenic

Hypovolemic Shock

This is a decrease in circulating volume. Hypovolemic shock is the most common form of shock in a trauma patient. If the patient has obvious signs of external hemorrhage, stop the bleeding. Hypovolemic shock, regardless of the cause, is characterized by a loss of preload. The decrease in preload results in decreased tissue perfusion, an increased response from the inflammatory cascade, a release of lactic acid, and change to coagulation (Khorsand et al., 2023).

- *Causes:* Hemorrhagic shock includes perioperative bleeding; gastrointestinal bleeding (ulcers, varices); obstetric bleeding (uterine atony or rupture, placental abruption, and ectopic pregnancy rupture); or traumatic bleeding from lacerations, burns, or amputations (Khorsand et al., 2023). Shock resulting from volume depletion is another form of hypovolemic shock. Viruses can lead to excessive vomiting and diarrhea, and decreased by mouth (PO) intake or a prolonged nothing by mouth (NPO) status can lead to hypovolemia (Khorsand et al., 2023). Diseases such as diabetes insipidus, an inappropriate secretion of antidiuretic hormone, or diabetes mellitus type 1 with polyuria increase the chances of hypovolemia because of a disproportionate increase in urine output (Khorsand et al., 2023).
- *Signs and symptoms:* Hypotension; tachycardia; tachypnea; cool, clammy skin with a pale pallor, an obvious sign of bleeding; and altered level of consciousness. Lab tests may reflect an elevated lactic level. Depending on the cause of the hypovolemia, the patient's acid–base findings may differ.
- *Interventions:* Treatment is based on the cause. If the patient has an obvious sign of bleeding, the airway, breathing, and circulation (ABC) acronym swiftly rearranges to circulation, airway, and breathing (CAB). In cases of hemorrhage, stop the bleeding. Once

the bleeding is controlled, assess the patient's airway and breathing. Establish IV access, attach the patient to the monitor, and prepare for possible mass transfusion. Be familiar with the hospital's equipment that is used for massive transfusion. Blood pressure and heart rate monitoring can indicate improvement or worsening of the patient's state while resuscitation is ongoing. While blood is infusing or fluids for nontraumatic hypovolemia, the physician may order vasopressors. Norepinephrine is suggested as the first-line vasopressor because of its mimicking of sympathomimetic properties (Khorsand et al., 2023). Anticipate admission to the ICU or operating room (OR), depending on the cause of the hypovolemia.

FAST FACTS

When performing massive transfusion, be aware of the hospital's protocol for the need to infuse calcium. Depending on the blood product component (whole blood, packed red blood cells, fresh frozen plasma, or platelets) and the quantities of each being infused, the patient is at increased risk for calcium depletion in their blood. This depletion could lead to cardiac abnormalities and alterations to the clotting cascade.

Cardiogenic Shock

In cardiogenic shock, the heart fails to pump blood effectively. Despite advances in diagnosis and treatment, mortality for cardiogenic shock is still 40% to 67% (Khorsand et al., 2023). End-organ dysfunction and damage result from systemic decompensation from cardiogenic shock and can damage cardiac muscle in the process (Khorsand et al., 2023).

- *Causes:* Approximately 81% of cardiogenic shock victims have acute coronary syndrome with resulting left ventricular dysfunction. This is then followed by acute decompensated heart failure (Khorsand et al., 2023). Other nonischemic causes include dilated cardiomyopathy, myocarditis, pregnancy-related heart disease, and stress-induced cardiomyopathy (takotsubo cardiomyopathy). Ischemic cardiogenic shock is the result of acute myocardial infarction (Khorsand et al., 2023).
- *Signs and symptoms:* "Cold and wet" is the hallmark presentation, indicating cold extremities due to compensatory peripheral vasoconstriction, along with wet lung sounds indicative of pulmonary congestion (Khorsand et al., 2023). Both symptoms show an inability to effectively pump blood throughout the cardiovascular system, allowing for vascular backup into the lungs (Khorsand et al., 2023). The patient may also have pulmonary rales, an S_3 heart sound, jugular vein distention, ascites, and peripheral edema (Sarma & Jentzer, 2024).
- *Interventions:* Assess the patient's ABC. Attach the cardiac monitor, establish IV access, and obtain a 12-lead EKG. If the patient is

experiencing an ST-elevation myocardial infarction (STEMI), prepare them to go to the catheterization lab for revascularization of the vessel (Sarma & Jentzer, 2024). Depending on the patient's vital signs and their overall stability, applying defibrillator pads in the event of sudden loss of pulses would not be inappropriate. Lab tests likely to be included are cardiac muscle cells (CMCs), comprehensive metabolic panel (CMP), serial troponins, brain natriuretic peptide (BNP), lactate, and imaging to include a chest x-ray. If the patient has moderate to significant respiratory compromise, prepare to assist the provider in application of bilevel positive airway pressure (BiPAP) or continuous positive airway pressure (CPAP), advancing to intubation if necessary. Fluids may be ordered, 3 to 4 mL/kg, but should be judiciously administered and the response closely monitored in patients with pulmonary congestion (Sarma & Jentzer, 2024). Remember, patients with pulmonary congestion and congestive heart failure are at greater risk for flash pulmonary edema during fluid resuscitation, posing a dangerous airway compromise. The physician may order norepinephrine or dobutamine, both of which require close monitoring and titration to the prescribed parameters. They may also order IV furosemide to decrease pulmonary congestion and facilitate movement of fluid into the kidney (Sarma & Jentzer, 2024).

Obstructive Shock: Cardiac Tamponade

This is fluid or blood buildup in the pericardial sac surrounding the heart. This form of shock is the least common, accounting for approximately 2% of all shock states (Khorsand et al., 2023). There is normally a small amount of fluid in the pericardial sac that allows for sliding and decreased friction between the outer structures of the heart and the sac. When tamponade occurs, a filling of the pericardial sac takes place that is disproportionate to its capacity. It could be related to infection, autoimmune diseases, cancer, or trauma (Stashko & Meer, 2023).

- *Causes:* Autoimmune diseases, cancers, penetrating chest trauma, infection such as tuberculosis or myocarditis (Stashko & Meer, 2023).
- *Signs and symptoms:* Chest pain; shortness of breath; palpitations; dizziness; syncope; Beck triad: hypotension, jugular vein distention, and muffled heart sounds; pulsus paradoxus; and in some severe cases, pulseless electrical activity in cardiac arrest (Stashko & Meer, 2023).
- *Interventions:* Attach continuous cardiac monitoring, apply oxygen therapy, obtain an EKG and IV access. Elevate the legs of the bed to encourage venous return. Be aware that positive pressure ventilation (CPAP or BiPAP) could be dangerous in these patients because of increased pressure on the heart, further decreasing venous return and cardiac output (Stashko & Meer, 2023). In patients who are unstable, prepare for a bedside pericardiocentesis. If they are pulseless, a thoracotomy is a possible treatment option to allow for rapid evacuation of the pericardial sac. Generally, blunt trauma cardiac arrest that results

in cardiac tamponade is considered nonsurvivable, and resuscitation efforts may be attempted but are not usually warranted (Stashko & Meer, 2023).

FAST FACTS

Lupus, an autoimmune disease, is a possible cause of cardiac tamponade. Because the tamponade is generally slow to accumulate, the compression on the heart is frequently better tolerated than rapidly progressing tamponades.

Obstructive Shock: Tension Pneumothorax

Tension pneumothorax is a life-threatening complication of pneumothorax. This occurs when trapped air increasingly accumulates in the pleural space, leading to collapse and compression, evidenced by a "tracheal shift" or "tracheal deviation" (Khorsand et al., 2023).
- *Causes:* Trauma, acute respiratory distress syndrome (ARDS), and existing pneumothorax (Khorsand et al., 2023).
- *Signs and symptoms:* Tracheal shift or deviation toward the unaffected lung, jugular vein distention, cyanosis, decreased breath sounds, subcutaneous emphysema, hypoxia, tachycardia, hypotension, tachypnea, and anxiety (Khorsand et al., 2023).
- *Interventions:* Treat ABCs; apply oxygen via nonrebreather (NRB) mask; place in high Fowler position; anticipate orders to prepare for needle thoracentesis and/or chest tube insertion (Khorsand et al., 2023); administer pain medications; arrange for chest x-ray.

Obstructive Shock: Pulmonary Embolus

A pulmonary embolus is a complete or partial thrombus blockage of the pulmonary artery that results in decreased oxygen saturation, cardiac output, and stroke volume (Khorsand et al., 2023).
- *Causes:* PEs are caused by venous thromboses. Risk factors for venous thromboses include but are not limited to atrial fibrillation, hip or leg fractures or joint replacements, major surgery or trauma, spinal cord injuries, central venous lines, congestive heart or respiratory failure, hormone replacement therapy or oral contraceptive use, cancer, immobility, recent pregnancy, obesity, and increased age (Duffett et al., 2020).
- *Signs and symptoms:* Dyspnea, pleuritic chest pain, cough, hemoptysis, presyncope, syncope, new-onset atrial fibrillation, calf swelling and tenderness, erythema, pedal edema, rales, decreased breath sounds, jugular vein distention, third heart sounds, cyanosis, hemodynamic collapse, and cardiac arrest (Vyas et al., 2024).
- *Interventions:* Attach continuous cardiac monitoring and pulse oximetry. Assess the patient's ABCs. Anticipate oxygen administration, with the route being determined by the patient's presentation and stability.

Prepare for possible BiPAP or CPAP attachment, or even intubation. Obtain IV access and verify with hospital policy or the imaging department the gauge necessary to obtain a CT pulmonary angiography (PA) study. CTPA studies may require a larger gauge IV (20 gauge or larger) to allow for accurate flow and timing of imaging contrast for an optimal study. Gather prescribed lab work. Depending on the results of the imaging studies, the patient may be started on anticoagulants such as a continuous heparin infusion. Patients with concern for submassive or massive PE may show right heart strain. These patients are at risk for sudden and significant decompensation and may require more drastic intervention such as thrombolytic medication such as tenecteplase, surgical embolectomy, or extracorporeal membrane oxygenation (ECMO; Vyas et al., 2024).

Distributive Anaphylactic Shock

Anaphylaxis is a result of mast cell activation. Left untreated, anaphylaxis can lead to anaphylactic shock. This is a rare occurrence but can be quickly fatal if not identified and treated in a timely manner.

- *Causes:* The patient may be allergic to certain foods such as nuts, seafood, or other allergens; bee stings or other insect venom; and some medications such as antibiotics, and these allergies may lead to anaphylaxis.
- *Signs and symptoms:* Rash, excessive sputum production, bronchospasm, status asthmaticus, edema, hypotension, poor capillary refill and other signs of significant venous dilation, tachycardia, third spacing of fluid resulting in hemodynamic collapse (Khorsand et al., 2023).
- *Interventions:* Administer oxygen and anticipate orders for intramuscular epinephrine. Administration should be in the middle third of the lateral thigh for the most effective results. Delay in administration could drastically increase the patient's mortality rate (Khorsand et al., 2023). Anticipate the need for a second dose in patients with persistent symptoms. Establish IV access and closely monitor the patient's response to treatment. Frequent ABC assessments should be completed to determine the need for additional interventions such as advanced airway management or a potential continuous infusion of epinephrine. High-volume fluid resuscitation or vasopressors may be required to offset shock. Additional medications such as steroids and antihistamines may be prescribed (Khorsand et al., 2023).

FAST FACTS

Be sure to verify the concentration of epinephrine prior to administration. For anaphylaxis, a 1:1,000 concentration is used for intramuscular or subcutaneous administration. Epinephrine is commonly used during cardiac arrest but at a different concentration. Mixing up these concentrations could be deadly.

DISTRIBUTIVE SEPTIC SHOCK

Septic shock is the result of a septic infection, hypotension despite fluid resuscitation that requires vasopressor support, and lactate level >2 mmol/L that is persistent after fluids (Font et al., 2020). Sepsis can lead to systemic inflammatory response syndrome (SIRS). SIRS is a somewhat predictive state and a useful bodily response to many infections. Determining whether the response is a life-threatening, dysregulated response versus a normal inflammatory response can complicate diagnosis and prognostication (Font et al., 2020).

- *Causes:* Typically caused by gram-negative or gram-positive bacteria. The infection usually stems from one source and then spreads to the rest of the body through the bloodstream. A massive SIRS is launched by the body, which results in vasodilation and hypotension.
- *Signs and symptoms:* Because this is a systemic response, almost every system can be affected. Table 16.1 identifies symptoms that may be exhibited based on the system.
- *Interventions:* Attach the patient to continuous cardiac monitoring, pulse oximetry, and blood pressure. Frequent blood pressure monitoring is vital to continuously assess the patient's status and response to treatment. Sepsis guidelines have set a standard of initiating antibiotics within 60 minutes of presentation. Establish IV access and obtain lab work as soon as possible. Anticipate orders for a "septic workup," primarily including blood cultures, in addition to standard lab work and imaging. Assess the patient's need for oxygen supplementation. Medications are likely to include initial fluid volume resuscitation of 30 mL/kg of body weight (Font et al., 2020). If the patient continues to be hypotensive despite fluid volume resuscitation, vasopressors are likely to be added to the treatment plan. Norepinephrine is the recommended first-line agent. Antibiotic choice is generally targeted toward coverage of gram-positive and gram-negative bacteria until test results can narrow down the pathogen (Font et al., 2020). After blood cultures have resulted, antibiotics may change depending on the discovery. Anticipate orders for ICU admission if the patient requires vasopressors or advanced airway management.

FAST FACTS

When obtaining blood cultures, obtain one set of cultures from two different sites. In patients where the provider has concern for endocarditis, a third set of blood cultures may be required per provider's orders.

Distributive Neurogenic Shock

Neurogenic shock results in disruption of sympathetic control over vascular tone. The decrease in tone leads to systemic hypoperfusion. This condition

TABLE 16.1

Distributive Septic Shock Symptoms Based on System

System	Symptoms
Cardiac	■ Arterial dilatation and vasodilation leading to hypotension, which can be profound ■ Patients may have mildly elevated troponins, and their increase can be linked to the severity of the septic infection. ■ Septic cardiomyopathy ■ Tachycardia
Respiratory	■ Increased permeability of alveolar and capillary endothelium, leading to noncardiogenic pulmonary edema, in turn leading to decreased oxygenation and ventilation ■ Tachypnea, preceded by hypoxia and metabolic acidosis
Renal	■ Acute kidney injury ■ Acute tubular necrosis ■ Hyperkalemia ■ Metabolic acidosis
Hematologic	■ Anemia ■ Leukocytosis ■ Neutropenia ■ Thrombocytopenia ■ DIC
Gastrointestinal	■ Liver failure, diagnosed by a bilirubin concentration >2 mg/dL and INR of 1.5 ■ Hepatic encephalopathy
Endocrine	■ Hyperglycemia ■ Adrenal insufficiency ■ Hypothyroidism
Neurological	■ Altered mental status ■ Hallucinations ■ Agitation

DIC, disseminated intravascular coagulation; INR, international normalized ratio.
Source: Font, M. D., Thyagarajan, B., & Khanna, A. K. (2020). Sepsis and septic shock—basics of diagnosis, pathophysiology and clinical decision making. *Medical Clinics of North America*, *104*(4), 573–585. https://doi.org/10.1016/j.mcna.2020.02.011.

is usually a result of a spinal cord injury due to a fracture or dislocation of vertebrae. Typically occurring within minutes of the trauma, the fracture or dislocation damages the lateral gray matter and anterior root of the spinal cord (Dave et al., 2023).

- *Causes:* Spinal cord injuries that occur in the cervical and upper thoracic spinal cord, especially above the level of T6; Guillain–Barré syndrome; toxins affecting the autonomic nervous system such as heavy metal toxicity and certain bacterial toxins such as botulism; transverse myelitis; and other neuropathies (Dave et al., 2023).

- *Signs and symptoms:* Hypotension; bradycardia; "warm, pink, and dry" skin—an important distinction when compared with hypovolemic shock, where patients are pale, cool, and diaphoretic (Dave et al., 2023).
- *Interventions:* Assess ABCs and maintain spinal precautions. Apply an appropriately sized C-collar to the patient and maintain C-spine and logroll precautions when moving this patient. Assist the provider in assessing palpable step-offs or deformities in the spinal column as part of a trauma assessment/survey. Hemodynamic stability is a priority in these patients. Like other forms of shock, fluid resuscitation is used as the first-line agent for hypotension. It is important to exercise caution with volume resuscitation, and frequent assessments are required to avoid fluid volume overload. Vasopressors are likely to be used in this patient population because of the pathophysiology of the injury. Norepinephrine is generally the preferred medication, and epinephrine can be a second-line agent. Although a second agent is rarely required, if the patient reaches maximum doses of norepinephrine, epinephrine is added if the patient has not achieved blood pressure and heart rate stability (Dave et al., 2023). Anticipate orders for imaging to determine the severity of a spinal cord injury. The patient will likely be admitted to the ICU for hourly neurological assessments, tight medication management, and vital sign frequency.

SUMMARY

Shock-related emergencies have been thoroughly discussed in this chapter. Shock is a frequent emergency seen in the ED, and determining timely and effective treatment is vital to decrease mortality. Although all shock states result in inadequate tissue perfusion, each type of shock has a completely different cause. Mortality rates are drastically improved by identifying and treating early stages of shock. Be observant for those subtle vital sign changes found in the early signs of shock. Early rapid responses save lives and preserve end organs.

REVIEW QUESTIONS

1) What criteria is required to be diagnosed with septic shock? Select all that apply
   a. Temperature >100.4°F
   b. Lactic acid >2 mmol/L
   c. Hypotension despite fluid resuscitation
   d. Vasopressors
2) Which assessment phenomenon is sometimes exhibited in patients experiencing cardiac tamponade?
   a. Tracheal deviation
   b. Cushing triad
   c. Chvostek sign
   d. Beck triad

REFERENCES

Duffett, L., Castellucci, L. A., & Forgie, M. A. (2020). Pulmonary embolism: Update on management and controversies. *BMJ, 370*, m2177. https://doi.org/10.1136/bmj.m2177

Font, M. D., Thyagarajan, B., & Khanna, A. K. (2020). Sepsis and septic shock—basics of diagnosis, pathophysiology and clinical decision making. *Medical Clinics of North America, 104*(4), 573–585. https://doi.org/10.1016/j.mcna.2020.02.011

Khorsand, S., Helou, M. F., Satyapriya, V., Kopanczyk, R., & Khanna, A. K. (2023). Not all shock states are created equal. *Anesthesiology Clinics, 41*(1), 1–25. https://doi.org/10.1016/j.anclin.2022.11.002

Koya, H. H., & Paul, M. (2023, July 24). *Shock*. In StatPearls [Internet]. StatPearls Publishing. Retrieved August 26, 2025, from https://www.ncbi.nlm.nih.gov/books/NBK531492/

Patel, S., Holden, K., Calvin, B., DiSilvio, B., & Dumont, T. (2022). Shock. *Critical Care Nursing Quarterly, 45*(3), 225–232. https://doi.org/10.1097/cnq.0000000000000407

Sarma, D., & Jentzer, J. C. (2024). Cardiogenic shock. *Critical Care Clinics, 40*(1), 37–56. https://doi.org/10.1016/j.ccc.2023.05.001

Stashko, E., & Meer, J. (2023, August 7). *Cardiac tamponade*. In StatPearls [Internet]. StatPearls Publishing. Retrieved August 26, 2025, from https://www.ncbi.nlm.nih.gov/books/NBK431090/

Vyas, V., Sankari, A., & Goyal, A. (2024, December 11). *Acute pulmonary embolism*. In StatPearls [Internet]. StatPearls Publishing. Retrieved August 26, 2025, from https://www.ncbi.nlm.nih.gov/books/NBK560551/

Traumatic Emergencies

Alexander Menard

> Trauma is defined as an injury caused by a sudden external force to bodily tissue. That external force can come in many different shapes and sizes, literally. Trauma is a common cause of presentation to the ED. From motor vehicle crashes, to falls from height or standing, to domestic violence and abuse. Whenever an injured person presents to the ED, the origin of the trauma can inform care of the patient.

In this chapter, you will learn to:
1. Discuss the common traumatic emergencies presenting to the ED
2. Identify the signs and symptoms of traumatic emergencies
3. Review the interventions to address traumatic emergencies

TRAUMATIC EMERGENCIES

In real life, the trauma team is performing several assessment steps simultaneously. However, if you were to take all the assessments and interventions and prioritize them in order of most important to least important, you would end up with the assessment that follows the airway, breathing, and circulation (ABCs). If your patient is arriving via emergency medical service (EMS), you have time to gather equipment and team members and prepare the room. Once the patient arrives, you should perform a quick across-the-room assessment: As you look across the room and see the patient, you should be looking for any uncontrolled hemorrhaging, alertness, color, and work of breathing. The trauma assessment is as easy as your ABCs. At any time, if you notice something is wrong during your assessment, stop and correct and reassess before moving on to the next part of your assessment.

Primary Survey
The primary survey is focused on rapid assessment of a patient's vital functions. The primary survey must include the ABCDEs (**A**irway, with

restriction of C-spine motion, **B**reathing, **C**irculation, **D**isability, and **E**xposure). Alterations in any of these elements must be addressed before moving on to the rest of the exam. The purpose of the primary survey (see Table 17.1) is to treat any instability in an attempt to prevent life-threatening deterioration.

Secondary Survey

The secondary survey, completed in the trauma bay, is a comprehensive head-to-toe assessment that seeks to identify other injuries that require urgent attention and intervention. Pertinent medical history leveraging the mnemonic AMPLE (**A**llergies and reactions, **M**edications **P**ast illnesses, pregnancy status, **L**ast meal, and **E**vents/environment related to injury) is collected (see Table 17.2). Adjunctive diagnostic testing ensues. Continuous monitoring and reassessment are essential during this phase. As injuries are diagnosed, decisions to transfer or treat are made. If the patient will stay, consultation with specialty services begins and comprehensive treatment plans are implemented. Now that your assessment is complete, you should be able to identify which diagnostic tests and interventions are needed and prepare to admit or transfer the patient.

TABLE 17.1

Primary Survey of the ABCDEs

ABCDE	Assessment
A = Airway (with restriction of C-spine motion)	■ Assess patency: Can the patient talk? ■ Inspect for blood or edema obstructing the airway. ■ Assess ability to maintain a patent airway. ■ Place cervical collar and maintain C-spine precautions.
B = Breathing and ventilation	■ Assess oxygen saturation. ■ Assess ability to take deep breaths.
C = Circulation with hemorrhage control	■ Assess skin perfusion. ■ Assess for decreased level of consciousness. ■ Observe heart rate for tachycardia. ■ Inspect for overt bleeding.
D = Disability	■ Assess neurologic status: Glasgow Coma Scale, movement, sensation.
E = Exposure	■ Completely undress the patient to ensure a complete evaluation of all surfaces. ■ Obtain temperature to identify any hypo- or hyperthermia.

ABCDEs, Airway, with restriction of C-spine motion, Breathing, Circulation, Disability, and Exposure.

TABLE 17.2
AMPLE Mnemonic

Mnemonic	Rationale
A = Allergies and reactions	Allergies are required to guide treatment. IV contrast may be needed during CT scans. Antibiotics may be required to treat open fractures or contaminated wounds.
M = Medications	Patients taking anticoagulants may require reversal agents. Beta-blockers or calcium channel blockers may blunt a patient's tachycardic response to injury.
P = Past illnesses, pregnancy status	Past medical history including neurologic deficits, cardiac history, and pulmonary diagnoses are especially important.
L = Last meal	Knowing the last meal is important, as trauma patients may need operative interventions. Help anesthesiologists gauge the risk of vomiting upon intubation and induction of anesthesia.
E = Events/environment related to injury	Pertinent events prior to or pertaining to the injury are helpful. Example: A patient who felt lightheaded or dizzy prior to falling may have had a medical event such as syncope or an arrhythmia precipitating a fall.

AMPLE, allergies and reactions medications past illnesses, pregnancy status last meal events/environment related to injury.

Trauma Triad of Death

If you have ever heard a colleague say "better to be warm and dead than cold and dead" during a trauma resuscitation, your colleague was right. Three components will cause a trauma patient to bleed out faster and spiral down quickly to an imminent death, and hypothermia is one of them. See Figure 17.1.

Avoid the "trauma triad of death" on all your trauma patients by:
- Keeping them warm
- Correcting acidosis
- Improving clotting formation by transfusing whole blood (platelets, plasma, and packed red blood cells [PRBCs])

Road Burn or Road Rash

Road burn/rash is a type of friction abrasion.
- *Causes:* Skin friction contact with the "road" or pavement or other abrasive material. It commonly occurs in motorcycle collisions when the patient is not wearing protective gear.
- *Signs and symptoms:* Painful abrasions or large areas of skin that are "rubbed off." Embedded debris or asphalt may be visible.

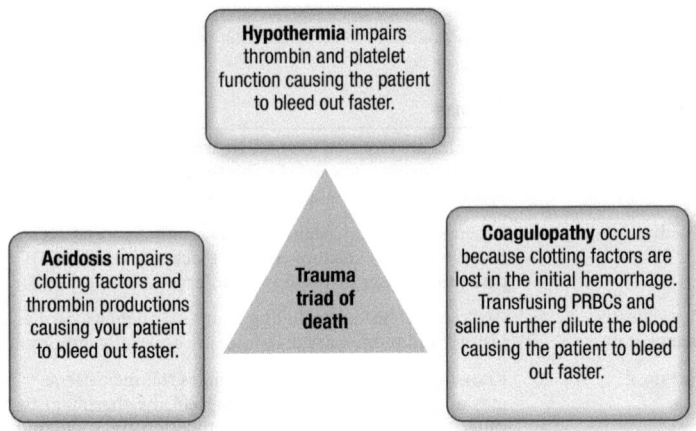

Figure 17.1 Trauma triad of death diagram. PRBCs, packed red blood cells.

- *Interventions:* Treat any life-threatening injuries first. Road rash is very painful; anticipate orders to apply local or topical anesthetics or administer pain medication prior to wound cleansing. Once the local or topical anesthesia has had the desired effect, the wound will need to be cleansed, removing any debris. Anticipate an order to apply antibiotic ointment and a nonadhesive dressing to the wounds.

Penetrating Trauma

Penetrating trauma is defined by a foreign object that penetrates body tissue. Most commonly this is from bullets, knives, industrial equipment, power tools, and other projectiles. The severity of the injury is directly related to the tissues and structures that are impacted. The amount of damage is also related to the force associated with the object. Higher-velocity penetrating objects will transfer more energy to the tissues compared with low-velocity objects; thus high-velocity projectiles cause more tissue damage.

- *Signs and symptoms:* Vary depending on the location, bleeding, tissue damage, organ damage, and signs of hypovolemic shock.
- *Interventions:* Note the size, length, and type of weapon used and location of injury; control bleeding with pressure and/or hemostatic dressing and tourniquet application as indicated; monitor cardiac rhythm and blood pressure. Contact local law enforcement according to state law and hospital policy. Place any removed clothing in a paper bag and maintain a chain of custody for forensic evidence. Anticipate orders to start two large-bore IVs; obtain type and crossmatch for blood transfusion; give emergency blood transfusion, as ordered, if the patient is in hypovolemic shock; and anticipate possible operating room and admission.

FAST FACTS

In the event of penetrating trauma with the foreign object still in place, stabilize the object and do not remove it until appropriate resources are readily available (operating room, surgeons, and other specialists).

THORACIC TRAUMA

These traumas may be the result of motor vehicle collisions, gunshot wounds, falls, blasts, blows to the chest, or crush injuries.

Pneumothorax
A pneumothorax is an air leak in the pleural space resulting in partial or total collapse of the lung.
- *Causes:* A traumatic lung injury or spontaneous rupture that results in an air leak into the pleural space.
- *Signs and symptoms:* Sucking chest wound; dyspnea; tachypnea; tachycardia; sudden, pleuritic chest pain; anxiety; restlessness; diminished or absent breath sounds on affected side; pallor; hypotension if severe; subcutaneous emphysema; palpitations; or asymptomatic if small.
- *Interventions:* Put patient in high Fowler position; give oxygen; cover open chest wounds with flap petroleum jelly (Vaseline), gauze dressing secured on three sides or a vented chest seal; anticipate orders to check pulse oximetry, connect to cardiac monitor, arrange for immediate chest x-ray, prepare to assist with needle or finger thoracostomy or chest tube insertion, administer pain medications, and obtain IV access.

FAST FACTS

Treatment for a sucking chest wound is a three-sided nonporous dressing. However, if the patient's respiratory status deteriorates after application of the three-sided dressing and signs of a tension pneumothorax (hypotension, distended neck veins, and tracheal deviation) are developing, try removing the three-sided dressing. Then reassess the respiratory status.

Hemothorax
A hemothorax is blood in in the pleural space that results in partial or total collapse of the lung.
- *Causes:* Penetrating chest trauma with bleeding into the lung.
- *Signs and symptoms:* Blood loss greater than 1,500 mL is considered a massive hemothorax: mediastinal shift (systolic blood pressure of less than 80 mmHg and capillary refill of more than 4 seconds); decreased

urine output; respiratory distress; hypotension; tachycardia; cyanosis; tracheal deviation; decreased or absent breath sounds; and flat neck veins due to hypovolemic shock.
- *Interventions:* Treat ABCs; assist with chest tube insertion; anticipate orders to prepare for emergency thoracotomy, open two large-bore IV accesses, administer IV fluid bolus, monitor cardiac performance, and prepare for emergency blood transfusion. If there is a large volume of blood loss, anticipate blood product administration or autotransfusion.

Flail Chest

A flail chest is a fracture of two or more ribs in two or more contiguous places, resulting in a free-floating segment of the chest wall.
- *Causes:* Chest trauma.
- *Signs and symptoms:* Paradoxical chest movement; chest pain; dyspnea; tachypnea; and crepitus.
- *Interventions:* Treat ABCs; anticipate orders to start IV access, monitor pulse oximetry, control pain, and prepare for possible intubation for ventilation assistance.

Diaphragmatic Injuries

Diaphragmatic injuries are rare but morbid complications of trauma. This is a tear or rupture of the diaphragm (Lee et al., 2025).
- *Causes:* Blunt or penetrating forces resulting in herniation of abdominal contents into the thoracic cavity.
- *Signs and symptoms:* Epigastric pain, chest pain, abdominal pain, bowel sounds in lower chest, dyspnea, dysphagia, and decreased breath sounds.
- *Interventions:* Anticipate orders to monitor cardiac performance and pulse oximetry, use nasogastric tube for stomach decompression, establish IV access, and prepare for surgery.

Spinal Cord Injuries

These traumas may result in spinal shock or neurogenic shock.
- *Causes:* Neck or back trauma.
- *Signs and symptoms:* Breathing difficulty; varying paralysis depending on injury location; bradycardia; hypotension; autonomic dysreflexia (hypertensive condition: headache, sweating, and bradycardia); warm and dry skin; may assume room temperature (poikilothermia); pain; loss of voluntary bowel or bladder control; and possible priapism.
- *Interventions:* Open airway maintaining cervical (C-spine) immobilization (use jaw-thrust maneuver); conduct a neurological assessment; prepare for possible endotracheal intubation; assist if ventilation assistance required; anticipate orders to administer IV fluids and insert a gastric tube and urinary catheter.

FAST FACTS

Assume an existing spinal injury on any trauma patient who has an altered level of consciousness or is intoxicated until proven otherwise. Maintain spinal immobilization until cleared with appropriate assessment, radiologic study results, and appropriate documentation of restrictions.

ABDOMINAL TRAUMA

Abdominal trauma can result in injuries to abdominal organs that can range from mild to lethal. Solid organ injuries are readily observed on CT scan, whereas other injuries, such as pancreatic or small bowel, may be more difficult to discover. Ongoing assessment and serial abdominal exams are essential to ensure all diagnoses are recognized and treated promptly.

Splenic Injuries
Splenic injuries are trauma or injuries to the spleen.
- *Causes:* Usually occurs with blunt left upper quadrant abdominal trauma.
- *Signs and symptoms:* Kehr sign (see Figure 17.2; left upper quadrant abdominal pain that may radiate to the left shoulder); absent or

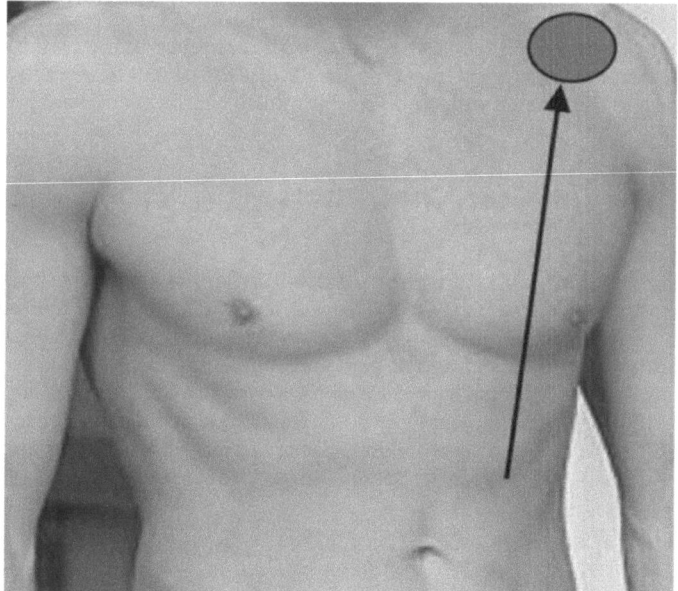

Figure 17.2 Kehr sign.
Source: Steve Han.

hypoactive bowel sounds; abdominal muscle rigidity; and hypovolemic shock.
- *Interventions:* Monitor frequent vital signs for the development of tachycardia, narrowing pulse pressure, tachypnea, pallor, and anxiety, indicating the patient is progressing into shock. Serial hemoglobin and hematocrit are essential to trend values to observe for stability versus ongoing bleeding. Anticipate orders to establish large-bore IV access. Indicate these patients as nothing by mouth (NPO) in the event the patient requires an intravascular embolization or surgical interventions. Ensure the patient has an active type and crossmatch with blood readily available in the blood bank.

Liver Laceration

The liver is the most commonly injured solid organ because of its size and location in the abdomen. Liver injuries commonly occur because of both blunt and penetrating injuries. Liver injuries are graded on a 1 to 5 scale, with 1 being least injured and 5 being the worst.
- *Causes:* Blunt or penetrating trauma.
- *Signs and symptoms:* Right upper quadrant pain, sometimes radiating to the back or shoulder.
- *Interventions:* Monitor frequent vital signs for the development of tachycardia, narrowing pulse pressure, tachypnea, pallor, and anxiety, which indicate that the patient is progressing into shock. Serial hemoglobin and hematocrit are essential to trend values to observe for stability versus ongoing bleeding. Anticipate orders to establish large-bore IV access. Keep this patient NPO in the event the patient requires an intravascular embolization or surgical interventions. Ensure the patient has an active type and crossmatch with blood readily available in the blood bank.

Pelvic Fractures

Pelvic fractures are either stable or unstable. With a pelvic fracture, a patient can lose several liters of blood.
- *Causes:* Pelvic trauma.
- *Signs and symptoms:* Pain; pelvic instability; rigidity; hypoactive bowel sounds; hypovolemic shock; and leg shortening or rotation. If the trauma is a urethral laceration, blood is at the urethral meatus. If the trauma is a bladder laceration, suprapubic pain and an inability to void are present.
- *Interventions:* Anticipate orders to apply a pelvic binder, establish large-bore IV access, administer IV isotonic fluid bolus, arrange for pelvic x-ray or CT scan, type and screen blood, prepare for possible blood product transfusion, and prepare for possible surgery or interventional radiology.

HEAD TRAUMA

Linear Skull Fracture

A linear skull fracture is a nondepressed skull fracture.
- *Causes:* Head trauma.

- *Signs and symptoms:* Pain over fracture, scalp laceration, headache, and possible decreased level of consciousness.
- *Interventions:* Elevate head of bed, obtain neurological assessment; clean and dress any wounds; arrange for skull x-rays or head CT scans.

Basilar Skull Fracture

A basilar skull fracture is a fracture to the bones at the base of the skull. Complications include infection and cerebrospinal fluid (CSF) leak.
- *Causes:* Head trauma to base of skull.
- *Signs and symptoms:* Altered level of consciousness; bruising behind the ear (Battle sign) 12 to 24 hours after injury; bruising around the eyes (racoon's eyes) 12 to 24 hours after injury; headache; rhinorrhea; otorrhea; and unilateral hearing loss (see Figure 17.3).

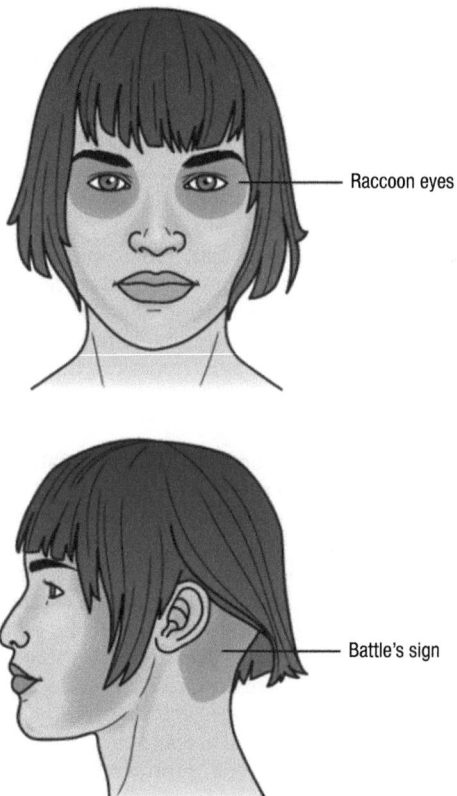

Figure 17.3 Raccoon eyes and Battle sign.

- *Interventions:* If there is a CSF leak, apply a dry, sterile, loose dressing below the drainage. Elevate the head of the bed, obtain frequent neurological assessments; anticipate orders to arrange for x-rays and head CT scan, establish IV access, administer antibiotics, and avoid nasogastric tube.

Depressed Skull Fracture
A depressed skull fracture is a concavelike skull fracture. It may be an open fracture; assess for CSF and bleeding.
- *Causes:* Direct blow to the head; head trauma.
- *Signs and symptoms:* Altered level of consciousness, head laceration, headache, and skull depression noted upon palpation.
- *Interventions:* Apply loose, sterile dressing; perform frequent neurological assessments; anticipate orders to establish IV access; administer antibiotics; arrange for operating room admission, x-rays, and head CT scan.

Concussion
A concussion is a closed head injury resulting in transient neurological changes.
- *Causes:* Blunt head or neck trauma.
- *Signs and symptoms:* Nausea; vomiting; dizziness; fatigue; headache; phonophobia; brief altered level of consciousness; anxiety; irritability; photophobia; poor concentration; normal head CT report; and possible amnesia.
- *Interventions:* Perform a neurological assessment; elevate head of the bed; anticipate orders for head CT scan and hospital admission if loss of consciousness lasts more than 5 minutes or patient remains confused and provide head injury discharge instructions. Sports activities should be restricted until cleared by the provider so that healing is promoted and postconcussive or second-impact syndromes can be avoided.

Subdural Hematoma
A subdural hematoma is bleeding between the dura mater (outermost brain covering) and the arachnoid layer (fine fibrous layer between dura and pia mater) of the meninges, resulting in direct pressure on brain tissue surface.
- *Causes:* Commonly caused by head trauma, acceleration and/or deceleration forces, or violent shaking resulting in a tear to the bridging veins.
- *Signs and symptoms:* Headache, nausea, vomiting, changes in level of consciousness; deteriorating mental status; fixed and dilated pupil on side of the injury; increased intracranial pressure; immediate and prolonged coma; and posturing (decorticate, toward the cord; decerebrate, away from the cord; see Figure 17.4).
- *Interventions:* Perform neurological assessment; anticipate orders for a head CT scan, take measures to reduce intracranial pressure, and prepare the patient for potential surgery.

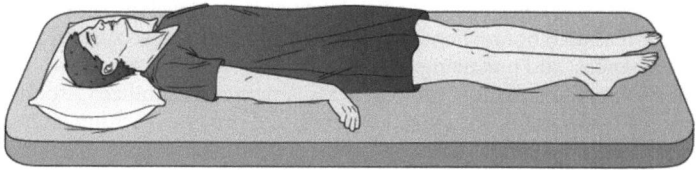

Decerebrate posturing

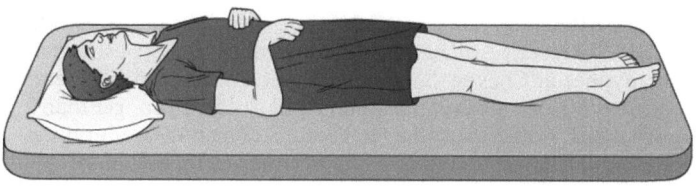

Decorticate posturing

Figure 17.4 Decerebrate and decorticate posturing.

Epidural Hematoma

An epidural hematoma is bleeding between the skull and dura mater.
- *Causes:* Head trauma. This condition commonly occurs with temporal and parietal skull fractures.
- *Signs and symptoms:* Transient loss of consciousness, ipsilateral pupil dilation, posturing, and hemiparesis.
- *Interventions:* Perform neurological assessment; anticipate orders for a head CT scan, take measures to reduce intracranial pressure, and prepare the patient for surgery.

Subarachnoid Hemorrhage

A subarachnoid hemorrhage is bleeding between the pia mater (delicate surface layer of brain) and arachnoid membrane.
- *Causes:* Head trauma. This injury is frequently associated with child abuse and has a high mortality rate.
- *Signs and symptoms:* Headache, nausea and vomiting, altered level of consciousness, neurological deficits, seizure, and posturing.
- *Interventions:* Prepare neurological assessment, anticipate order to arrange for head CT scan, and prepare for surgery.

Contusion

A contusion is a bruise to the brain surface.
- *Causes:* Direct blow to the head.

- *Signs and symptoms:* Neurological deficits, altered level of consciousness for more than 6 hours, nausea and vomiting, amnesia, seizure, visual disturbances, and posturing.
- *Interventions:* Perform neurological assessment, immobilize C-spine, arrange for head CT scan when ordered, and provide teaching on head injury upon discharge.

Increased Intracranial Pressure
- *Causes:* Head trauma, electrolyte imbalances, and meningitis.
- *Signs and symptoms:*
  - *Early:* Altered level of consciousness; headache, nausea/vomiting.
  - *Late:* Nonreactive, dilated pupils; unresponsiveness; posturing; bradypnea or Cheyne–Stokes respirations; bradycardia; widening pulse pressure; and bulging fontanels in children younger than 2 years.
- *Interventions:* Anticipate orders to administer mannitol, administer sedatives, and maintain intracranial pressure less than 15 mmHg, elevate head of bed to 30 degrees, avoid hypotension, and avoid Valsalva maneuver.

SUMMARY

Major trauma emergencies are always critical situations. You should be able to differentiate among the various types of basic trauma and know how to respond. Remember to control any hemorrhaging because it is one of the most preventable causes of death in a trauma patient. Complete your trauma assessment and avoid the trauma triad of death. Finding time to chart during a critical emergency is difficult. Most of the time, you need another nurse to help. All ED nurses must be team players. Notify your team and volunteer or ask someone to document as care is provided. Rapid responses save lives. After a trauma, it is good to debrief with the team and talk about what went well and any areas of opportunity.

REVIEW QUESTIONS

1) A 25-year-old male is brought to the ED after a motor vehicle collision. The patient is unresponsive with shallow breathing and a weak pulse. What is the next best nursing intervention?
   a. Assess airway patency and prepare for possible intubation.
   b. Establish IV access and begin fluid resuscitation with normal saline.
   c. Perform a focused neurological exam to assess for traumatic brain injury.
   d. Obtain a full set of vital signs and initiate secondary assessment.
2) A 45-year-old patient arrives at the ED after a fall from a two-story building. The patient is pale, diaphoretic, tachycardic (HR 128), and hypotensive (BP 85/50 mmHg). What is the nurse's next action
   a. Administer vasopressors to stabilize blood pressure.

b. Place the patient in Trendelenburg position to improve blood pressure.
c. Monitor urine output before initiating fluid resuscitation.
d. Place two large-bore IVs and prepare for blood transfusion.

REFERENCE

Lee, K., Kashyap, S., & Atherton, N. S. (2025, January). *Diaphragm injury* [Updated 2023 July 25]. In Statpearls [Internet]. StatPearls Publishing. Retrieved August 26, 2025, from https://www.ncbi.nlm.nih.gov/books/NBK482207/

Substance Abuse and Toxicologic Emergencies

Alexander Menard

> *Substance misuse and abuse and toxicologic emergencies can be a primary reason for presentation to the ED or can be a complicating factor of the primary reason for presentation. As an ED nurse you must have a high suspicion of intoxication, whether it be intentional or accidental. Being able to identify patterns associated with toxicologic and substance use and misuse is essential.*

In this chapter, you will learn to:
1. Discuss the substance abuse and toxicologic emergencies seen in the ED
2. Identify the clinical patterns associated with substance abuse and toxicologic emergencies
3. Review the interventions to address substance abuse and toxicologic emergencies

SUBSTANCE ABUSE AND TOXICOLOGIC EMERGENCIES

Substance abuse and toxicologic conditions, which are seen regularly in the ED, can be fatal. The death rate related to drug overdose has risen incrementally by the tens of thousands year over year for the last decade. Many types of substance abuse and poisonous materials exist, and remembering them all is difficult. Increasingly, teenagers and young adults are vaping various substances and finding creative inexpensive ways to get high. These may include synthetic drugs or household substances such as nutmeg, poisonous flowers, cough syrups, and family members' prescribed home medications. A detailed assessment and patient history are key to identifying the substance taken. Be sure to include feedback from any witnesses, friends, or family members who may be willing to disclose what was taken (Hoffman, 2025). This chapter provides a simple and easy-to-use substance abuse and toxicology table (Table 18.1).

TABLE 18.1

Substance Abuse and Toxicology

Drug/Substance	Signs and Symptoms	Interventions/Anticipated Orders
Acetylcholinesterase inhibition (cholinergics) Insecticides, organophosphates, carbamates, and nerve agents.	Remember **SLUDGE**: **S**aliva, **L**acrimation, **U**rination, **D**efecation, **GI** upset, and **E**mesis. Early on, tachycardia; lethargic; paralysis; shock; anxiety; bronchospasms; ataxia; pulmonary edema; bradypnea; seizure; and coma. Bradycardia in late stages.	Wash toxins off the patient. If oral ingestion within 1 hour, consider 1 g/kg charcoal. Atropine may reverse central nervous system effects. Ipratropium bromide (Atrovent)–nebulized treatment may dry secretions. Administer pralidoxime or obidoxime as ordered. Pralidoxime should *not* be administered without concurrent atropine.
Alcohol abuse Liquors, beers, wines, moonshine, rubbing alcohol, and even mouthwash. Vaping or use of alcohol-soaked tampons are also methods of ingesting alcohol.	Slurred speech; unsteady gait; hypoglycemia, and alcohol odor. The patient may go into withdrawal.	Obtain alcohol level. Benzodiazepines such as lorazepam (Ativan) are used to treat and prevent further progression of withdrawal.
Anticholinergic overdose Antihistamines, antidepressants, dicyclomine, tropicamide, alkaloids cyclopentolate, homatropine, phenothiazines, *Amanita muscaria*,	Mnemonic: Blind as a bat, mad as a hatter, red as a beet, hot as hare, dry as a bone, the bowel and bladder lose their tone, and the heart runs along. Respectively, pupillary dilation—	Consider charcoal 1 g/kg within 1 hour of ingestion. Supportive measures, benzodiazepines for agitation and seizures. Antidote: Physostigmine in cases with both peripheral and central signs of

jimsonweed or deadly nightshade, belladonna, atropine, and tricyclics.	blurred vision; delusions, hallucinations, or delirium; hyperthermia; dry mucosa and skin; GI and bladder paralysis; and tachycardia. Cardiovascular collapse; seizure; hypertension; thirst.	anticholinergic poisoning and 1 g/kg charcoal if ingestion was <1 hour ago.
Anticoagulants—oral Direct thrombin inhibitor Dabigatran (Pradaxa)	Bleeding.	Antidote: idarucizumab (Praxbind)—life-threatening bleeding or emergency/invasive procedure. IV 5 g (administered as 2 separate 2.5-g doses no more than 15 minutes apart). Hemodialysis.
Factor Xa inhibitor Rivaroxaban (Xarelto) Apixaban (Eliquis) Edoxaban (Savaysa) Betrixaban (Bevyxxa)	Bleeding.	Antidote: Andexanet alfa (Andexxa) Only for severe life-threatening bleeding (e.g., intracranial hemorrhage); off-label use for edoxaban and betrixaban. Kcentra (PCC) IV 2,000 units × 1 or 25–50 units/kg × 1.

(continued)

TABLE 18.1

Substance Abuse and Toxicology (continued)

Drug/Substance	Signs and Symptoms	Interventions/Anticipated Orders
Warfarin (Coumadin, Jantoven)	Bleeding.	Obtain prothrombin time and INR level and give phytonadione (vitamin K); onset of action: PO 6–10 hours; IV 1–2 hours. PCC for acute major bleeding or urgent surgery/invasive procedure. Onset of action: within 10 minutes.
Anticoagulants—parenteral LMWH Enoxaparin (Lovenox)	Bleeding.	Antidote: Protamine partial reversal agent.
Heparin	Bleeding.	Obtain partial thromboplastin time level and antidote: protamine sulfate.
Benzodiazepines Depressants and sedatives such as diazepam (Valium), oxazepam (Serax), alprazolam (Xanax), lorazepam (Ativan), clonazepam (Klonopin), midazolam (Versed), and flunitrazepam (Rohypnol) (aka "roofies"), which are 10 times as potent as diazepam.	Drowsiness; amnesia; confusion; bradypnea; cool, clammy skin; dilated pupils; sedation; and hypotension.	Support measures; fluids and/or vasopressors for hypotension. Respiratory depression/failure intubation. Antidote: flumazenil (Romazicon) Only use in acute life-threatening ingestion. Do NOT use in patients who are chronically on benzodiazepines. Reversal may cause life-threatening seizures and withdrawal.

Beta-blockers
Atenolol, metoprolol, propranolol, and sotalol.

Bradycardia; hypotension; shock; and cardiac arrest.

Hypotension: fluids and vasopressors. Glucagon 3–10 mg IV bolus. IV calcium chloride or gluconate. Hyperinsulinemia-euglycemia therapy. Atropine for symptomatic bradycardia and prepare pacemaker.

Caffeine powder/capsules
Concentrated OTC caffeine.
2 tsp = **(10,000 mg)** lethal dose (like drinking 70 Red Bulls at one time).

Tachycardia, seizures, hypertension, dysrhythmias, coma, and death in high doses.

If recent ingestion, charcoal may be helpful. IV fluids, EKG, beta-blockers (esmolol), procainamide, lidocaine, bicarbonate. Vasopressin or phenylephrine if hypotension occurs. Dialysis or intralipid therapy may be helpful.

Calcium channel blockers
Verapamil, nifedipine (Procardia), and diltiazem.

Bradycardia; hypotension; lethargy; confusion; bradypnea; nausea and vomiting; shock; hyperglycemia; and cardiac arrest.

Calcium chloride 10–20 mg/kg (max 2 g) or calcium gluconate 60 mg/kg (max 3–6 g) IV over 5 minutes until response seen. Significant hypercalcemia may be necessary before severely intoxicated patients respond. Give normal saline bolus and vasopressors for hypotension. Hyperinsulinemia-euglycemia therapy.

Carbon monoxide poisoning
Carbon monoxide displaces oxygen on the hemoglobin.

Hypoxia; confusion; headache; nausea and vomiting; dizziness; coma; seizures; cyanosis; and death.

Give oxygen via nonrebreather mask; provide hyperbaric oxygen treatment; and obtain carbon dioxide levels.

(*continued*)

TABLE 18.1

Substance Abuse and Toxicology (*continued*)

Drug/Substance	Signs and Symptoms	Interventions/Anticipated Orders
Cardiac glycosides Digoxin, digitoxin, oleander, and foxglove.	Visual yellow-green halos; nausea and vomiting; headache; bradycardia; hyperkalemia and hypokalemia, ventricular arrhythmias; shock; and cardiac arrest.	Obtain digoxin level; charcoal 1 g/kg within 1 hour of ingestion. Give digoxin (Digibind) immune fab; dose dependent on digoxin dose ingested; 1 mg/kg lidocaine IV for arrhythmias, and atropine for bradycardia.
DXM Cough suppressant found in OTC cold medications. Street names: triple C; CCC; dexing; skittles; velvet; poor man's PCP; rojo; and robo tripping.	Confusion; hallucinations; lethargy; slurred speech; hypertension; eye spasms; paranoia; tachycardia; vomiting; seizures; coma, and death.	Many cold medications have other medications such as acetaminophen, pseudoephedrine, and guaifenesin to consider. Treatment is supportive. Antidotes and screening for DXM are currently unavailable.
Ethylene glycol (antifreeze)	First 1–12 hours: slurred speech; inebriated; coma; seizure; and death. Next 12–24 hours: tachycardia; hypertension; tachypnea; congestive heart failure; acute respiratory distress syndrome; and cardiac collapse. Next 24–72 hours: nephrotoxicity; flank pain; renal failure; and hypocalcemia.	Lab tests: Determine serum ethylene glycol level; prepare basic metabolic panel; and obtain urinalysis. Consider gastric lavage (charcoal is ineffective). Antidote: Give fomepizole therapy immediately; seizure control: benzodiazepines, hypocalcemia-induced seizures 10% 10–20 mL calcium gluconate IV. Metabolic acidosis 50 mEq IV sodium bicarbonate; cofactor

GHB acid

Depressant sold as liquid or dissolvable white powder. Street names: Easy Lay, G, Georgia Home Boy, Goop, Grievous Bodily Harm, Liquid XTC, Liquid X, and Scoop.

Low doses produce euphoria, lethargy, reduced anxiety, confusion, and memory loss. High doses produce bradycardia, bradypnea, hypothermia, nausea, vomiting, seizures, unconsciousness, coma, and death.

therapy: pyridoxine IV 100 mg; 2 g IV magnesium; 100 mg IV thiamine; 15 mg/kg IV fomepizole (Antizol); and prepare for dialysis.

Support ABCs and treat the symptoms. No toxicologic screening or current antidote exists. GHB analogues can cause liver and kidney damage, check liver function tests and metabolic panel. Supportive therapy; withdrawal symptoms: tachycardia, anxiety, tremors, hypertension, insomnia, and psychotic thoughts.

Hallucinogens

Mushrooms; ketamine; XTC/MDMA; PCP; LSD abuse and perennial herb *Salvia divinorum*.

Street names: acid, blotter, Shrooms, Mind Candy, Doses, Fry, Special K, Sally D, and vitamin K.

Agitation; hallucinations; dilated pupils; hyperthermia; hypertension; bradypnea; seizures; tachycardia; and respiratory arrest.

Reassure and reorient to reality; instruct patient to keep eyes open; and provide good lighting to decrease shadows. Give benzodiazepines for agitation.

Insulin

Weakness; lethargic; syncope; and blood sugar <80.

Monitor blood sugar; give 1-amp dextrose (D50) IV, if alert, feed the patient a meal; give IM glucagon as ordered if IV access is unobtainable; persistent hypoglycemia may require dextrose continuous infusion (D10).

(continued)

TABLE 18.1

Substance Abuse and Toxicology (continued)

Drug/Substance	Signs and Symptoms	Interventions/Anticipated Orders
Iron	Initially: hypotension; nausea; vomiting; and bloody stools. Late (2–3 days): coagulopathies; metabolic acidosis; hemorrhage; renal failure; liver failure; and shock.	Deferoxamine mesylate (Desferal) binds with iron and is excreted via the kidneys.
Marijuana concentrates 4–6× stronger than top-shelf marijuana. Street names: 710 (oil flipped and backwards) wax, earwax, honeycomb, budder, butane hash oil, BHO shatter, dabs, black glass, and errl; e-cigarettes, and vaporizers make it odorless and smokeless. THC can legally be purchased in some states in the form of gummies and unknowingly overdose.	Paranoia, anxiety, panic attacks, nausea, abdominal pain, cyclic vomiting, hallucinations, psychosis, tachycardia, asthma exacerbation, hypertension. Withdrawal, addiction, and cyclic vomiting problems may occur.	Support ABCs. No antidotes exist; treatment is supportive. Benzodiazepines may help anxiety. IV fluids and antiemetics may be used for nausea and abdominal pain. Haldol may help with cyclic vomiting.

MDMA

Colorful pills, powder, or liquid stimulant/psychedelics: Street names: XTC, X, STP, Hug drug; Lover's Speed; Beans; Disco Biscuit, E; Go; Eve; and XTC Ecstasy, Molly.

Euphoria; increased trust; tachycardia; hypertension; **hyperthermia;** sweating; muscle cramps; sexual arousal; chills; confusion; depression; and blurred vision. SIADH.

Treatment is supportive. Treat ABCs first. Cooling blanket or device may be ordered to regulate temperature. Check metabolic panel. Treat any electrolyte imbalances (hyponatremia). Head CT. Consider activated charcoal if recent ingestion.

Nonspecific or unknown

Varies. Complete a thorough assessment and patient history for any clues.

Treat symptoms. Consider activated charcoal in water or 1 g/kg sorbitol.

Narcotics (opioids)

Morphine, methadone, DXM, heroin, (synthetic opioid) meperidine (Demerol), codeine, diphenoxylate, propoxyphene, and synthetic opioids fentanyl (100× more potent than morphine) and carfentanil (10,000× more potent than morphine).

Fentanyl and Demerol can be negative in UDS.

Pinpoint pupils (miosis), central nervous system depression, depression, bradycardia, flushed face, hypotension, constipation, cool clammy skin, and bradypnea.

Protect airway and provide rescue breaths as needed. IV 0.4–2 mg **naloxone (Narcan)** q2–3 min, if no response observed after 10 mg total, consider other causes of respiratory depression. If no IV access can also be IM, IN, or nebulized. Naloxone action is shorter than most opioids; **repeat doses or continuous infusion may be required.** Can be obtained over the counter and may have been given on scene. Can lead to agitation and withdrawal symptoms.

(continued)

TABLE 18.1

Substance Abuse and Toxicology *(continued)*

Drug/Substance	Signs and Symptoms	Interventions/Anticipated Orders
Neuroleptics Metoclopramide, haloperidol, thioxanthenes, and phenothiazines.	EKG changes (prolonged QT segments); dysrhythmias; and altered level of consciousness.	Consider activated charcoal within 1 hour of ingestion. Supportive therapy: extrapyramidal symptoms: Diphenhydramine or benztropine (Cogentin) blocks dopamine reuptake. Neuroleptic malignant syndrome: benzodiazepines; IV crystalloid fluids.
NSAIDs (e.g., ibuprofen, naproxen, ketorolac, meloxicam)	Nausea; vomiting; abdominal pain; drowsiness; tarry or bloody stools; hemoptysis; shallow breathing; syncope; or coma.	Consider activated charcoal within 1–2 hours post ingestion; supportive care; maintain ABCs; gastric lavage if acute ingestion of massive amounts; hemodialysis to correct acidosis; benzodiazepines for seizures; metabolic acidosis: sodium bicarbonate.
Salicylates Aspirin	Nausea and vomiting; tinnitus; diaphoresis; acidosis; altered mental status; seizures; and shock.	Consider charcoal within 1 hour of ingestion. However, salicylates are absorbed erratically. Charcoal may be beneficial beyond 1 hour. Fluid resuscitation. Serum and urine alkalization: sodium bicarbonate bolus 1–2 mEq/kg, then

Stimulants (sympathomimetics) Aminophylline, amphetamines, cocaine, ephedrine, caffeine, methylphenidates, methamphetamines, and PCP. Yaba: Meth + Caffeine Wasping: Meth + bug spray.	Hypertension; dilated pupils; tachycardia; paranoia; vasoconstriction; hyperthermia; seizures; chest pain; acute myocardial infarction; coma; stroke; (hypotension with caffeine); altered mood; and death.	continuous infusion to maintain 1–2 mL urine/kg/hr. Monitor hypokalemia and cautiously replace. Seizure: benzodiazepines; hypoglycemia: dextrose; dialysis for enhanced elimination. Activated charcoal within 1 hour of ingestion. Agitation, anxiety, psychosis, and seizure control: benzodiazepines or haloperidol. Hypertension: sedation with benzodiazepines, nitroglycerin, or nitroprusside (Nipride) for hypertension. Avoid beta-blockers.
Synthetic cannabinoids Inhaled synthetic marijuana is commonly marketed as herbal incense or potpourri. Street names: K-2, Spice, Crazy Clown, Blaze, Demon, Black Magic, Ninja, Smoke, Skunk, Yucatan, Fire, and Red X Dawn.	Relaxation; euphoria; anxiety; tachycardia; hypertension; pallor; diaphoresis; delusions; paranoia; psychosis; hallucinations; seizures; nausea and vomiting; loss of consciousness; and aggressive or violent behavior toward self or others. May lead to renal failure.	Antidotes and routine toxicology screening for synthetic cannabinoids are currently unavailable. Treatment is supportive. Benzodiazepines may be ordered for agitation or seizures. Antiemetics may be ordered for nausea. IV fluids may be ordered to correct any electrolyte imbalances.

(continued)

TABLE 18.1

Substance Abuse and Toxicology (continued)

Drug/Substance	Signs and Symptoms	Interventions/Anticipated Orders
Synthetic cathinones Oral, inhaled, or injectable synthetic stimulants known as bath salts, alpha-PVP, and Flakka. Street names: Ivory wave, Pure Ivory, Red Dove, Vanilla Sky, White Dove, White Lightning, Cloud Nine, Ocean Burst, and Purple Wave.	Stimulant effects; sweating; palpitations; tachycardia; hallucinations; dilated pupils; paranoid; psychosis; aggressive violent behavior toward self or others; anxiety; agitation; hyperthermia; hypertension can lead to renal failure or myocardial infarction.	Antidotes and routine toxicology screening for synthetic cathinones are currently unavailable. Treatment is supportive. Benzodiazepines can help with agitation and seizures. Restraints may be ordered for safety. Antipsychotics may be given with caution as they tend to lower seizure thresholds.
TCA Amitriptyline, desipramine, nortriptyline, and imipramine.	Tachycardia; nausea; vomiting; tachydysrhythmias; hypotension; seizures; shock; and cardiac arrest.	Activated charcoal within 1 hour of ingestion. Antidote: None. Supportive therapy: Impaired cardiac conduction. Give IV sodium bicarbonate for TCA to obtain serum pH of 7.50–7.55 to alter protein binding; refractory cardiac conduction: hypertonic saline; hypotension: fluid resuscitation and norepinephrine (Levophed). Seizures: benzodiazepines.

Tylenol (acetaminophen) overdose Can lead to liver failure and death. Toxic doses destroy hepatocytes resulting in liver damage and necrosis. A dose of 140 mg/kg is toxic. Tylenol can also be mixed or cut in OTC or street drugs such as "cheese" (heroin cut with Tylenol PM).	First 24 hours: asymptomatic; minor GI upset. Next 24–72 hours: elevated liver function test or renal failure. Next 72–96 hours: jaundice; renal failure; coagulopathy; and liver necrosis. Next 4 days to 2 weeks: symptoms resolve, or patient dies.	Lab tests: check acetaminophen level 4 hours after ingestion and use the Rumack-Matthew nomogram. Activated charcoal within 1 hour of ingestion. Antidote: Administer NAC (Acetadote Mucomyst, available IV and PO, respectively), the sooner the better; may be useful up to 72 hours after ingestion. Monitor for anaphylactic reactions to NAC, which is more common in the IV formulation and in people with asthma.
Venom of rattlesnakes, cottonmouth/water moccasins, and copperheads.	Bite/fang marks with redness/bruising; pain; and swelling.	Antidote: Antivenom, CroFab initial dose 4–6 vials or 8–12 vials in life-threatening effects (shock serious active bleeding). Repeat doses of 4–6 vials if control not achieved. Maximum initial dose: 12 vials. Maintenance dose: 2 vials every 6 hours up to 18 hours. Normal saline for mild symptoms.

ABCs, airway, breathing, and circulation; BHO, butane honey oil; CCC, Coricidin HBP cough and cold; CroFab, crotalidae polyvalent immune Fab; DXM, dextromethorphan; GHB, gamma-hydroxybutyric acid; GI, gastrointestinal; IM, intramuscular; IN, intranasal; INR, international normalized ratio; IV, intravenous; LMWH, low-molecular-weight heparin; LSD, D-lysergic acid diethylamide; MDMA, 3,4-methylenedioxy-methamphetamine; NAC, N-acetylcysteine; NSAIDs, nonsteroidal anti-inflammatory drugs; OTC, over-the-counter; PCC, prothrombin complex concentrate; PCP, phencyclidine; PO, by mouth; PVP, pyrrolidinopentiophenone; SIADH, syndrome of inappropriate antidiuretic hormone; SLUDGE, saliva, lacrimation, urination, defecation, GI upset, and emesis; STP, serenity, tranquility, and peace; TCA, tricyclic antidepressants; THC, tetrahydrocannabinol; UDS, urine drug screen; XTC, ecstasy.

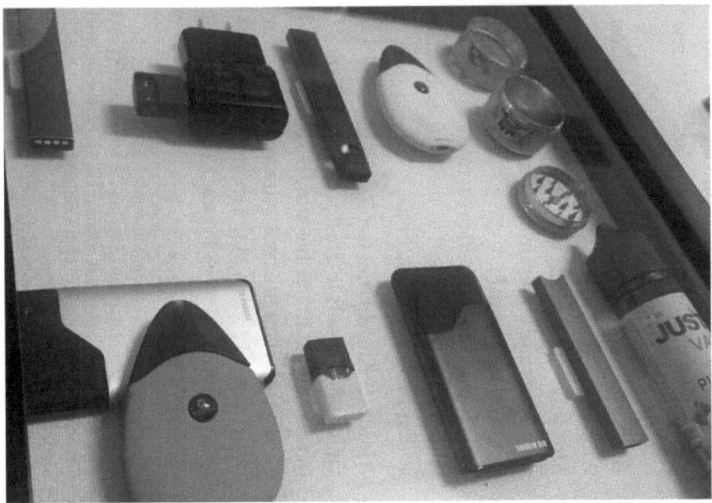

Figure 18.1 Different types of vaping devices.

Even with access to this table, you must still always consult with poison control after the patient is triaged. Poison control will give you vital individualized suggestions that are based on the patient's weight, circumstances, amount of drug intake, and the time frame in which the drug was taken. Document and communicate the suggestions provided by poison control with the ED provider to obtain any necessary immediate orders.

FAST FACTS

Detailed patient assessment and history taking is vital to aid in the identification of the substance taken.

Many controlled substances are being inhaled via electronic cigarettes or vaping devices. These vaping devices can be disguised as other small objects such as plug or outlet connections or universal serial bus (USB) devices. See Figure 18.1 for various types of vaping devices.

SUMMARY

You now have a stronger knowledge base for substance abuse and toxicology emergencies. You should be able to differentiate the types of substance abuse and toxicology emergencies and know how to respond. Because a urine drug screen (UDS) does not screen everything, get an accurate history and complete physical assessment. Check for contents such as pills, bottles, illicit substances, pipes, or any additional information to help identify the causative agent. Tablets and capsules can be identified with drug references, poison control, or the pharmacy department. Each overdose case is different. Many factors will affect the treatment, including time of ingestion, amount of substance, patient's weight, and current vital signs. Be sure to contact poison control for every case. They will help you and the provider come up with the proper individualized treatment course needed.

REVIEW QUESTIONS

1) A patient presents with flushed skin, dry mucous membranes, dilated pupils, urinary retention, and altered mental status. Which toxidrome is most consistent with these findings?
   a. Cholinergic
   b. Anticholinergic
   c. Opioid
   d. Sympathomimetic
2) Which of the following orders from a provider would the nurse expect for a patient suspected of opioid overdose presenting with respiratory depression?
   a. Flumazenil
   b. Atropine
   c. Naloxone
   d. Activated charcoal

REFERENCE

Hoffman, R. J., & Nillas, A. (2025). Toxidromes and a general approach to poisoning. *Archives of Disease in Childhood, 110*(9), 681–686. https://doi.org/10.1136/archdischild-2024-326969. Archdischild-2024-326969. Epub ahead of print. PMID: 39978865.

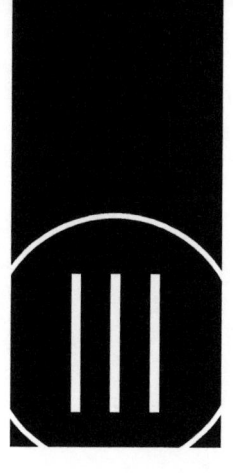

SPECIAL POPULATIONS IN ED NURSING CARE

19

Geriatric Emergencies

Alexander Menard

> As the baby boomer generation ages, we are encountering an even higher volume of ED patients. The normal physiological changes of the aging process leave patients more vulnerable to illness, injuries, and complications.

In this chapter, you will learn to:
1. Discuss the geriatric emergencies seen in the ED
2. Identify the red flag warnings for geriatric emergencies
3. Review the interventions to address geriatric emergencies

GERIATRIC EMERGENCIES

Aging decreases physiological reserve, rendering older adult patients unable to recover from what may seem relatively minor ailments. Additionally, multiple comorbidities impact their ability to tolerate acute illness, being acute or acute on chronic. Many geriatric patients have decreased renal function, decreased circulation, thinner skin, weaker bones, less muscle mass, decreased hearing, decreased gastric motility, brain atrophy, and visual impairments. It is always important to take these age-related changes into consideration when caring for older patients (Li et al., 2023).

Elder Maltreatment

Elder maltreatment can take several different forms, including physical, sexual, financial, and psychological; it can also include neglect. Abuse or maltreatment is physical harm, pain, or mental anguish; neglect is the failure to provide services or goods needed to prevent physical harm and mental anguish. Elder abuse is an international problem that can be difficult to detect. Females are more commonly abused than males. You must report all suspected cases of abuse.

- *Causes:* Not always known. Elder maltreatment/abuse can occur in any socioeconomic group. Lack of resources and stressed or burned-out caregivers can contribute to the problem.
- *Signs and symptoms:* Conflicting stories describing how an injury occurred; patient not given an opportunity to speak; time lapse between injury and presentation to the ED; disinterested caregiver; history of similar injuries; hand marks; bite marks; multiple bruises; multiple fractures in various healing stages; altered ambulation from sexual assault; malnourishment; dehydration; poor hygiene; withdrawal; and agitation.
- *Interventions:* Treat injuries and illness; accurately document and photograph injuries or neglect per policy; ascertain whether a report needs to be filed; notify social services as soon as possible; obtain supportive services through community referrals; consider hospitalization to ensure patient safety; and refer to adult protective services.

Falls

Falls are the leading cause of hospital admissions and injury-related death in the geriatric population. Complications often include soft tissue injuries, hip fractures, Colles fracture (wrist), subdural hematoma, and hot water burns from falls in the bathtub. First, assess the reason for the fall. Document any symptoms prior to the fall (e.g., dizziness, chest pain, and loss of consciousness). What was the activity during the fall? The location? Were there any witnesses? Any history of falls or alcohol intake? Finally, assess whether the patient fell at ground level. If not, how many feet did the patient fall?

- *Causes:* They are multifactorial and can be attributed to impaired vision, sensation, neurocirculatory system, gait, and balance.
- *Signs and symptoms:* Depends on the fall and injuries.
- *Interventions:* Give nothing by mouth; consider cervical injury and immobilization (rest, ice, splint, and elevate injury); clean and apply sterile dressing to wounds; assess pain; administer pain medications as ordered; arrange neurological exams; monitor extremity movement; and check circulation. Prepare for diagnostic studies. Educate patients and families on fall prevention.

FAST FACTS

If elder abuse is suspected, it must be reported in accordance with your local and state laws.

Syncope

Syncope is transient loss of consciousness with a spontaneous recovery (von Alvensleben, 2020).

- *Causes:* Identifying the cause may prove to be more valuable than treating the sustained injuries. Assess the patient's activity just before the syncopal event.
  - Temporary, abrupt decrease in cardiac output caused by aortic stenosis, mitral valve disease, cardiomyopathy, dysrhythmias, and sick sinus syndrome.
  - Volume depletion resulting from hemorrhage/anemia, diuresis, dehydration, and third-space fluid shift.
  - Hypersensitive carotid sinus caused by neck turning, constrictive collars, and drugs (digitalis, propranolol hydrochloride, and alpha-methyldopa).
  - Vasovagal response with hypotension resulting from cough, defecation, or urination.
  - Hypoglycemia or hypoxia.
- *Signs and symptoms:* Dizziness, chest pain, dyspnea, weakness, confusion, loss of consciousness, witnesses to the fall, and previous history.
- *Interventions:* Anticipate orders to obtain serum glucose and complete basic metabolic panel; administer oxygen through nasal cannula; check pulse oxygen; perform EKG and CT scan.
  - If caused by hypoglycemia, treat IV with dextrose 50% injection (D50; 1 amp) or give oral or intramuscular injection of glucose. Then feed patients once they are alert and oriented to person, place, and time.

FAST FACTS

Determining the underlying cause of the syncopal event is a necessity and can prevent future visits to the ED.

Dehydration

Dehydration is a lack of required serum fluid levels. Older adults are more prone to dehydration because of normal physiological changes that occur with aging.
- *Causes:* Altered sense of thirst; decrease in total body fluid; decreased kidney function; and decreased effectiveness of antidiuretic hormone, which helps conserve water.
- *Signs and symptoms:* Confusion; seizure; dry oral mucosa; dry skin; sunken eyes; lethargy; headache; constipation; hyperthermia; weak, rapid pulse; orthostatic hypotension; altered respiration; concentrated urine; and decreased urine output.
- *Interventions:* Anticipate orders to administer fluids IV or by mouth, assess mental status, check vital signs, and measure intake and output. Diagnostic studies may include metabolic panel, hematocrit, blood urea nitrogen, and complete blood count (CBC).

Dementia

Dementia is commonly mistaken for normal age-related cognitive changes. However, with dementia, the onset is more severe with an abrupt onset compared to normal aging.

- *Causes:* Multifactorial. Not always known, but may be attributed to electrolyte imbalance, dehydration, infection, and stroke. This assessment requires input from caregivers to determine the patient's normal cognitive baseline.
- *Signs and symptoms:* Alert with impaired orientation; impaired recent memory; impoverished thinking; difficulty finding words; confused speech; and poor sleep.
- *Interventions:* Provide a safe environment; put bed in low, locked position; monitor patient closely (place close to nurses' station); and assess for any new causes of confusion. Anticipate orders for IV access, IV fluids, CBC with differential, metabolic panel, urinalysis, toxicology screen, chest x-ray, and head CT, and, if possible, have family or sitter available at the bedside to redirect or reorient the patient.

Alzheimer Disease

Alzheimer disease affects one in eight people older than 65 years. It is a chronic, progressive, irreversible, degenerative dementia that has no preventive measures or cure.

- *Causes:* Unknown, with focus studies on loss of synapses in the brain.
- *Signs and symptoms:* Forgetfulness; memory loss; paranoia; delusions; irritability; depression; aphasia; apraxia; and history of progressively deteriorating mental functioning.
- *Interventions:* Prevent patients from injuring self or others; provide supervised safe environment with minimal stimulation; give short explanations and simple instructions; involve supportive services (social services); and provide healthcare resources and community referrals.

Pneumonia

Pneumonia is a bacterial, viral, or fungal infection below the bronchi resulting in inflammation of lung parenchyma.

- *Causes:* Bacterial, viral, or fungal lung infection. Contributing factors include a weak immune system; general debilitated condition; decreased mobility; chronic cardiac disease; chronic pulmonary disease; weak cough reflex; decreased lung capacity; aspiration; late diagnosis; and diabetes.
- *Signs and symptoms:* Confusion; change in normal activity; anorexia; tachypnea; dyspnea; fever or subnormal temperature; dehydration; productive or nonproductive cough; chills; weakness; chest pain; nausea and vomiting; abdominal distention; diaphoresis; cyanosis; and diminished lung sounds or crackles.
- *Interventions:* Anticipate orders for chest x-ray, CBC, blood cultures, and arterial blood gases. Monitor and document work of breathing. Start IV

access, maintain bed rest, and give fluids IV; pulse oximeter monitoring, along with oxygen and antibiotics as ordered.

Urosepsis

Urosepsis is an infection caused by a urinary tract infection that is more common in females than in males. In general, urinary infections are one of the most common bacterial infections in older adults. Urosepsis may lead to septic shock.

- *Causes:* Predisposing factors include an indwelling catheter and kidney stones.
- *Signs and symptoms:* Confusion; lethargy; altered mental status; tachycardia; tachypnea; fever or subnormal temperature; urinary frequency; urinary urgency; incontinence; nausea and vomiting; abdominal tenderness; and hypotension.
- *Interventions:* Anticipate orders to obtain urinalysis, administer fluids and antibiotics IV, and monitor urinary output. Prepare for possible admission.

FAST FACTS

The older adult presenting to the ED with confusion should be evaluated for an acute infection.

SUMMARY

You now have a better understanding of the diseases most commonly associated with older adults in the ED. Age-related physiological changes in older adults will affect their condition and can lead to complications. Be sure to assess and document these patients carefully. Obtain histories from them and their caregivers, when available.

REVIEW QUESTIONS

1) An 82-year-old female is brought to the ED by her daughter after falling at home. The patient denies hitting her head but reports hip pain. Her medical history includes osteoporosis and hypertension. What should the ED nurse do next?
    a. Encourage the patient to ambulate to assess mobility.
    b. Perform a focused musculoskeletal assessment and prepare for imaging.
    c. Administer opioid pain medications.
    d. Administer oral pain medication before assessing for fractures.
2) A 90-year-old female resident of a long-term care facility is brought to the ED for increased confusion and agitation over the past 24 hours. She has a history of dementia, hypertension, and osteoarthritis. Her vital

signs are stable, and she has no fever but reports dysuria and flank pain. What is the nurse's next action to help the patient?
  a. Assess for recent medication changes and monitor for worsening confusion.
  b. Obtain a urine sample for urinalysis and culture.
  c. Initiate fall precautions and reorient the patient as needed.
  d. Encourage oral fluids and reassess hydration status.

REFERENCES

Li, N., Liu, G., Gao, H., Wu, Q., Meng, J., Wang, F., Jiang, S., Chen, M., Xu, W., Zhang, Y., Wang, Y., Feng, Y., Liu, J., Xu, C., & Lu, H. (2023, September 15). Geriatric syndromes, chronic inflammation, and advances in the management of frailty: A review with new insights. *BioScience Trends, 17*(4), 262–270. https://doi.org/10.5582/bst.2023.01184. Epub 2023, August 23. PMID: 37612125.

von Alvensleben, J. C. (2020, October). Syncope and palpitations: A review. *Pediatric Clinics of North America Journal, 67*(5), 801–810. https://doi.org/10.1016/j.pcl.2020.05.004. Epub 2020 August 11. PMID: 32888682.

OB/GYN Emergencies

Sarah Berry

> Obstetrical (OB) and gynecological (GYN) emergencies occur regularly in the ED. As a nurse, you must be familiar and comfortable with the various types of OB/GYN emergencies. This chapter reviews common types of OB/GYN issues, including sexual assault, that a nurse could see in the ED.

In this chapter, you will learn to:
1. Discuss the possible OB/GYN conditions and emergencies that present to the ED
2. Understand the psychological implications and complexities of patients who have been sexually assaulted or are in danger of being abused
3. Anticipate the interventions

INTRODUCTION

When caring for these patients, be sure to always respect their privacy by closing doors and curtains and providing blankets for covering up. Patients may be uncomfortable talking about OB/GYN matters. It is also true that some females are not well educated about their bodies. Thus, the nurse must be sure to document a full, accurate triage and primary and secondary assessment to find the source of the patient's complaint. The ED nurse may have to ask a lot of questions to get the necessary patient history. Always be prepared for the possibility and challenges of caring for two patients in one package: mother and baby or babies.

Endometriosis

Endometriosis is a chronic disease that affects approximately 10% of females worldwide. When endometrial cells exist outside the uterus, it can have long-standing, debilitating effects on those affected. Despite this being a gynecological disease, if left untreated, it can affect other systems in the

body such as gastrointestinal, immunological, neurological, cardiovascular, and mental health (Horne & Missmer, 2022).
- *Causes:* Although the causes are not entirely known, there are studies suggesting a genetic component or a DNA variation. A common hypothesis is reflux of endometrial fragments, and "protein rich fluid through the fallopian tubes into the pelvis during menstruation is considered the most likely explanation for why endometriotic lesions form within the peritoneal cavity" (Horne & Missmer, 2022). There are also studies that support changes in brain chemistry that are associated with increased pain perception, leading to "chronic pain that is unresponsive to conventional treatment, including surgery" (Horne & Missmer, 2022).
- *Signs and symptoms:* Chronic pelvic pain (with or without relation to the patient's menstrual cycle), dysmenorrhea, pain during sex, pain with bowel movements, cancers, and pain with urination (Horne & Missmer, 2022). Additionally, patients may experience symptoms outside of the pelvis including fibromyalgia, migraines, and various types of arthritis (Horne & Missmer, 2022). Irritable bowel syndrome is a common co-occurring disease, as well as interstitial cystitis (Horne & Missmer, 2022).
- *Interventions:* Although diagnosis may take time and several interventions, in the ED, pain and symptom management should be the priority. Treatment is generally personal, requires multiple disciplines, and is taking place from multiple angles. Management should be directed by OB/GYN providers and is dependent on the severity of the patient's presenting symptoms.

Bartholin Cyst

Bartholin cyst is an obstruction/abscess of the Bartholin gland. The Bartholin gland is responsible for vaginal secretions during sexual arousal.
- *Causes:* The ducts to the gland can be blocked because of mucus, edema from infection, or trauma to the area (Illingworth et al., 2020). Possible types of trauma include an episiotomy or childbirth (Lee & Wittler, 2023). The cysts can sometimes evolve into an abscess, which is typically filled with nonpurulent fluid that is contaminated with *Staphylococcus*, *Streptococcus*, or *Escherichia. coli* (Lee & Wittler, 2023).
- *Signs and symptoms:* Although many Bartholin gland cysts are asymptomatic and are incidental findings on pelvic exams, patients may experience symptoms. They may experience pain or discomfort during activity like walking, sitting, standing, or sex. They may also experience drainage from the area (Lee & Wittler, 2023).
- *Interventions:* Inquire about duration of symptoms and any tenderness the patient may experience during activity. Additional symptoms to inquire about are any drainage, vaginal bleeding or discharge, or concern about possible sexually transmitted diseases (STDs; Lee & Wittler, 2023). Anticipate chaperoning the pelvic exam and participating in collection

of any samples that may be collected. Be sure to document participation in the pelvic exam appropriately, as well as labeling and handling any samples collected during the exam. Cysts generally do not require additional treatment. If abscesses form and drain spontaneously, sitz baths and over-the-counter analgesics are the mainstay for treatment (Lee & Wittler, 2023). Patients may require an incision and drainage, with or without the insertion of a catheter, to allow for the abscess to drain. Nurses may be asked to prepare the tools needed for this procedure and any local anesthetics that may be prescribed such as lidocaine. After completion of the procedure, nurses should educate the patient on how to care for the area and any antibiotics that may need to be completed (Lee & Wittler, 2023).

Vaginitis

"Vaginitis" is a general term for an altered vaginal flora pH and encompasses several subcategories of infection, with the most common being bacterial vaginosis (BV; Marnach et al., 2022).

- *Causes:* Vaginitis can be caused by many things such as cancers, pelvic inflammatory disease (PID), ulcerative conditions such as herpes simplex virus, vaginal fistulas, trauma, or other dermatological diseases, but it is most often caused by BV. Common pathogens for BV include *Candida vulvovaginitis*, *Trichomonas vaginalis*, or a mix of these pathogens potentially also including *Mycoplasma* or *Ureaplasma* (Marnach et al., 2022). Furthermore, cervicitis, which may be independent or concomitant with BV, is commonly caused by *Neisseria gonorrhea* and *Chlamydia trachomatis* (Marnach et al., 2022).
- *Signs and symptoms:* Odor, irritation, burning, pruritus, dysuria, pain with intercourse, or changes to vaginal discharge (Marnach et al., 2022).
- *Interventions:* Prepare for pelvic exam with culture specimen collection as ordered; be sure to document participation in the exam appropriately as witness and assistant. Administer antibiotics or other medications as prescribed. Educate the patient on the importance of completing antibiotic therapy and having active partners tested if concerns for sexually transmitted diseases arise.

Pelvic Inflammatory Disease

PID is a vaginal bacterial infection that ascends into and beyond the cervix, involving the uterus, fallopian tubes, ovaries, and peritoneum. If left untreated, PID can lead to serious long-term consequences such as ectopic pregnancies, infertility, and chronic pain (Shroff, 2023).

- *Causes:* Typically caused by *C trachomatis*, *N gonorrhoeae*, and other bacteria-associated pathogens of the vagina (Shroff, 2023).
- *Signs and symptoms:* Many females are asymptomatic prior to being diagnosed with PID through a vaginal exam. When symptoms occur, they include vaginal discharge, intermittent bleeding between menses

or following sexual intercourse, dysuria, or pain during intercourse. Additionally, once infection spreads further past the vagina and cervix, patients may experience fevers; lower back, abdominal, or pelvic pain; nausea or vomiting;, or right upper quadrant pain, though this is less common (Shroff, 2023).
- *Interventions:* Prepare for a pelvic exam and collection of cultures. Document participation in pelvic exam as witness and assistant as appropriate. Anticipate and administer orders for antibiotics to be given both by IM injection and by mouth (PO). If the patient is experiencing significant symptoms such as fever, nausea, or vomiting and is unable to be discharged, anticipate the patient being admitted to undergo IV antibiotic therapy until the patient can be transitioned to PO (Shroff, 2023). Educate the patient on the importance of antibiotic therapy completion and abstaining from sexual intercourse until 1 week after antibiotic therapy (Shroff, 2023). Encourage them to reach out to sexual partners they have had within the last 60 days to be tested for infections, and inform the patient that anonymous disclosure is possible through the help of the local Department of Public Health (Shroff, 2023).

FAST FACTS

More than 1.5 million cases of chlamydia and gonorrhea were reported in the United States in 2020.

Sexual Assault

"Sexual violence" as defined by the Centers for Disease Control and Prevention (CDC) is a "sexual act that is committed or attempted by another person without freely given consent of the victim or against someone who is unable to consent or refuse" (Yemane & Sokkary, 2022). Healthcare providers are in an important position to assess and help those who may be victims of sexual or intimate partner violence. Screening for all patients is important because it helps to identify those at risk or in need of assistance. Screening for domestic violence may be part of a hospital's triage protocol and should be completed in private. Depending on the presenting complaint or who the patient is accompanied by, the triage or bedside nurse may have to be creative in their approach to this set of questions.

The following statistics from the National Sexual Violence Resource Center were found regarding sexual assault in the United States (Statistics, n.d.):
- One in five females experienced completed or attempted rape during their lifetime.
- A reported 24.8% of males experience some form of contact sexual violence in their lifetime.

- In 2018, an estimated 734,630 people in the United States reported threatened, attempted, or completed rape.
- About 51% of females report being raped by an intimate partner and 40.8% by an acquaintance; males report 52.4% of rape being perpetrated by an acquaintance and 15.2% by a stranger.

FAST FACTS

Victims of rape have an estimated cost of $122,461 as a result of lifelong effects.

If a sexual assault victim presents to the ED, hospitals may or may not have a sexual assault nurse examiner (SANE) available to conduct the sexual assault kit. In addition to the kit itself that is used to collect specimens and possible evidence, the SANE provides support and crisis intervention, resources for after the ED visit to support medical and emotional needs, and treatment if necessary (Torregosa & Benavides, 2025). In the absence of this resource, there is a chance that the bedside nurse caring for that patient will be asked to assist in a sexual assault exam, or "rape kit." It is important to remember that simply because patients present to the ED with a chief complaint of sexual assault, they may not want a kit completed or not understand that it is even an option. If the patient decides to participate in a kit for evidence collection, it is important to remember and educate the patient that each step of the kit is voluntary, meaning they can opt out of any portion or the entire exam if they so choose (Ladd & Seda, 2023). If they refuse a full or partial kit for evidence collection, bloodwork, some pelvic swabs, and urine can be collected to test for HIV, hepatitis B and C, syphilis, pregnancy, gonorrhea, chlamydia, *Trichomonas*, and urine drug screen. Be sure to reinforce education about prophylactic treatment for pregnancy (emergency contraception), antibiotics (sexually transmitted infection [STI]/STD exposure), and antivirals (HIV prophylaxis; Farahi & McEachern, 2021).

Although the focus may fall on evidence collection and treatment of potential complications such as acquired disease or unwanted pregnancy, be sure to do a thorough assessment of any other medical needs that may need tending to. If the patient sustained physical violence beyond the sexual nature or has additional medical needs that require treatment, these also need to be addressed in a timely manner (Ladd & Seda, 2023). Education regarding follow-up after the patient's ED presentation is also vital in the recovery process. This allows for additional testing to ensure any and all STIs are treated and repeat pregnancy and HIV testing is completed, as well as hepatitis C. Furthermore, appointments as far as 12 to 24 weeks out may need to be scheduled for follow-up of HIV and hepatitis C screening to allow time for viral loads to mount (Ladd & Seda, 2023). These follow-up appointments also allow for check-ins from a psychological standpoint to see how the patient is coping with the incident and if intervention is needed.

Sex or Human Trafficking

Human trafficking "involves the use of force, fraud, or coercion to obtain some type of labor or commercial sex act" (U.S. Department of Homeland Security, 2022). Human trafficking is a $150 billion industry internationally, with an estimated 40.3 million victims being involved in what is considered modern-day slavery (Toney-Butler et al., 2023).

- *Causes:* Adverse childhood experiences (ACEs) are thought to increase risk-taking behavior. This behavior predisposes people to be sought out by traffickers. When people are victims of ACEs, evidence shows their neurodevelopment is disrupted or stunted. Social, emotional, and cognitive impairments can lead to high-risk behavior (Toney-Butler et al., 2023). This high-risk behavior can further lead to disease, disability, and social problems (Toney-Butler et al., 2023). Victims of sexual abuse often grow to participate in substance abuse, have mental health issues, and lack social norms (Toney-Butler et al., 2023). Traffickers are often seen as rescuers of this developmental group because victims are often promised a better life and security (Toney-Butler et al., 2023).
- *Signs and symptoms:* Bruising, lacerations, or hematomas in various stages of healing; poor dentition and oral hygiene; trouble hearing; signs of dehydration through dry mucous membranes; signs of strangulation or other trauma such as cigarette burns. Patients may also have concerning tattoos such as "Daddy," "Property of . . . " or "For Sale." Some may have barcodes or QR codes. Concerns of OB/GYN problems such as STIs, unplanned or unwanted pregnancies, repeated or forced abortions, changes to menstruation cycles, injuries sustained from forced sex, and retained foreign bodies may also tip off hospital staff (Toney-Butler et al., 2023). Signs of anorexia, bulimia, malnutrition, and electrolyte abnormalities could lead to cardiac problems (Toney-Butler et al., 2023).
- *Interventions:* It is important to establish a private, quiet, safe environment to assess these patients further. Using opportunities such as bathroom trips, going for testing, or requiring privacy for examination can help to create these environments. Maintain eye contact, speak slowly and clearly, and ask open-ended nonconfrontational questions (Toney-Butler et al., 2023). It is of utmost importance for the patient to feel that they are in a safe, judgement-free zone. Before opening the dialogue, ask the patient if it is safe. Simply being separated from a possible trafficker does not automatically imply safety. The patient may have a device such as a cell phone or recording device somewhere on their person that could tip off the trafficker (Toney-Butler et al., 2023). Do not make false promises. Be sure that the hospital has strategies and resources in place to use prior to encouraging them to disclose their situation. Use phrases such as "We are here to help you," "Your safety is our priority," "Help us so this does not happen to anyone else," and "You have rights, and you deserve to feel

safe and not be afraid" (Toney-Butler et al., 2023). If they are insistent on not wanting action at the time of the visit, supply them with the National Human Trafficking Hotline phone number: 1-888-373-7888. Educate the patient that they do not have to give their name to the hotline, and it is available 24/7 (Toney-Butler et al., 2023).

Ectopic Pregnancy

An ectopic pregnancy is defined as a gestational sac that implants in a location that is not the uterus. Possible implantation sites include tubal, interstitial, cesarean scar, heterotopic, cervical, ovarian, and abdominal, with the highest incidence being tubal at 95% (Mullany et al., 2023). Ectopic pregnancies are the leading cause of maternal mortality in the first trimester, accounting for 5% to 10% of pregnancy-related death (Mullany et al., 2023).

- *Causes:* Although the cause is not entirely known, almost half of patients have no known risk factors. Those who do have risk factors include prior ectopic pregnancies; damage to the fallopian tubes from prior surgery or disease; prior pelvic surgery; smoking; age >35 years; and a history of PID, endometriosis, abnormal reproductive anatomy, or pregnancies that occur in the presence of a contraceptive intrauterine device (Mullany et al., 2023).
- *Signs and symptoms:* Abdominal pain, pelvic pain of varying degrees and locations, syncope, vomiting, diarrhea, shoulder pain, urinary tract symptoms, rectal pressure, or pain with defecation. The patient may have physical findings of hemodynamic instability such as hypotension or tachycardia if the ectopic pregnancy has ruptured (Hendriks et al., 2020).
- *Interventions:* Anticipate orders to obtain either urine or serum samples for a pregnancy test, as well as a type and screen and other baseline lab tests. Monitor for sudden changes in hemodynamics and vital signs that could indicate rupture or impending instability. Once an ectopic pregnancy is confirmed through imaging, usually ultrasound, the patient may receive treatment through either medical or surgical management. Management largely depends on the estimated gestational age, size of ectopic pregnancy, impending complications, or concern for rupture. Patients may receive either an intramuscular (IM) injection of methotrexate or surgical intervention. The number of injections may depend on the beta human chorionic gonadotropin (beta-hCG) trends, and the type of surgery is dependent on several factors (Mullany et al., 2023).
- *Complications:* Rupture of the fallopian tube is a surgical emergency, and significant, uncontrolled bleeding may lead to hypovolemic shock. States of hypovolemic shock, as discussed in previous chapters, is a life-threatening condition that if left unmanaged or not managed properly could quickly result in death.

Spontaneous Abortion (Miscarriage)

Miscarriage is diagnosed as the loss of an intrauterine pregnancy before viability (Quenby et al., 2021). Viability is determined at different times in different countries, but in the United States, and according to the American Society of Reproductive Medicine, viability is defined as gestation of 20 weeks (Quenby et al., 2021). Types of miscarriages are discussed in Table 20.1.

- *Causes:* Risk factors are advanced maternal age of 45 years or older at 65%, a male partner of 40 years or older, increased body mass index, and Black ethnicity. Lifestyle choices that increase the risk of miscarriage include those who smoke and consume alcohol while pregnant, are exposed to air pollution or pesticides, have persistent stress, and work a night shift (Quenby et al., 2021). Several bacterial and viral infections have been linked to increased probability of miscarriage. *Lactobacillus organisms* deplete microbiota and are most often associated with miscarriage, though the direct cause remains unclear (Quenby et al., 2021).

RhoGAM may be ordered for Rh-negative females demonstrating signs and symptoms of ectopic pregnancy or spontaneous miscarriage when there is possibility of fetal Rh-positive blood mixing with maternal Rh-negative blood (Alves et al., 2023). Such mixing of positive and negative blood could cause a hemolytic reaction, similar to mismatched blood transfusions.

Rachel's Gift (www.rachelsgift.org) and your labor and delivery department are great resources to help provide patients with infant loss and grief support. Be sure to verify hospital policy for administration and observation of the patient following administration.

FAST FACTS

In some hospital systems, RhoGAM is considered a blood product, though nontraditional when compared with packed red blood cells, whole blood, fresh frozen plasma, or platelets, and sometimes needs the same style of postadministration observation requiring vital signs and allergic reaction.

Placenta Previa

Placenta previa occurs when the placenta implants itself in the lower uterus, covering the cervical os (Jain et al., 2020). Knowing where the placenta implants is of utmost importance for either method of delivery, vaginal or cesarean. A placenta covering the cervical os could prove problematic as the baby descends into the cervix because it may block their passage. This could increase the chances of hemorrhage as the fetal head pushes through the cervix, taking the placenta with it. Alternatively, if the patient undergoes a cesarean delivery, the potential for hemorrhage during incision (Kerr incision) increases significantly (Jain et al., 2020). Because of the abnormal placement, all females with placenta previa have an inherent increased risk of morbidly adherent placenta, meaning the placenta adheres abnormally deep into the uterus (Jain et al., 2020). Additionally, they are at inherent increased risk of vasa previa, especially if the cord is inserted inappropriately close to

TABLE 20.1

Types of Miscarriages

Diagnosis	Symptoms	Physical Findings	Treatment
Threatened pregnancy loss	■ Bleeding ■ Cramping	■ Cervical os is closed.	■ Serial ultrasounds and beta-hCG levels if further bleeding occurs or until location of the gestation can be verified. ■ Progesterone supplementation in patients with a history of miscarriage or short cervical length (<25 mm) may be recommended.[1]
Incomplete pregnancy loss	■ Moderate to severe bleeding ■ Cramping ■ Expulsion of tissue/clots	■ Cervical os is open. ■ POC may be visible at the cervical os.	■ Management of hemorrhagic hypovolemia and fever (concerning for septic miscarriage) ■ Expectant, medical, and surgical approaches ■ Expectant: allowing the natural process of miscarriage to progress without intervention, as long as the patient is not showing signs of infection ■ Medical: vaginal misoprostol, with potential additional doses between 3 hours and 7 days later ■ Surgical: indicated in patients who are hemodynamically unstable, those at risk of hemorrhage or septic miscarriage, or those who failed other miscarriage pathways[2]
Complete pregnancy loss	■ Resolution of bleeding and cramping ■ Reported passage of tissue/clots by patient	■ Cervical os is closed.	■ No treatment is required, pregnancy tissue has already evacuated the uterus.[3]
Septic miscarriage	■ Bleeding ■ Cramping pelvic pain ■ Fever ■ Attempted self-induced abortion	■ Significant uterine tenderness to palpation ■ Purulent discharge ■ Signs of sepsis	■ Hemodynamic stability and appropriate emergency resuscitation ■ Empiric broad-spectrum antibiotics ■ Surgical intervention to remove POC

POC, products of conception.

Source: [1]Mouri, M., Hall, H., & Rupp, T. (2024, February 12). *Threatened miscarriage.* In StatPearls [Internet]. StatPearls Publishing. Retrieved August 26, 2025, from https://www.ncbi.nlm.nih.gov/books/NBK430747/; [2]Redinger, A., & Nguyen, H. (2024, February 12). *Incomplete miscarriage.* In StatPearls [Internet]. StatPearls Publishing. Retrieved August 26, 2025, from https://www.ncbi.nlm.nih.gov/books/NBK559071/; [3]Nankoo, M., & Chorro-Mari, V. (2022, May 27). Miscarriage: Causes, prevention and counselling. *The Pharmaceutical Journal.* https://pharmaceutical-journal.com/article/ld/miscarriage-causes-prevention-and-counselling#types.

the cervical os (Jain et al., 2020). The placenta is an organ that develops during gestation, and with it comes many functions, responsibilities, and risks. Although significant knowledge of the detail of the placenta is not necessary to function in the ED, knowing possible risks if a patient shows up with an imminent birth can help to prepare the ED team, or the hospital's OB team, to anticipate the needs of that patient and their unborn baby.

- *Causes:* Although the true cause is unknown, risk factors for placenta previa include prior spontaneous abortion, prior induced abortion, a male fetus, smoking, advanced maternal age, previous C-section, and assisted reproductive techniques such as in vitro fertilization (Jenabi et al., 2022).
- *Signs and symptoms:* Painless vaginal bleeding during the second and third trimester. Bleeding may be preceded by intercourse, vaginal exams, labor, or sometimes without cause (Anderson-Bagga & Sze, 2023).
- *Interventions:* If the patient presents to the ED and is in labor where birth is imminent, notify labor and delivery as soon as possible. Anticipate the possibility of a postpartum hemorrhage and activate any postpartum hemorrhage protocol that the hospital has in place. Attempt to avoid digital or speculum cervical exams when bright red blood is present to decrease risk of hemorrhage. Patients diagnosed with placenta previa are generally scheduled for an elective C-section between 36 and 37 weeks' gestation. Fetal heart monitoring should be initiated. Establish IV access and draw baseline lab tests, including a complete blood count (CBC), type and screen, and coagulation studies. If significant bleeding is already present, a type and crossmatch for 2 to 4 units of blood should be prepared (Anderson-Bagga & Sze, 2023). If the patient's delivery is <36 weeks' gestation, they should receive magnesium sulfate for fetal neuroprotection and steroids for lung development (Anderson-Bagga & Sze, 2023).

Abruptio Placentae

Abruptio placentae, or placental abruption, is when the placenta separates from the wall of the uterus prior to delivery of the fetus (Brandt & Ananth, 2023).

- *Causes:* Although there is no direct correlation, chronic processes of thrombosis, inflammation, infection, and vasculopathy can trigger abruption (Brandt & Ananth, 2023). Abdominal trauma could also lead to abruption because of mechanical or shearing forces. Rapid decompression of the uterus can also lead to an abruption after the birth of the first of twins or multiple fetuses (Brandt & Ananth, 2023). Other risks for abruption are preeclampsia (increased by fourfold to sixfold), pregestational and gestational diabetes, premature rupture of membranes, chorioamnionitis, oligohydramnios, iron deficiency anemia, infection, folate deficiency, and hyperhomocysteinemia (Brandt & Ananth, 2023).
- *Signs and symptoms:* Vaginal bleeding; abdominal pain; several variations of abnormal fetal heart patterns; signs of hemorrhage shock such as

hypotension and tachycardia. The degree of abruption is classified as acute versus chronic, which is characterized by color of, number of episodes of, and amount of blood lost during bleeding (Brandt & Ananth, 2023).
- *Interventions:* Maternal stabilization is first and foremost. Establish IV access and anticipate fluid resuscitation. Obtain lab work consistent with a CBC, type and cross, and coagulation studies. If the patient is hemorrhaging, anticipate emergency administration of uncrossed O-negative blood products (Brandt & Ananth, 2023). Contact labor and delivery and initiate the hospital protocol for postpartum hemorrhage if one is in effect. Establish fetal heart monitoring to establish potential distress. Take note of the characteristics of contractions such as duration, frequency, and uterine characteristics during labor such as tetany, or high-frequency, low-amplitude contractions (Brandt & Ananth, 2023). After delivery of the fetus and placenta, if the patient remains in the ED, be observant and recognize signs of disseminated intravascular coagulation (DIC) early for a more favorable outcome (Brandt & Ananth, 2023).

PREGNANCY-INDUCED HYPERTENSION OR GESTATIONAL HYPERTENSION

Preeclampsia is a leading cause of maternal mortality worldwide (Karrar et al., 2024). Eclampsia, an exacerbation of preeclampsia, is a life-threatening complication in pregnancy (Magley & Hinson, 2024).

Preeclampsia

Preeclampsia is new-onset hypertension in the setting of pregnancy that is usually accompanied by proteinuria (Karrar et al., 2024). This complication is often diagnosed after 20 weeks' gestation. A spectrum of hypertensive diseases are encompassed by the term *preeclampsia,* including gestational hypertension, preeclampsia with severe features, then advancing to eclampsia and hemolysis, elevated liver enzymes, and low platelets (HELLP) syndrome (Karrar et al., 2024). The "mild range" is determined by a blood pressure of >140/90, and "severe range" is a blood pressure >160/110 (Karrar et al., 2024). The classic triad of hypertension, edema, and proteinuria is often seen in patients prior to potential end-organ dysfunction in the absence of treatment (Karrar et al., 2024).
- *Causes:* The cause is not entirely understood. The overall concept is related to uteroplacental ischemia from diffuse vasculopathy. It is thought to be related to a defective placenta with decreased blood flow, evident by numerous infarcts and arterial sclerosis (Karrar et al., 2024).
- *Signs and symptoms:* New-onset headache with no alternative diagnosis, with or without visual disturbance, that does not respond to medication. Right upper quadrant or epigastric pain with nausea and vomiting. Shortness of breath and increased swelling that is increased from baseline

may also be reported. In addition to these symptoms, two readings at least 4 hours apart of blood pressure >140/90 should raise suspicion of preeclampsia (Karrar et al., 2024). Lab values of proteinuria (24-hour urine collection) of >300 mg, thrombocytopenia (l<100 K/mm), impaired liver function (enzymes >2 times the upper normal limit), and renal insufficiency (>1.1 mg/dL, or 2 times greater than baseline) may also be present (Karrar et al., 2024).

- *Interventions:* Determine the hospital's policy on where the patient should be stabilized. If the hospital policy is to transport the patient to the labor and delivery unit, transport them following the protocol. If the policy dictates to treat the patient in the ED, monitor the patient's blood pressure. Establish IV access. Anticipate the need for continuous fetal heart monitoring and contact labor and delivery. Determine if the patient is being treated as an outpatient with antihypertensives and if they are taking them as prescribed. Anticipate orders for antihypertensives such as beta-blockers, calcium channel blockers, or vasodilators. Administer medications as prescribed, and observe closely for alleviation of symptoms or progression of preeclampsia. Antiseizure medications may also be prescribed if the preeclampsia is associated with severe features. This is generally in anticipation of the preeclampsia progressing to eclampsia (Karrar et al., 2024). The provider may consult obstetrics for further interventions or discharge parameters, as well as follow-up instructions and outpatient management.
- *Complications:* If the patient is near or at term and delivery is delayed, the patient is at increased risk for development of further complications such as "eclampsia, HELLP syndrome, pulmonary edema, myocardial infarction, acute respiratory distress syndrome, stroke, renal or retinal injury, and fetal complications including fetal growth restrictions, placental abruption, or fetal or maternal death" (Karrar et al., 2024).

Eclampsia

Sudden onset of seizures from hypertensive disorders in pregnancy is a life-threatening complication of gestation. The highest risk of eclampsia is in the first week postpartum, but it can occur at any point before, during, or after labor (Magley & Hinson, 2024). Seizures can lead to hypoxia, trauma, and aspiration, although long-term neurological damage is rare in these cases (Magley & Hinson, 2024).

- *Causes:* Preeclampsia, maternal infections, and inflammation such as periodontal disease and urinary tract infections. Maternal obesity, gestational diabetes, and other metabolic disorders are thought to be significant contributors (Magley & Hinson, 2024).
- *Signs and symptoms:* Seizure activity, with or without hypertension, because it is not always present in patients with eclampsia. If hypertension is present, >140/90 is generally the hallmark blood pressure measurement. Additionally, patients may experience severe headaches,

visual disturbances such as double or blurred vision, flashes of light, transient blindness, and epigastric pain (Magley & Hinson, 2024).
- *Interventions:* Assess the patient's airway, breathing and circulation (ABC) and establish an airway if necessary. Enable end-tidal capnography to evaluate ventilation and pulse oximetry to assess oxygenation. Position the patient in the lateral decubitus position to decrease pressure on the major vessels of the abdomen and increase blood flow. Place the patient on continuous cardiac monitoring and establish IV access. Determine if the patient is still actively pregnant or if they are postpartum because this could change the medical teams requiring notification. Notify OB and labor and delivery, and make sure the neonatal ICU (NICU) is available in the event of an imminent birth. Magnesium sulfate is the overall gold standard for antiseizure management. The recommended loading dose is 6 g IV over 15 to 20 minutes, followed by a maintenance dose of 2 g/hr. If the team is unable to establish IV access, 10 g IM is an alternative. Recurrent seizures may require additional doses of magnesium or benzodiazepines. After administration of any of these medications, be sure to monitor for respiratory depression or cardiac arrest (Magley & Hinson, 2024).

Prolapsed Cord

The cord is prolapsed when a pregnant female comes into the ED in active labor and you see the cord hanging out. **Get her to the birth center immediately.** Cord prolapse has different classifications, depending on where the cord is in relation to the cervix and whether or not the membranes are ruptured or intact. Cord prolapse has increased risk of fetal mortality and poor outcomes because of hypoxia (Wong et al., 2021).
- *Causes:* Certain risks increase development of umbilical cord prolapse. Risks include fetal malpresentation, multiple gestations, polyhydramnios, preterm rupture of membranes without proper engagement of the fetal head with the cervical os, intrauterine growth restriction, preterm delivery, and cord abnormalities; attempting external cephalic version with ruptured membranes; placement of a fetal scalp electrode for monitoring; or cervical ripening balloon (Wong et al., 2021).
- *Signs and symptoms:* Fetal bradycardia, visible cord in the cervix before or with a fetal presenting part, and recent rupture of membranes (Wong et al., 2021).
- *Interventions:* Prepare for expedient delivery, likely through a C-section. Management of the umbilical cord until delivery is possible and is of utmost importance. Funic decompression relieves pressure on the cord by elevating the fetal presenting part (Wong et al., 2021). Decompression should be done manually by using a finger or hand in the vaginal vault and gently elevating the presenting part of the cord. Place the mother in a steep Trendelenburg or knee-to-chest position. Do not try to reduce the cord back into the uterus through the os because this has been associated with increased fetal mortality. If the cord is largely present outside the

vaginal vault, keeping the cord warm and moist is important to decrease the risk of vasospasm, leading to fetal hypoxia. One method is inserting a moist tampon into the vagina after putting the presenting umbilical cord in the vaginal vault (Wong et al., 2021).

TRAUMA DURING PREGNANCY

Trauma is the "leading cause of nonobstetric maternal death" (Downing & Sjeklocha, 2023). Pregnant trauma can be significantly more complex because the team is now protecting two lives, not just one. This increase, especially in a significant trauma or unstable trauma, could require additional teams and coordination by the ED staff. Other teams to consider activating are OB/labor and delivery and anesthesiology, along with notification to the OR, NICU, and a pediatrician/pediatric surgeon (Downing & Sjeklocha, 2023).

- *Causes:* Blunt force trauma (motor vehicle accidents, falls) is the most common, followed by penetrating trauma (gunshot wounds), then burns. Interpersonal or domestic violence is also a candidate for cause (Downing & Sjeklocha, 2023).
- *Signs and symptoms:* Dependent on the type of trauma sustained.
- *Interventions:* Assess ABCs and stabilize the airway as soon as possible.
    - Anticipate a potentially difficult airway because of normal physiological changes that take place during gestation (increased mucosal edema, rhinitis, and congestion) and be prepared to assist the lead provider in intubation if requested. Keep in mind that normal physiological changes during pregnancy can alter the blood gas values if lab tests are obtained. A baseline respiratory alkalosis can be expected and does not necessarily need to be corrected, as this happens to sustain fetal development (Downing & Sjeklocha, 2023).
    - Position the patient optimally by manually displacing the uterus to the left laterally to allow for decompression of the major vessels in the abdomen (Downing & Sjeklocha, 2023). Do this while maintaining C-spine precautions and as much lower spinal precautions as possible.
    - Hypervolemia is an expected change during pregnancy, which increases the maternal blood volume in anticipation for postpartum bleeding. Patients may inadvertently mask signs of hemorrhage or shock and should be considered for massive transfusion protocol (MTP) early. Because of vasopressors reducing uterine blood flow, it is important to establish adequate blood/fluid resuscitation, then reevaluate the need for additional vasopressor management (Downing & Sjeklocha, 2023).
    - Traumatic cardiac arrest and perimortem cesarean delivery (PMCD) (Downing & Sjeklocha, 2023).
        - Advanced cardiovascular life support (ACLS, including CPR, defibrillation, and drug administration) guidelines are

consistent whether the adult patient is pregnant or not and therefore should not be altered.
- Recognition of reversible causes and rapid intervention (hemo/tension pneumothorax, cardiac tamponade, hemorrhage) are instrumental in survival.
- PMCS may prove beneficial to both mother and fetus if standard resuscitative measures fail.
  - PMCD should not be delayed more than 5 minutes if initial resuscitation is failing and the fetus is "deemed potentially viable." History, bedside fundal exam (fundus is palpable >2 cm above the umbilicus), or ultrasound may be used to determine gestational age, therefore determining viability
  - This is generally not intended to be sterile, but lifesaving. The goal is to deliver the fetus, begin resuscitation, and, in turn, increase the likelihood of maternal survival upon the evacuation of added stress (gestation) on the mother. Studies support the return of spontaneous circulation in the mother after delivery and after 15 minutes of arrest (Downing & Sjeklocha, 2023).
- Once the immediate threats have been stabilized, the secondary survey should unfold as normal, with added questions and exams regarding pregnancy. Diagnostic studies such as lab work should include a CBC, comprehensive metabolic panel (CMP), type and screen, and a Kleihauer–Betke test to determine if the maternal and fetal blood has mixed as a result of the trauma indicating a fetomaternal hemorrhage. Imaging requiring radiation (x-rays and CT scans) is the gold standard for patients with trauma. The exposure of radiation to the fetus is "dose dependent." Fetal development and risk for exposure, though a consideration, should not be a deterrent from obtaining potentially necessary imaging in a timely fashion. Obtaining imaging in the setting of pregnancy is supported by multiple organizations including the Eastern Association for the Surgery of Trauma (EAST), American College of Gynecology (ACOG), and Society of Obstetricians and Gynaecologists of Canada (SOCG) (Downing & Sjeklocha, 2023).
- Anticipate admission to the appropriate level of care after the patient has been stabilized and a disposition has been met.

FAST FACTS

Intimate partner violence is estimated to be >8% during pregnancy but may be sorely underreported or underrecognized because of a decreased likelihood to seek out medical treatment.

DELIVERY IN THE ED

An aspect of working in the ED is the possibility of a prehospital or ED delivery taking place. If a patient shows up stating they are close to delivery, consider a rapid evaluation in the ED. If the patient does not have signs of imminent birth, consider taking them to labor and delivery expeditiously and notify the unit of concern for impending birth.

- *Causes:* The patient arrives in the ED instead of the labor and delivery area, or they are unaware they are pregnant and are in labor.
- *Signs and symptoms:* A strong, reflexive urge to push or defecate that is uncontrollable (fetal ejection reflex), intense contractions at intervals of <2 minutes apart, a bulging perineum, or a crowning head or presenting fetal part (umbilical cord, buttocks, foot, and arm; Beaird et al., 2023).
- *Interventions:* Evaluate the patient for signs of imminent birth. If these signs are present, anticipate delivery in the ED. Establish access and evaluate contractions for duration, frequency, and uterine characteristics. Obtain as much of a history as possible regarding the patient's pregnancy such as gestational age; number of fetuses; prior pregnancies; and complications of pregnancy such as gestational diabetes, preeclampsia or gestational hypertension, Rh incompatibility, anemia, placenta previa, or known fetal positioning (such as the fetus is breech). Notify the labor and delivery team, and prepare the ED team to care for the newborn. Encourage the patient to push when they feel the urge and to rest in between contractions. As the head descends, encourage the patient to breathe naturally and moan low to keep the airway open. If the patient holds their breath, it encourages the Valsalva maneuver, which does not have supportive evidence (Beaird et al., 2023). Assist the provider in delivery of the fetus, while offering verbal encouragement to the patient as much as possible.
- *Following delivery:* After the infant is born, place them on the mother's chest. This initiates the start of the "golden hour": 60 minutes of bonding that allows the infant to acclimate to the world while using the mother's body heat to assist in thermoregulation. Dry the infant to stimulate crying and to decrease risk of hypothermia through evaporation. Assess the infant for breathing and adequate respiratory effort, heart rate, color, tone, and irritability. If both the mother and infant are stable and do not require immediate intervention, delay cord clamping. The cord should not be clamped until it stops pulsating, about 30 to 60 seconds following delivery (Beaird et al., 2023). Assess the cord and clamp accordingly. Suction the airways, oral then nasal.
  - If the infant does not respond to manual stimulation (drying) or demonstrate adequate respiratory effort or either patient is unstable, move the infant to the warmer to begin resuscitation.
  - Anticipate delivery of the placenta and observe for postpartum complications.
- *Provide oxygen:* Assess the infant's oxygen status and respiratory effort. If the infant requires support, use the T-piece at room air to provide pressure to open the alveoli (Nguyen et al., 2024; see Table 20.2).

TABLE 20.2
Target Neonatal Room Air Oxygen Levels Postdelivery

Time Postdelivery	Pulse Oxygen Levels
1 minute	60%–65%
2 minutes	65%–70%
3 minutes	70%–75%
4 minutes	75%–80%
5 minutes	80%–85%
10 minutes	85%–95%

Source: Nguyen, T. C., Madappa, R., Siefkes, H. M., Lim, M. J., Siddegowda, K. M., & Lakshminrusimha, S. (2024). Oxygen saturation targets in neonatal care: A narrative review. *Early Human Development*, *199*, 106134. https://doi.org/10.1016/j.earlhumdev.2024.106134.

TABLE 20.3
The Apgar Score

Sign	0	1	2
Color	Cyanotic/blue	Body pink, blue extremities	Whole body pink
Muscle tone	Limp	Some flexion	Active movement
Respirations	Absent	Slow, irregular	Good (30–60 bpm)
Heart rate	Absent	Slow (<100 bpm)	Good (100–180 bpm)
Reflex irritability (tactile stimulation)	No response	Facial grimace	Cry, cough, and sneeze

- The Apgar score is used to determine fetal status. Use Table 20.3 to determine the baby's score. You want the baby to score a perfect 10 by the 10th minute postdelivery.

Neonatal resuscitation is a specific science and can be daunting and challenging. The Neonatal Resuscitation Program (NRP) may also benefit the ED nurse on the assessment, interventions, and specific care needs of infants intradelivery and postdelivery and during the neonatal stage of life (0–30 days). Inquire with the educator of the department and see if NRP is an option.

Postpartum Hemorrhage
Postpartum hemorrhage (PPH) is defined as cumulative blood loss of 1,000 mL or more, regardless of delivery route, or blood loss with associated signs of hypovolemia (hypotension, tachycardia). Signs of hypovolemia

may not be visible in the postpartum state because of the normal physiological increase in blood volume related to gestation (Bienstock et al., 2021). Generally, symptoms do not start to appear until approximately >1,500 mL of blood has been lost as a result of this change in hemodynamics. PPH is still the leading cause of preventable illness and death globally (Bienstock et al., 2021). Despite advances in many areas of healthcare and overall development in the United States, it still has one of the highest maternal mortality rates in the developed world, with approximately 11% being contributed to PPH.

- *Causes:* The 4 Ts—uterine atony (70%), trauma (lacerations or uterine rupture, 20%), tissue (retained placenta, 10%), and thrombin (clotting-factor deficiency, DIC, <1%) (Bienstock et al., 2021).
  - *Uterine atony:* Often preceded by chorioamnionitis, use of magnesium sulfate, prolonged labor or precipitous birth, induction of labor or augmentation, uterine fibroids, uterine distention caused by multiple fetuses, fetal macrosomia, polyhydramnios, cesarean delivery, advanced maternal age, and history of more than four pregnancies (Bienstock et al., 2021).
  - *Trauma:* Lacerations can be caused by operative vaginal delivery (forceps or vacuum), precipitous birth, or episiotomy (Bienstock et al., 2021).
  - *Tissue:* Caused by placenta accreta, placenta increta, or placenta percreta (Bienstock et al., 2021).
  - *Thrombin:* Severe preeclampsia, eclampsia, HELLP syndrome, intrauterine fetal death, placental abruption, or amniotic fluid embolism (Bienstock et al., 2021).
- *Signs and symptoms:* Tachycardia, hypotension, lack of uterine tone (atony or a "boggy uterus"; Wormer et al., 2024).
- *Interventions:* Intervention is targeted toward the cause of the hemorrhage. Stabilization of hemodynamics is first. Remember ABC? In the situation of PPH, consider rearranging to circulation, airway, and breathing (CAB) to intervene on circulation first if the patient is breathing. If the patient's airway or breathing is unstable, ABCs will likely be happening simultaneously. Establish IV access. Anticipate early orders for MTP because postpartum patients do not generally show signs of hypovolemic shock from hemorrhage until over 1,500 mL of blood has been lost. Contact labor and delivery, relaying concern for PPH and a need for intervention. Measures that can be taken in the interim, especially for uterine atony, include bimanual uterine massage (fundal massage), which can be performed to encourage the uterus to contract (Bienstock et al., 2021). Monitor output of estimated blood loss.

SUMMARY

This chapter encompassed a more detailed knowledge of OB/GYN emergencies. Be sure to locate and be familiar with all OB/GYN equipment, to know how to contact labor and delivery efficiently, and to find out if there are any policies or procedures at the facility related to OB rapid response. Nothing is worse than running around trying to find supplies during an emergency. Be sure to practice assisting with a couple of pelvic examinations during orientation. Obtain a good history and ensure privacy and a safe environment. This means asking questions, such as: When did it start? Does anything make the pain worse? How many pads did you go through today? With pregnant patients, consider the fact that there may be two or more patients. Always be professional and respect every patient's privacy.

REVIEW QUESTIONS

1) In the stable newborn, how long should cord clamping be delayed?
   a. 30 to 60 seconds or until pulsatility subsides
   b. It should not; cut the cord immediately
   c. 5 minutes
   d. For however long the provider feels like
2) What is the definition of an ectopic pregnancy?
   a. A pregnancy of >20 weeks' gestation
   b. A pregnancy that is implanted outside the uterus
   c. A pregnancy that is at risk for spontaneous miscarriage
   d. A pregnancy where more than one fetus is seen on ultrasound

REFERENCES

Alves, C., Jenkins, S., & Rapp, A. (2023, October 12). *Early pregnancy loss (spontaneous abortion)*. In StatPearls [Internet]. StatPearls Publishing. Retrieved August 26, 2025, from https://www.ncbi.nlm.nih.gov/books/NBK560521/

Anderson-Bagga, F. M., & Sze, A. (2023, June 12). *Placenta previa*. In StatPearls [Internet]. StatPearls Publishing. Retrieved August 26, 2025, from https://www.ncbi.nlm.nih.gov/books/NBK539818/

Beaird, D. T., Ladd, M., Jenkins, S., & Kahwaji, C. (2023, October 26). *EMS prehospital deliveries*. In StatPearls [Internet]. StatPearls Publishing. Retrieved August 26, 2025, from https://www.ncbi.nlm.nih.gov/books/NBK525996/

Bienstock, J. L., Eke, A. C., & Hueppchen, N. A. (2021). Postpartum hemorrhage. *New England Journal of Medicine*, 384(17), 1635–1645. https://doi.org/10.1056/nejmra1513247

Brandt, J. S., & Ananth, C. V. (2023). Placental abruption at near-term and term gestations: Pathophysiology, epidemiology, diagnosis, and management. *American Journal of Obstetrics and Gynecology*, 228(5), 1313–1329. https://doi.org/10.1016/j.ajog.2022.06.059

Downing, J., & Sjeklocha, L. (2023). Trauma in pregnancy. *Emergency Medicine Clinics of North America*, 41(2), 223–245. https://doi.org/10.1016/j.emc.2022.12.001

Farahi, N., & McEachern, M. (2021, February 1). *Sexual assault of women*. American Family Physician. https://www.aafp.org/pubs/afp/issues/2021/0201/p168.html#collection-of-evidence

Hendriks, E., Rosenberg, R., & Prine, L. (2020, May 15). *Ectopic pregnancy: Diagnosis and management*. American Family Physician. https://www.aafp.org/pubs/afp/issues/2020/0515/p599.html

Horne, A. W., & Missmer, S. A. (2022). Pathophysiology, diagnosis, and management of endometriosis. *BMJ, 379*, e070750. https://doi.org/10.1136/bmj-2022-070750

Illingworth, B., Stocking, K., Showell, M., Kirk, E., & Duffy, J. (2020). Evaluation of treatments for Bartholin's cyst or abscess: A systematic review. *BJOG: An International Journal of Obstetrics and Gynaecology, 127*(6), 671–678. https://doi.org/10.1111/1471-0528.16079

Jain, V., Bos, H., & Bujold, E. (2020). Guideline No. 402: Diagnosis and management of placenta previa. *Journal of Obstetrics and Gynaecology Canada, 42*(7), 906–917. https://doi.org/10.1016/j.jogc.2019.07.019

Jenabi, E., Salimi, Z., Bashirian, S., Khazaei, S., & Ayubi, E. (2022). The risk factors associated with PLACENTA PREVIA: An umbrella review. *Placenta, 117*, 21–27. https://doi.org/10.1016/j.placenta.2021.10.009

Karrar, S. A., Martingano, D., & Hong, P. (2024, February 25). *Preeclampsia*. In StatPearls [Internet]. StatPearls Publishing. Retrieved August 26, 2025, from https://www.ncbi.nlm.nih.gov/books/NBK570611/

Ladd, M., & Seda, J. (2023, January 29). *Sexual assault evidence collection*. In StatPearls [Internet]. StatPearls Publishing. Retrieved August 26, 2025, from https://www.ncbi.nlm.nih.gov/books/NBK554497/

Lee, W., & Wittler, M. (2023, July 5). *Bartholin gland cyst*. In StatPearls [Internet]. StatPearls Publishing. Retrieved August 26, 2025, from https://www.ncbi.nlm.nih.gov/books/NBK532271/

Magley, M., & Hinson, M. (2024, October 6). *Eclampsia*. In StatPearls [Internet]. StatPearls Publishing. Retrieved August 26, 2025, from https://www.ncbi.nlm.nih.gov/books/NBK554392/

Marnach, M. L., Wygant, J. N., & Casey, P. M. (2022). Evaluation and management of vaginitis. *Mayo Clinic Proceedings, 97*(2), 347–358. https://doi.org/10.1016/j.mayocp.2021.09.022

Mullany, K., Minneci, M., Monjazeb, R., & CoiadoC. K. (2023). Overview of ectopic pregnancy diagnosis, management, and innovation. *Women's Health, 19*. https://doi.org/10.1177/17455057231160349

Nguyen, T. C., Madappa, R., Siefkes, H. M., Lim, M. J., Siddegowda, K. M., & Lakshminrusimha, S. (2024). Oxygen saturation targets in neonatal care: A narrative review. *Early Human Development, 199*, 106134. https://doi.org/10.1016/j.earlhumdev.2024.106134

Quenby, S., Gallos, I. D., Dhillon-Smith, R. K., Podesek, M., Stephenson, M. D., Fisher, J., Brosens, J. J., Brewin, J., Ramhorst, R., Lucas, E. S., McCoy, R. C., Anderson, R., Daher, S., Regan, L., Al-Memar, M., Bourne, T., MacIntyre, D. A., Rai, R., Christiansen, O. B., … Coomarasamy, A. (2021). Miscarriage matters: The epidemiological, physical, psychological, and economic costs of early pregnancy loss. *The Lancet, 397*(10285), 1658–1667. https://doi.org/10.1016/s0140-6736(21)00682-6

Shroff, S. (2023). Infectious vaginitis, cervicitis, and pelvic inflammatory disease. *Medical Clinics of North America, 107*(2), 299–315. https://doi.org/10.1016/j.mcna.2022.10.009

Statistics. (n.d.). *National sexual violence resource center*. https://www.nsvrc.org/statistics

Toney-Butler, T., Ladd, M., & Mittel, O. (2023, June 11). *Human trafficking*. In StatPearls [Internet]. StatPearls Publishing. Retrieved August 26, 2025, from https://www.ncbi.nlm.nih.gov/books/NBK430910/

Torregosa, M. B., & Benavides, M. D. R. (2025). Becoming a sexual assault nurse examiner. *The Clinical Teacher, 22*(2), e70059. https://doi.org/10.1111/tct.70059

U.S. Department of Homeland Security. (2022, September 22). *What is human trafficking?* https://www.dhs.gov/blue-campaign/what-human-trafficking

Wong, L., Kwan, A. H., Lau, S. L., Sin, W. T., & Leung, T. Y. (2021). Umbilical cord prolapse: Revisiting its definition and management. *American Journal of Obstetrics and Gynecology, 225*(4), 357–366. https://doi.org/10.1016/j.ajog.2021.06.077

Wormer, K., Jamil, R., & Bryant, S. (2024, July 19). *Postpartum hemorrhage.* In StatPearls [Internet]. StatPearls Publishing. Retrieved August 26, 2025, from https://www.ncbi.nlm.nih.gov/books/NBK499988/

Yemane, R. E. H., & Sokkary, N. (2022). Sexual assault/domestic violence. *Obstetrics and Gynecology Clinics of North America, 49*(3), 581–590. https://doi.org/10.1016/j.ogc.2022.02.020

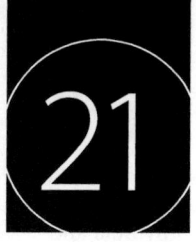

Mental Health Emergencies

Alexander Menard

> *Mental health emergencies are happening everywhere. The ED is a likely location where nurses will engage with patients with mental health emergencies. This chapter reviews some common mental health emergencies and provides some simple interventions to make these patient encounters safe and beneficial for the patient and nurse.*

In this chapter, you will learn to:
1. Discuss the common mental health emergencies presenting to the ED
2. Identify the signs and symptoms of mental health emergencies
3. Review the interventions to address mental health emergencies

MENTAL HEALTH

Mental health emergencies may not be everyone's favorite topic. We can all empathize; everyone experiences anxiety, stress, anger, and depression in their lives, but some people become suicidal, violent, or psychotic. Mental health patients may be difficult to treat at times, particularly when they engage in disruptive behavior. At times, security, antianxiety medication, seclusion, and restraints may be necessary for short periods to maintain patient safety. However, restraints should be a last resort after the least restrictive measures have been attempted. Restraint legal documentation requirements can be intense and vary according to the purpose (medical/nonviolent vs. violent behavior). Take the time to learn the various restraint documentation requirements at your facility. Be aware that state suicide intent documentation does not always necessitate restraints and vice versa. Your priority must always be to maintain safety for yourself, your staff members, your patient, and other patients. However, you will find that most mental health patients respond better if you listen, respect their personal space, and educate them on all procedures clearly and early on (Buettner, 2022).

Anxiety
Anxiety is a vague feeling of apprehension, tension, and uneasiness that can be divided into four levels: mild, moderate, severe, and panic.
- *Causes:* Usually some sort of stressor, but it varies with the individual and their circumstances.
  - *Signs and symptoms by level:*
    - *Mild:* Minimal muscle tension; normal vital signs; constricted normal pupils; random controlled thoughts; and appearance of calm.
    - *Moderate:* Normal to slightly elevated vital signs; tension; excited behavior; alertness; optimum state for problem-solving and learning; attentiveness; and energization.
    - *Severe:* Flight-or-fight response; tachycardia; tachypnea; hypertension; diaphoretic; urinary urgency; diarrhea; dry mouth; dilated pupils; difficulty in problem-solving; feeling overwhelmed; and decreased appetite.
    - *Panic:* Faint feeling or syncope from sympathetic nervous system release; pallor; hyperventilation; hypertension; pain; weakness; lack of coordination; choking or gasping sensation; chest pressure or lump in throat; helplessness; and shortness of breath; may become angry, combative, withdrawn, or tearful.
- *Interventions:* Maintain calm and private environment; reduce stimulation; stay with the patient or have a support person stay; use simple repetitive communication; encourage verbalization of feelings; administer antianxiety/analgesic medications; evaluate effectiveness of medications; and teach relaxation/breathing techniques.

Posttraumatic Stress Disorder
The disorder is a reaction to overwhelmingly traumatic events.
- *Causes:* A traumatic or overwhelming event such as military combat, rape, and natural or manufactured disaster.
- *Signs and symptoms:* Signs of anxiety, hyperarousal, or stress; recurring dreams or flashbacks, which may be accompanied by dissociative reactions; explosive anger; increased substance abuse; sleep disturbances; difficulty concentrating; avoidance of activities surrounding the event; and feelings of guilt.
- *Interventions:* Assess suicidal/homicidal ideations; assess anxiety levels; provide therapeutic listening; avoid judgment; and provide referrals for group or individual counseling.

Depression
Depression is a state of sadness or hopelessness that affects one mentally and physically. Short periods of depression following a specific event, such as divorce or death, are natural and resolve in time. However, clinical depression related to chemical or hormonal imbalances may require medication and therapy for either a certain period or a lifetime.

- *Causes:* Vary by individual and circumstances. May be the natural result of a specific event, such as divorce or death, or may be more situational. If, however, it is the result of hormonal or chemical imbalances, the condition may require prolonged treatment.
- *Signs and symptoms:* Sad mood; lack of interest in or pleasure from activities; insomnia or hypersomnia; fatigue; feelings of guilt or worthlessness; inability to think or concentrate; inability to make decisions; anorexia; and suicidal ideation or attempt.
- *Interventions:* Assess suicide risk; discuss patient's emotional state; show interest and concern; and provide choices. Antidepressants are rarely administered in the ED; they are not usually effective for the first week or two.

FAST FACTS

Depression is a state of sadness or hopelessness that affects one mentally and physically.

Suicide

Suicide is an intentional self-inflicted death. Suicidal actions include suicidal thoughts, threats, gestures, and attempts.

- *Causes:* Vary by individual and circumstance. There are, however, common risk factors: male; age older than 65 years; White; substance, physical, sexual, mental, or emotional abuse; depression; family history of or prior suicide attempt; terminal or chronic illness; psychosis; living alone; recent change/loss in life; and low self-esteem.
- *Signs and symptoms:* Previous suicide attempts; verbal statements of suicidal thoughts; giving away favorite items; writing a will; depressed mood; isolated; and withdrawn.
- *Interventions:* Create a safe room for the patient; have security scan the patient with a metal detection device and remove any potentially dangerous objects or contraband from the patient and the room. Dress the patient in a suicidal safe gown and secure any personal belongings. Document according to hospital policy for high-risk or suicidal patients. Engage in one-on-one observations; encourage verbal expression of feelings and thoughts; promote hope; obtain lab tests as ordered for medical clearance; and obtain mental health evaluation. Assessment questions are listed as follows:
    - Are you having thoughts about ending your life?
    - If you had a way, would you try to take your own life?
    - Have you ever had specific thoughts or plans about ending your own life?
    - Have you set a time or place?
    - What are these plans?

- Do you have access to _____ [this method]?
- Have you done anything or made preparations to take your own life?

Another option for assessment is the SAD PERSONS Scale (Table 21.1). This tool is a clinical assessment to determine suicide risk.

Violent or Aggressive Behavior

This is behavior that has harmed or may result in harm to the patient or others.

- *Causes:* Many factors can trigger aggressive behavior, including alcohol, drugs, or long waiting times in the ED.
- *Signs and symptoms:* Loud/threatening speech; yelling profanities; bragging about past violence; demanding personality; pacing; acting tense; clenching fists; slamming, pushing, or throwing objects; alcohol odor; or other unusual behavior.
- *Interventions:* Stay calm; speak softly, slowly, and clearly; respect the patient's personal space; provide brief and honest facts; be an empathetic listener; encourage the patient to verbalize feelings; provide "show of force" with security if needed; restrain as last resort; administer medications as ordered and as necessary; and document all interventions and behaviors.

TABLE 21.1

SAD PERSONS Scale

Risk Factors	Points
S—Sex	1 point if male; 0 if female
A—Age	1 point for age <20 or >44
D—Depression	1 point if present
P—Previous attempt	1 point if present
E—Ethanol abuse	1 point if present
R—Rational thinking loss	1 point if present
S—Social support lacking	1 point if present
O—Organized plan	1 point if plan is made and lethal
N—No spouse	1 if divorced, widowed, separated, or single
S—Sickness	1 if chronic, debilitating, and severe
Total Points	**Risk Assessment**
0–5	Low: may be safe for discharge
5–8	Moderate: possible mental health consult required
8–10	High: possible mental health admission

> **FAST FACTS**
>
> There are some people you cannot make happy no matter what you do. When you have tried everything listed previously, tell the person you will find someone to help and calmly *walk away*. Then chart the person's behavior and your interventions. Notify your charge nurse or supervisor that you require assistance. Safety first!

Psychosis

Psychosis is defined as a grossly impaired sense of reality. It is commonly associated with schizophrenia, which usually includes "negative symptoms," such as difficulty forming social and coherent conversations.

- *Causes:* Origin may be unknown, but the patient must be medically cleared. Some brain injuries, chemical imbalances, loss, separation, rejection, and use of illicit drugs can also cause psychosis.
- *Signs and symptoms:* Delusions; hallucinations; disorganized speech or behavior; catatonia; paranoia; poverty of speech; and flat affect.
- *Interventions:* Reorient to reality; maintain calm professional manner; explain unseen noises, voices, and activities clearly and simply; give haloperidol (Haldol) as ordered; and respect the patient's personal space.

Manic Behavior

Manic behavior is an elevated, unstable, or irritable mood. Bipolar disorder includes manic and depressive behaviors.

- *Causes:* Bipolar disorder and drug use are common.
- *Signs and symptoms:* Euphoria; grandiosity; insomnia; flight of ideas; aggression; easily distracted; impulsive; increased motor activity; and pressured speech (i.e., very talkative). It can be difficult to get one word in with these patients.
- *Interventions:* Reduce stimuli; obtain urine drug screen and lithium level as ordered; reorient to reality; use "show of force" as needed with security personnel for aggressive behavior; set limits on manipulative/negative behavior; and restrain as needed for safety according to policy.

> **FAST FACTS**
>
> Manic behavior is an elevated, unstable, or irritable mood.

SUMMARY

You should now have a better understanding of mental health emergencies and how to handle them. From sad and suicidal patients to loud and schizophrenic patients, you never know what kind of mental health challenge you will face. Nevertheless, your mental health patients will respond better when you remain calm, speak concisely, respect personal space, and inform patients of upcoming procedures. Document carefully and become familiar with your state's and facility's legal forms and policies regarding suicide, restraints, and seclusion. In addition, know how to get a hold of security personnel if you need them right away.

REVIEW QUESTIONS

1) A 22-year-old female is brought to the ED by her roommate, who reports that the patient has been isolating herself, giving away personal belongings, and recently mentioned "everyone would be better off without me." What should the nurse do?
   a. Encourage the patient to express her feelings and schedule outpatient counseling.
   b. Assess the patient's suicide risk, including intent, plan, and means.
   c. Provide reassurance and contact a family member for emotional support.
   d. Give the patient time alone to reflect on her emotions.
2) A 40-year-old male with a history of schizophrenia is brought to the ED by police for aggressive behavior in public. Upon arrival, the patient is agitated, pacing, shouting, and refusing to answer questions. What is the nurse's best initial approach?
   a. Stand close to the patient and use direct eye contact to establish authority.
   b. Restrain the patient to prevent harm to staff and others.
   c. Immediately administer a sedative to prevent escalation.
   d. Speak calmly, offer space, and use de-escalation techniques.

REFERENCE

Buettner, J. R. (2022). *Fast facts for the ER nurse: Guide to a successful emergency department orientation*. Springer Publishing Company.

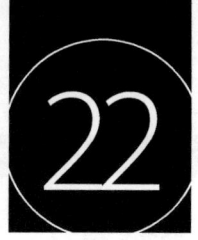

Pediatric Emergencies

Sarah Berry

> Pediatric patients are a population unto their own. *"This is not [emergency medicine] in miniature. These are the tiny humans. These are children. They believe in magic. They play pretend. There is fairy dust in their IV bags. They hope, and they cross their fingers, and they make wishes. And that's what makes them more resilient than adults. They recover fast, survive worse, they believe. In Peds., we have miracles and magic. In Peds., anything is possible . . ."*
> —*Arizona Robbins, Grey's Anatomy*

In this chapter, you will learn to:
1. Identify the common pediatric conditions and their treatments performed in the ED
2. Better understand how to participate in the care of children
3. Understand when pediatric vital signs are abnormal

INTRODUCTION

Children can be some of the most delightful and yet scariest patients. Why scary? For two reasons. First, children cannot always explain what is wrong. Assessing thoroughly, asking age-appropriate questions, and listening to the parents can establish a decent baseline. Although sometimes challenging, family-centered care is crucial, and parents generally know when something is wrong with their babies. Second, children may look okay when they are actually in distress because they are good at compensating. When they can no longer compensate, they deteriorate rapidly. This does not leave the ED staff much time to resuscitate them. Therefore, treating children aggressively at the early signs of distress is critical, which include tachycardia and increased respirations. Hypotension is a late sign, which is followed by rapid deterioration. Inquire about taking a pediatric advanced life support class during orientation. Pediatric emergency nursing really is a specialty of its own, but this chapter provides some of the basic pediatric emergency nursing tools needed to succeed.

> **FAST FACTS**
>
> According to the Centers for Disease Control and Prevention (CDC), firearm-related deaths of children and adolescents in the United States in 2020 reached an all-time high of 45,222, making it the leading cause of death (Goldstick et al., 2022).

Normal Pediatric Vital Signs

Table 22.1 lists all of the pediatric vital signs according to age group. Become familiar with these vitals during orientation. Reference cards are available for purchase to keep attached to badges for quick reference. Basically, the younger the child, the lower the blood pressure and higher the heart rate and respirations will be. When obtaining vital signs from pediatric patients, remember to use age-appropriate terms. Examples could include "listen for the birdie" when waiting for the thermometer to result with the chirp, "we're going to light your finger like Rudolph" for the pulse oximeter, and "I'm going to give your arm a big squeeze" to obtain a blood pressure. For kids who move a lot, consider the "statue game." Ask the patient to "sit as still as a statue" and also sit motionless during the time interval to increase chances of compliance in the game.

Fever

A fever is defined as a temperature >100.4°F. While the numerical value is helpful, the actual appearance and behavior of the child are more telling about their status. Concerning findings of serious illness are altered levels of consciousness, irritability, and lethargy in addition to fever. When inquiring about temperature, be sure to verify the route it was obtained. In infants and young children, rectal temperatures are the most accurate. As the child ages, axillary temperatures are more feasible. Oral temperatures could be skewed with mouth breathing or with recent ingestion of a hot or cold beverage (Rose, 2021). In children, the leading cause of fever is viral illness (Rose, 2021). Patients of this population, especially young infants (younger than 3 months), are at increased risk for serious bacterial infections and require special attention (Rose, 2021).

- *Causes:* Viral infections that are generally self-limiting, respiratory syncytial virus (RSV), influenza, herpes simplex virus, *Escherichia coli*, group B streptococcus (GBS), *Staphylococcus aureus*, and *Klebsiella*. Urinary tract infections; "*S pneumoniae* and *Neisseria meningitidis* are the most common causes of bacterial meningitis in children older than 1 month. The most common causes of sepsis in older infants/children include *Streptococcus pneumoniae*, *N meningitidis*, *S aureus* (including MRSA), and gram-negative enteric bacteria" (Rose, 2021).
- *Signs and symptoms:* Poor feeding; rectal temperature >100.4°F; irritability; lethargy; dry mucous membranes; decreased tear production; sunken or bulging fontanel; tachycardia; and tachypnea.

TABLE 22.1
Age-Specific Normal Vital Signs

Age	Newborn	Infant	Toddler	Preschooler	School Age	Adolescent	Adult
Respirations	40–60	30–55	22–38	22–30	16–22	12–20	12–20
Heart rate	110–170	100–160	80–150	70–120	60–100	60–100	60–100
Systolic blood pressure	55–85	65–90	70–105	95–110	100–120	110–135	130

- *Interventions:* Anticipate orders to give antipyretic medications (acetaminophen [Tylenol] = 15 mg/kg, ibuprofen [Motrin] = 10 mg/kg) by mouth or suppository, administer IV fluids for dehydration, and monitor temperature. In patients with a fever of unknown origin, anticipate a possible lumbar puncture and lab work including a blood culture, complete blood count (CBC), comprehensive metabolic panel (CMP), C-reactive protein (CRP), erythrocyte sedimentation rate (ESR), lactic acid, a respiratory panel, and urine sample. Patients may also be prescribed antibiotics for empiric coverage for possible bacterial infections. Encourage by mouth (PO) intake of fluids such as Popsicles or various juices. If the patient is unable to tolerate PO intake, IV fluids may be required. Patients who are exhibiting sepsis symptoms may require 10 to 20 mL/kg (Weiss & Fitzgerald, 2023).

FAST FACTS

When assisting a lumbar puncture, be sure to assess for bradycardia or apneic episodes that may be exacerbated by the patient's lateral decubitus position.

Epiglottitis

Epiglottitis is a rapid swelling and inflammation of the epiglottis that can lead to a life-threatening airway obstruction. This can ultimately lead to asphyxia and respiratory arrest (Sutton et al., 2024).

- *Causes:* Primarily infectious, from bacterial pathogens. More than 90% of pediatric epiglottitis is caused by *Haemophilus influenza* type b. However, several bacterial infections could lead to epiglottitis. Although viruses do not immediately cause epiglottitis, a viral infection can later lead to a bacterial superinfection, which then leads to epiglottitis. Viruses that allow a superinfection include varicella-zoster, herpes simplex, and Epstein–Barr. Noninfectious causes include trauma, thermal injuries, blind finger sweeps to remove foreign bodies in choking victims, and acute leukemia (Sutton et al., 2024).
- *Signs and symptoms:* Rapid onset of symptoms. Sore throat, dysphagia, fever, stridor, labored breathing, refusal to eat or drink, hoarseness, and anxiety. The **3 Ds—drooling, dysphagia, distress**. Use of accessory muscles, cyanosis, and tripod positioning (Sutton et al., 2024).
- *Interventions:* Avoid laying the patient flat, causing undue anxiety or stress that may lead to crying and therefore airway agitation, and imaging that requires them to lie flat. **Never use a tongue blade** to examine their throat if epiglottitis is a concern. Anticipate the need to secure the airway. Blow-by oxygen administration is viable until a further airway is needed. After securing the airway, draw the ordered lab tests and administer antibiotics and steroids as prescribed (Sutton et al., 2024).

Bronchiolitis

Bronchiolitis is a viral infection of the bronchioles, characterized by inflammation and obstruction with mucus to the smaller airways. This leads to lung hyperexpansion, alterations in lung function, atelectasis, and wheezing (Dalziel et al., 2022).

- *Causes:* Most commonly caused by RSV. Other possible causes are rhinovirus, human metapneumovirus, adenovirus, parainfluenza, influenza, human bocavirus, coronaviruses HCoV NL63 and HKU1, and *Bordetella pertussis* (Dalziel et al., 2022).
  - *Risk factors in this population:* Gestational age <37 weeks, chronological age at time of the exam <10 weeks, exposure to cigarette smoke, breastfeeding for <2 months, failure to thrive, chronic lung disease, heart or neurological conditions, and disadvantaged socioeconomic status (Dalziel et al., 2022).
- *Signs and symptoms:* Recent viral illness, rhinorrhea, fever, cough, tachypnea, increased work of breathing, use of accessory muscles and intercostal retractions, grunting or nasal flaring, and wheezing (Dalziel et al., 2022).
- *Interventions:* Interventions are symptom based, unless an investigation for sepsis is on the differential or the patient is exhibiting signs of severe respiratory distress or impending respiratory arrest. Anticipate supportive therapy such as oxygen delivery through blow-by unless the patient requires pressure support. High-flow nasal cannula or continuous positive pressure therapy may be prescribed for respiratory distress. Suction may be helpful to remove mucus, but saline nasal drops have not been shown to improve outcomes. Chest physiotherapy, including vibration and percussion, may be beneficial to mobilize deep mucus and allow for postural drainage to remove mucus. Hydration is key and can be established either PO if the patient can tolerate it or through nasogastric hydration if dehydration is severe (Dalziel et al., 2022). Prepare nebulized medications as prescribed and steroids for inflammation.

Croup

Croup is inflammation and edema of the larynx, trachea, and bronchi. It is the most common cause of acute airway obstruction in pediatric patients between the ages of 6 months and 3 years, with it peaking around 18 months (Quraishi & Lee, 2022).

- *Causes:* A viral illness (generally 24–48 hours of nasal congestion and rhinorrhea prior to cough development), with parainfluenza being the most likely culprit. Nonviral croup, also known as spasmodic croup, can be found in patients as well. Recurrent croup, with or without a viral cause, warrants a workup to determine if there is an underlying condition (Quraishi & Lee, 2022).
- *Signs and symptoms:* Low-grade fever, barking cough, stridor, hoarseness, and potential respiratory distress (Quraishi & Lee, 2022). Steeple sign

(50% of cases). Severity of croup is based on a system called the Westley score, which uses assessment findings to calculate a score (Sizar & Carr, 2023). See Table 22.2.

- *Interventions:* Treatment is generally based on exam findings, vital signs, patient presentation, and Westley score. Patients with mild scores should be given a dose of steroids. Children with moderate to severe croup may benefit from nebulized epinephrine (racemic epinephrine) and steroids. Supplemental oxygen may be required to maintain adequate oxygen saturation. Consider blow-by oxygen for patients who do not tolerate nasal cannula or are congested and breathing through their mouth. Involve parents in oxygen administration and demonstrate how to administer blow-by oxygen to their child. More than one dose of racemic epinephrine may be required if symptoms return. Moderate to severe cases should be observed for at least 4 hours for rebound symptoms once the racemic epinephrine wears off. If symptoms persist and the patient does not show improvement, admission may be warranted. Unless absolutely necessary, try to avoid agitating the patient through interventions like IV insertion. This could cause an acute exacerbation of breathing difficulty due to crying. X-ray has not been shown to make

TABLE 22.2

Westley Score for Evaluating Severity of Croup

Inspiratory stridor	- None—0 - When agitated—1 - At rest—2
Retractions	- None—0 - Mild—1 - Moderate—2 - Severe—3
Air entry	- Normal—0 - Decreased—1 - Markedly decreased—2
Cyanosis	- None—0 - When crying—4 - At rest—5
Level of consciousness	- Alert—0 - Disoriented—5
Totals	- ≤2—mild (85% of presentations) - 3–5—moderate - 6–11—severe croup - >12—impending respiratory failure (<1% of presentations)

Source: Adapted from Sizar, O., & Carr, B. (2023, July 24). *Croup*. In StatPearls [Internet]. StatPearls Publishing. Retrieved August 26, 2025, from https://www.ncbi.nlm.nih.gov/books/NBK431070/.

a difference in outcome, although about 50% of patients exhibit a steeple sign on imaging that can further confirm diagnosis (Sizar & Carr, 2023).

FAST FACTS

Pediatric intramuscular (IM) injection tips:
- Infants to 3 years—vastus lateralis (anterolateral thigh)
- 3 years and older—deltoid
- Depending on the volume, medications may need to divided into multiple sites.
  - Recruit a coworker to help administer multiple injections simultaneously.

Ask parents prior to the injection if they feel comfortable helping to hold the patient. Emphasize the importance of a strong, steady hold to ensure the patient does not move, thus decreasing the risk of injury, complication, or further pain for the patient.

New-Onset Type 1 Diabetes Mellitus

Type 1 diabetes mellitus (T1DM) is one of the most common autoimmune diseases diagnosed in childhood (Primavera et al., 2020). It is a disease that is based on the destruction of beta cells in the pancreas, leading to hyperglycemia and lifelong insulin dependence. Once children have symptoms, they have already reached a critical level of destruction of these cells, showing late stages of disease development (Primavera et al., 2020).

- *Causes:* There are several theories about risk factors, including genetics, infection, dietary, and humoral, with about 50% of predisposition being attributed to genetics.
- *Signs and symptoms:* **the 3 P's—polyuria, polydipsia, polyphagia**; additionally, nocturia (due to excessive urination), unexplained weight loss, altered mental status, dehydration/dry mucous membranes, tachycardia, hypotension, abdominal pain, nausea, vomiting, blurred vision, lethargy, decreased appetite, ketones in urine, fruity breath, and irregular breathing pattern (Kussmaul respirations) (Gomez & Sanchez, 2024).
- *Interventions:* Take a thorough history of the patient's symptoms, recent illness, and familiar predisposition. Obtain a point-of-care glucose level and report the results to a provider. Determine patient acuity based on the child's presentation and vital signs. Approximately 25% to 40% of patients with new-onset T1DM present with diabetic ketoacidosis (DKA; Calimag et al., 2023), and depending on the advancement of the disease, it could be an emergency. Patients who are showing concerning vital signs and are ill appearing should be roomed and evaluated as soon as possible. Attach cardiac monitoring; establish IV access; and obtain lab work consistent with a CBC, CMP, hemoglobin A1c, lactic acid, blood

gas, and beta-hydroxybutyrate (Calimag et al., 2023). Depending on the concern of the provider, a septic workup may be added to include blood cultures and imaging. Anticipate orders for fluid resuscitation (10 mL/kg normal saline) and then maintenance fluids, serial point-of-care testing (POCT) finger sticks to monitor response to insulin infusions (dependent on provider order but generally starts at 0.05 units/kg/hr to 0.1 units/kg/hr), CMPs to check serum potassium levels as treatment progresses, and monitoring of urine output (Calimag et al., 2023). Be mindful of changes in orders for fluids or medications because they may be altered as lab results come back or as treatment progresses. Anticipate admission to either a pediatric ICU or pediatric medical/surgical floor, depending on the severity of the patient's symptoms and response to treatment.

Child Maltreatment

The World Health Organization defines child maltreatment as "all forms of physical and emotional ill-treatment, sexual abuse, neglect, and exploitation that results in actual or potential harm to the child's health" (Gonzalez et al., 2024). There are four types of abuse: neglect, physical, psychological, and sexual. Neglect includes inadequate healthcare, education, supervision, protection from hazards, and unmet basic needs like clothing or food; neglect is the most common form of child abuse. Physical abuse is just as it sounds: beating, shaking, burning, and biting. Rib fractures are the most common finding associated with abuse. Psychological abuse consists of verbal abuse, humiliation, and acts to terrorize the child. Sexual abuse is not limited to physical acts including penetration of any nature but may include exposure to sexually explicit materials or inappropriate physical sexual contact (Gonzalez et al., 2024).

- *Causes:* Although a "cause" is not necessarily identified, risk factors exist. Child disability, unmarried mothers, maternal smoking, parental depression, domestic violence or more than two siblings at home, lack of recreational facilities, poverty, and living with an unrelated relative at home are among these risk factors (Gonzalez et al., 2024).
- *Signs and symptoms:* Injury in an infant who has not started moving independently yet, injuries in nonverbal children, or injuries inconsistent with that child's physical abilities (developmental milestones). If the mechanism of reported injury does not match the injury acquired, abuse should be investigated. The TEN 4—bruising on **T**orso, **E**ars, and **N**eck and **4** years old/younger than 4 months old is a helpful mnemonic (Gonzalez et al., 2024). Bruising in areas other than the knees and shins as well as bony prominences like the forehead should raise concern for abuse. Burns are a common form of abuse as well. Sexually inappropriate behavior exhibited by children should be a point of exploration by healthcare professionals. Additionally, if the patient appears exceptionally dirty, lacking appropriate clothes for the season, or malnourished, reporting to child protective services (CPS) should be initiated (Gonzalez et al., 2024).

- *Interventions:* Ensure stability of the patient hemodynamically and establish a safe environment. Once safety has been ensured, complete a physical exam with the provider and note any areas of injury. File a report with CPS and determine if any lab tests or imaging needs to be obtained. Document all findings, and reference numbers for cases filed with CPS in the patient's healthcare record to ensure continuity of care at follow-up appointments.

Nursemaid's Elbow (Radial Head Subluxation)

Nursemaid's elbow is a subluxation of the elbow. It is characterized by the radial head slipping under the annular ligament, leading to pain and the inability to supinate the forearm (Nardi & Schaefer, 2023).

- *Causes:* Commonly occurs when a child younger than 5 years is swung around by the arms or lifted by one arm. Pulling on a child's arm to keep them from falling can actually lead to the subluxation (Nardi & Schaefer, 2023).
- *Signs and symptoms:* The child may appear anxious or be supporting or guarding the affected arm with the opposite hand. Signs of trauma such as ecchymosis or swelling are generally absent. The arm may be partially or completely extended and pronated (Nardi & Schaefer, 2023).
- *Interventions:* Assess circulation, motor, and sensation distal to the injury, though circulation is expected to be intact with this type of injury. Anticipate orders for x-rays if fracture is suspected or if there are additional signs of trauma. Generally, a closed reduction can be completed within a few seconds without the need for conscious sedation. Explain to the patient and caregivers that a brief period of discomfort may happen, but the pain the patient is currently feeling should be resolved after just a few minutes. Encourage the parents to hold the patient to reduce stress and anxiety. No additional interventions are generally needed following reduction such as a sling or medication (Nardi & Schaefer, 2023).

Sudden Infant Death Syndrome

Sudden infant death syndrome (SIDS) is the "sudden death of an infant under one year of age which remains unexplained after a thorough case investigation, including performance of a complete autopsy, examination of the death scene, and review of the clinical history" (Willinger et al., 1991). It is the leading cause of death in children younger than 1 year (Kim & Pearson-Shaver, 2023). A massive decline in incidents has been noticed since the "Back to Sleep" campaign has been initiated (Jullien, 2021).

- *Causes:* Although a clear cause is unknown, it is suggested that suboptimal physiological responses to hypoxemia and hypercarbia, in addition to both intrinsic and extrinsic factors, are attributed (Kim & Pearson-Shaver, 2023). Supine sleeping is the number one measure to prevent SIDS (Kim & Pearson-Shaver, 2023).
- *Signs and symptoms:* Generally, infants who die of SIDS are found deceased. It is estimated that >80% of SIDS deaths occur between 12 p.m.

and 6 a.m. Loose-fitting bed clothing or blankets that cover the head are present in a large percentage of scene investigations where infants have died of SIDS (Kim & Pearson-Shaver, 2023).
- *Interventions:* Educate parents on the "Back to Sleep" campaign. A safe sleep environment of a supine position, a firm surface, no soft objects (e.g., stuffed animals) or loose bedding (ill-fitted sheets), no head coverings, no overheating (use of a fan, cool temperature room, appropriate level of clothing for sleep according to room temperature), room-sharing without bed-sharing, breastfeeding on demand (when mother is able), and use of a pacifier are all recommended to decrease the risk of SIDS (Jullien, 2021). If the parents present to the ED with a deceased child and a concern for SIDS is the underlying condition, provide comfort for the parents while resuscitative attempts or investigations are underway. If a genetic cause is of concern, advise genetic testing in the future (Kim & Pearson-Shaver, 2023).

Intussusception

Intussusception occurs when a segment of the intestines folds over on itself like a telescope. It usually involves the small bowel and, rarely, the large bowel of children ages 6 to 18 months old (Jain & Haydel, 2023).
- *Causes:* Unknown; risk factors include infections, cystic fibrosis, and intestinal polyps (Jain & Haydel, 2023).
- *Signs and symptoms:* Intermittent abdominal pain, vomiting, bloating feeling, red currant jelly stools, lethargy, and pulling the patient's knees to their chest (Jain & Haydel, 2023).
- *Interventions:* Imaging can be challenging because of its intermittent nature. Ultrasound is the most effective method of imaging for pediatric patients. Anticipate orders for an enema (type of enema is provider dependent). If the enema is unsuccessful or the intussusception is recurrent, a surgical consult may be indicated (Jain & Haydel, 2023).

SUMMARY

Pediatric emergency nursing is its own specialty. Be sure to always take account of differences between children and adults. Pediatric patients have different vital signs, deteriorate more rapidly than adults, become dehydrated more easily, and can run higher fevers. All pediatric patient medication doses are based on weight in kilograms. Remember that children cannot always tell healthcare providers what is wrong. Therefore, it is up to the nurse to obtain an accurate history and detailed physical assessment. Sometimes, the toughest challenge is defusing the hysterical parent's anger or anxiety. Parents do not always realize they are hindering or delaying care when they panic. If the situation cannot be defused, do not waste time. Have another coworker or manager handle the parent, leaving the primary nurse to care for the child. Be mindful that pediatric patients are a special group and should be treated as such.

REVIEW QUESTIONS

1) What is the recommended fluid resuscitation in children experiencing new-onset diabetes with DKA features?
   a. 2 L over 1 hour
   b. 0.05 mL/kg/hr
   c. 10 mL/kg
   d. Encourage the patient to take PO fluids to avoid having to put an IV in.
2) What is the most common form of child abuse?
   a. Sexual abuse
   b. Physical abuse
   c. Psychological abuse
   d. Neglect

REFERENCES

Calimag, A. P., Chlebek, S., Lerma, E. V., & Chaiban, J. T. (2023). Diabetic ketoacidosis. *Disease-a-Month*, *69*(3), 101418. https://doi.org/10.1016/j.disamonth.2022.101418

Dalziel, S. R., Haskell, L., O'Brien, S., Borland, M. L., Plint, A. C., Babl, F. E., & Oakley, E. (2022). Bronchiolitis. *The Lancet*, *400*(10349), 392–406. https://doi.org/10.1016/s0140-6736(22)01016-9

Goldstick, J. E., Cunningham, R. M., & Carter, P. M. (2022). Current causes of death in children and adolescents in the United States. *New England Journal of Medicine*, *386*(20), 1955–1956. https://doi.org/10.1056/nejmc2201761

Gomez, P., & Sanchez, J. (2024). Type 1 diabetes screening and diagnosis. *Endocrinology and Metabolism Clinics of North America*, *53*(1), 17–26. https://doi.org/10.1016/j.ecl.2023.09.008

Gonzalez, D., Mirabal, A. B., & McCall, J. D. (2024, July 4). *Child abuse and neglect*. In StatPearls [Internet]. StatPearls Publishing. Retrieved August 26, 2025, from https://www.ncbi.nlm.nih.gov/books/NBK459146/

Jain, S., & Haydel, M. J. (2023, April 10). *Child intussusception*. In StatPearls [Internet]. StatPearls Publishing. Retrieved August 26, 2025, from https://www.ncbi.nlm.nih.gov/books/NBK431078/

Jullien, S. (2021). Sudden infant death syndrome prevention. *BMC Pediatrics*, *21*(S1), 320. https://doi.org/10.1186/s12887-021-02536-z

Kim, H., & Pearson-Shaver, A. L. (2023, July 24). *Sudden infant death syndrome*. In StatPearls [Internet]. StatPearls Publishing. Retrieved August 26, 2025, from https://www.ncbi.nlm.nih.gov/books/NBK560807/

Nardi, N. M., & Schaefer, T. J. (2023, August 14). *Nursemaid elbow*. In StatPearls [Internet]. StatPearls Publishing. Retrieved August 26, 2025, from https://www.ncbi.nlm.nih.gov/books/NBK430777/

Primavera, M., Giannini, C., & Chiarelli, F. (2020). Prediction and prevention of type 1 diabetes. *Frontiers in Endocrinology*, *11*, 248. https://doi.org/10.3389/fendo.2020.00248

Quraishi, H., & Lee, D. J. (2022). Recurrent croup. *Pediatric Clinics of North America*, *69*(2), 319–328. https://doi.org/10.1016/j.pcl.2021.12.004

Rose, E. (2021). Pediatric fever. *Emergency Medicine Clinics of North America*, *39*(3), 627–639. https://doi.org/10.1016/j.emc.2021.04.011

Sizar, O., & Carr, B. (2023, July 24). *Croup*. In StatPearls [Internet]. StatPearls Publishing. Retrieved August 26, 2025, from https://www.ncbi.nlm.nih.gov/books/NBK431070/

Sutton, A., Guerra, A., & Waseem, M. (2024, October 5). *Epiglottitis*. In StatPearls [Internet]. StatPearls Publishing. Retrieved August 26, 2025, from https://www.ncbi.nlm.nih.gov/books/NBK430960/

Weiss, S. L., & Fitzgerald, J. C. (2023). Pediatric sepsis diagnosis, management, and sub-phenotypes. *Pediatrics, 153*(1), e2023062967. https://doi.org/10.1542/peds.2023-062967

Willinger, M., James, L. S., & Catz, C. (1991). Defining the sudden infant death syndrome (SIDS): deliberations of an expert panel convened by the National Institute of Child Health and Human Development. *Pediatric Pathology, 11*(5), 677–684. https://doi.org/10.3109/15513819109065465

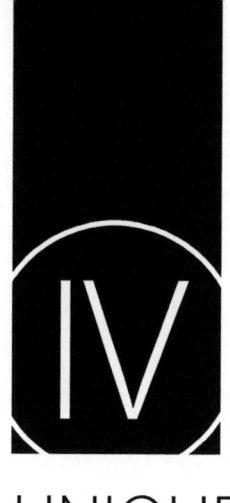

UNIQUE CIRCUMSTANCES IN ED NURSING

Disaster Management

Sarah Berry

> *Disasters happen. Whether you are in a major city or a small town, any sudden influx of patient flow either from an event or a major accident can bring the department (and the hospital) to a screeching halt. This can be anything from a multivehicle car accident, a building collapse, a mass shooting or stabbing incident, to things such as bioterrorism and chemical warfare.*

In this chapter, you will learn to:
1. Understand what to anticipate in the initial phases of a mass casualty incident (MCI)
2. Triage patients based on the START triage system
3. Recognize the signs and symptoms of different disasters, diseases, and contaminants that could be used for terrorism, leading to possible MCIs

INTRODUCTION

Any ED can become the epicenter of an MCI. Whether patients arrive via emergency medical service (EMS) or they are loaded to capacity into private vehicles and come that way, the staff has to be able to triage and manage a massive influx of patients at a moment's notice. Although there may be some warning by EMS, depending on the location of the incident in comparison to the hospital, the warning may be a large group of people limping to the entrance, screaming for help. At this point, the department must activate the protocols set in place by the hospital, develop a command center, enact appropriate personal protective equipment (PPE) for staff, and prepare a decontamination area if necessary. Then, hard work begins: triaging the sick, wounded, and broken and treating them, while still maintaining the current census in the ED, whatever that may be.

IMMEDIATE RESPONSE TO WALK-IN PATIENTS

When a sudden influx of patients come to the ED, either by EMS or by walk-in, a strategy needs to be prepared and executed immediately. Whoever is the first person to see this influx, likely through the main entrance, should notify the charge nurse and attending physician(s). The charge nurse and attending physician(s) should then activate the "mass casualty plan" or "mass influx plan" that is established at the facility. Generally, this activates a cascade of events. Administration is notified of the disaster, resources are reallocated, and staff is redirected to areas of high need, whether that be the ED, the operating room (OR), or other areas of the hospital. A command center should be set up in a large space, such as the cafeteria, to house incoming family and friends who are searching for loved ones. This helps to decompress the ED waiting room, hallways, and areas outside the ED in the hospital and centrally locates everyone for when reuniting them with their family is feasible. Registration is a vital role in this part of the initial place because hospital staff are getting wristbands and identification for everyone, getting them in the system and making them available electronically for orders and results. Many EDs keep a large dry-erase board somewhere as a working floor plan.

FAST FACTS

Consider the use of the hospital chaplain in times of crisis to connect patients to their family and friends when the patient is able to have visitors.

Patients who are already in the ED prior to the influx may need to be reevaluated for the severity of their condition. Can these patients be moved from rooms with cardiac monitors to the hall? Can they tolerate a seated position, and therefore be moved to a chair? If they are admitted and waiting for a bed, can the staff in other parts of the hospital relax on their ratios to encompass a stable patient from the ED to make room for someone who is unstable and needs the resources? Elective or nonemergency operations may be stopped or rescheduled to handle any acute surgical cases that may present. If float nurses, physicians, advanced practitioners, or nursing assistants are available who can come to the ED to be extra hands, they may be sent to facilitate moving patients upstairs or elsewhere in the hospital, answering bells or calls for help, writing orders, and seeing patients. Every little bit helps.

Setting up zones for treatment may be a viable option. Later, disaster triage is discussed. An area for each color may be helpful so everyone of that caliber is clustered together. Red tags would ideally be roomed immediately or near trauma bays or resuscitation areas. Yellow tags may be in other rooms where cardiac monitors are available. Green tags may be clustered in a room of chairs or in hallways because they require the least intervention.

Constant, open communication with the charge nurse and hospital supervisor is key. Assign an employee to track movement of patients through the flow of treatment; for example: All traffic that leaves the ED goes through one exit into the hospital. Those patients are moved either electronically or otherwise by the assigned employee so that they do not get lost in the system.

MASS CASUALTY INCIDENT TRIAGE

Preparation is key. If the department has a plan, encourage MCI drills. If the hospital never needs it, that is great. But if and when the time comes, the department can be confident in its ability to expand, adapt, and overcome in the face of disaster.

MASS CASUALTY INCIDENT TRIAGE

The World Health Organization defines MCIs as "disasters and major incidents characterized by quantity, severity, and diversity of patients that can rapidly overwhelm the ability of local medical resources to deliver comprehensive and definitive medical care" (Clarkson & Williams, 2023).

Although a few different triage systems are available, START triage is the most widely used currently in the United States (Clarkson & Williams, 2023). Commercial tags are available that some systems have on hand, but any form of identification of each category is a viable option in a pinch (Figure 23.1). Something as rudimentary as using a colored marker or writing the word on a piece of paper and stapling it to the patient's shirt can be used. See Table 23.1.

This triage process is not as extensive as other triage processes in the ED. Although traditional triage training is recommended to not be completed until 1 year of experience in the ED, the measures used to identify each

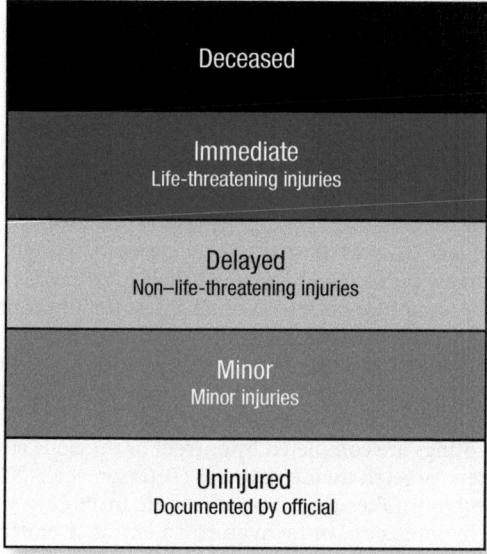

Figure 23.1 START triage card that may be used to differentiate categories of patients and be attached to them prior to treatment.
Source: New Jersey Division of Health Emergency Preparedness & Response. (n.d.). *New Jersey disaster triage tag*. https://www.nj.gov/health/ems/documents/ems-task-force/disaster_tag_presentation.pdf.

TABLE 23.1
START Triage Categories

Black	Deceased/expected to die: injuries are incompatible with life	No spontaneous respirations after repositioning the airway
Red	Immediate: severe injuries but high potential of survival, transport should be expedited	Respiratory rate >30, absent radial pulse or capillary refill >2 seconds, unable to follow simple commands
Yellow	Delayed: transport can be delayed but includes serious injuries	Respiratory rate <30, radial pulse present or capillary refill <2 seconds, able to follow commands
Green	Minor: relatively uninjured; "walking wounded," unlikely to deteriorate	Able to walk

Source: Data from Yancey, C. C., & O'Rourke, M. (2023, August 28). *Emergency department triage*. In StatPearls [Internet]. StatPearls Publishing. Retrieved August 26, 2025, from www.ncbi.nlm.nih.gov/books/NBK557583/

group in START triage are predetermined and require little investigation. Following the parameters given, any person able to perform an assessment can complete this type of triage.

MASS SHOOTING

Mass shooting has a different definition depending on the source. The victim fatality threshold is generally the determining factor, but additional criteria, including time and place, play a role. Relatively speaking, a mass shooting is defined as a shooting where three to four or more victims, possibly including the offender, are killed (Peterson et al., 2024). Mass shootings commonly take place in areas of work or commerce. Although school shootings are more largely publicized because of their high-profile victims (children), they only account for about 7% of all cases. Retail shooting accounts for 20% of all cases (Peterson et al., 2024).

- *Causes:* A total of 44% of mass shootings are completed by "insiders"—perpetrators who are current or former employees of either the establishment or the school where the shooting occurs. A total of 88% of school shootings are completed by current or previous attendees, and 30% of shooters targeted their employers (Peterson et al., 2024).
- *Signs and symptoms:* Bleeding, hemodynamic instability such as tachycardia, hypotension, or tachypnea; an entrance and/or exit wound.
- *Interventions:* Stop the bleeding. Apply a tourniquet if the wound is on an extremity; note the time the tourniquet was placed. If the wound is in a place where a tourniquet cannot be placed, such as the chest, abdomen, or head, pack the wound with gauze and apply pressure to tamponade the

bleeding. Assess for airway compromise and vital signs and determine the need for immediate intervention. Management of multiple gunshot patients can quickly deplete resources such as transfusable blood or blood products, ventilators, tranexamic acid (TXA), dressings, and OR space. Consideration of the patient's probable outcome (survivable versus nonsurvivable) may be a determining factor of intervention and resource allocation.

BIOTERRORISM

Bioterrorism is "the deliberate release of viruses, bacteria, toxins, or fungi with the goal of causing panic, mass casualties, or severe economic destruction" (Rathjen & Shahbodaghi, 2021). Thirty-seven bioterrorist attacks have taken place between 1981 and 2018. The Centers for Disease Control and Prevention (CDC) includes anthrax, botulism, the plague, smallpox, tularemia, and viral hemorrhagic fevers as category A concerns (Rathjen & Shahbodaghi, 2021).

- **Anthrax**
  - *Causes:* The release of anthrax, a naturally occurring disease—gram-positive, rod-shaped bacterium, *Bacillus anthracis*.
  - *Signs and symptoms:* Cutaneous anthrax—the most common form of infection, and the least dangerous. Mostly seen on the head, neck, forearms, and hands are areas of small, itchy blisters or bumps with edema. They are painless sores with a black center. Inhalation anthrax—fever and chills, excessive sweating, chest pain, cough, shortness of breath, altered mental status, nausea, vomiting, headache, body aches, and excessive fatigue. Gastrointestinal anthrax—fever, chills, swelling of neck or neck glands, sore throat, hoarseness, painful swallowing, nausea, bloody vomit, diarrhea, headache, red face and eyes, abdominal pain and swelling, and syncope (Centers for Disease Control and Prevention, 2025).
  - *Interventions:* Decontaminate the patient in a controlled environment ("decon shower") and bag the patient's clothing in a plastic bag. Assess vital signs and airway, breathing, and circulation (ABCs), then triage and treat appropriately. Establish IV access. Patients with concern for inhaled anthrax should receive IV ciprofloxacin and clindamycin. Cutaneous anthrax should receive oral ciprofloxacin or doxycycline, unless extensive edema or head and neck involvement are present, for which the IV regimen is recommended (Simonsen & Chatterjee, 2023).
- **Botulism:** A neurotoxin that leads to a neuroparalytic syndrome caused by *Clostridium botulinum*. It is the most potent poison known to humans, with its simplicity to produce, store, and disperse (Jeffery et al., 2024).
  - *Causes:* A neurotoxin that is gram-positive, rod-shaped, spore-forming, and an obligate anerobic.
  - *Signs and symptoms:* Diplopia, ptosis, ophthalmoparesis, dysphagia, dysphonia, dysarthria, fixed and dilated pupils, and cranial nerve

palsies (bulbar symptoms—effects on muscles involving speaking, swallowing, and facial expressions). This progresses symmetrically downward, with weakness into the trunk, extremities, and smooth muscles, ultimately leading to flaccid paralysis. The time frame of symptom onset is directly related to the amount of the toxin ingested. Eventually, the paralysis may reach the diaphragm, leading to respiratory failure, constipation, and urinary retention (Jeffery et al., 2024).

- *Interventions:* Assess the patient's ABCs and monitor their respiratory status closely. Obtain a history and try to ascertain how the patient interacted with the toxin, whether it was through food or a wound, and so forth. Discuss a Foley catheter for urinary retention. Establish IV access and anticipate orders for bloodwork and administration of botulism antitoxin. For wound botulism, debridement and antibiotic therapy of IV penicillin G or metronidazole should be administered (Jeffery et al., 2024).

- **Plague:** The plague has been infecting humans for thousands of years. It includes subtypes of bubonic, septicemia, and pneumonic, all of which result from gram-negative bacillus *Yersinia pestis* (Dillard & Juergens, 2023). It has caused three pandemics historically, including the "black death" of the 14th century in Europe. The most recent pandemic began in the 19th century and continues today in Africa after having swept through Asia and India (Dillard & Juergens, 2023).
  - *Causes:* Typically, through a bite from an infected vector (mostly rats). Transmission of pneumonic plague can be spread from person to person, with higher prevalence in warm climates (Dillard & Juergens, 2023).
  - *Signs and symptoms:* Skin lesions, but they are often not noticed. Patients then experience high fever, chills, headache, and generalized weakness. Once a bubo develops, there is intense pain near the lymph nodes, specifically inguinal, then axillary, and then cervical lymph nodes. Patients eventually progress to a shock state with hypotension and tachycardia. Other signs of plague involve cough, chest pain, and hemoptysis (Dillard & Juergens, 2023).
  - *Interventions:* Treatment is based on symptoms, and antibiotic therapy is crucial for the decrease in spread. Gentamicin is the first-line agent. Doxycycline is also a treatment option (Dillard & Juergens, 2023). The outcome of plague is generally poor and increases exponentially if left untreated with a 50% to 90% mortality rate, with pneumonic plague being >50% fatal, even with early intervention. Proper diagnosis and timely treatment decrease mortality to 5% to 15% (Dillard & Juergens, 2023).
- **Smallpox:** Variola major, also known as smallpox, is one of several viruses in the Poxviridae family. Although the other viruses in the family can cause significant illness, variola is the major human-to-human illness (Rathish et al., 2023).

- *Signs and symptoms:* Around 8 days after transmission, a sudden fever begins. By days 12 to 14, a high-grade fever, fatigue, and headache can occur. Some patients may exhibit a maculopapular rash in the mouth, pharynx, and face, which then spreads to the torso and limbs. The rash is most prominent on the face, limbs, palms, and soles of the feet (Rathish et al., 2023).

FAST FACTS

Hemorrhagic smallpox leads to petechiae and bleeding, with a high mortality rate. Flat-type smallpox has a slower onset of skin lesions and is associated with toxemia, which also has a high mortality rate (Rathish et al., 2023).

- *Interventions:* Since its eradication in 1980, routine smallpox vaccinations have been stopped, therefore leaving the general public unprotected in the event of an outbreak. If concern for smallpox arises, isolate the patient in airborne precautions to limit air transmission of the virus. Swab any open lesions for confirmatory testing and treat any presenting symptoms. There are no current antivirals or specific treatments for smallpox. If the patient presents within 4 days of a known exposure but is without symptoms, vaccinating at that time may be effective against smallpox (Rathish et al., 2023).
- **Tularemia:** *Francisella tularensis* is a gram-negative coccobacillus organism that is highly infectious. It can be inhaled, ingested, or absorbed through the skin or mucous membranes (Rathish et al., 2023).
  - *Signs and symptoms:* Ulcerations on the skin and nearby lymphadenopathy. Inhalation results in pneumonia. Ingestion leads to tonsillitis or pharyngitis (Rathish et al., 2023).
  - *Interventions:* Treatment is based on symptoms. Antibiotic regimens include IV gentamicin, and ciprofloxacin is an option in mild disease if caught early (Rathish et al., 2023).
- **Hemorrhagic fevers:** Hemorrhagic fevers encompass an extensive family of viruses that manifest in bleeding to various degrees. Four branches of the family exist: Arenaviridae (eight viruses included), Bunyaviridae (10 viruses included), Filoviridae (five viruses included), and Flaviviridae (four viruses included; Rathish et al., 2023). Although most of these viruses carry high mortality rates, the ones most recognized by the public are Ebola, which carries an extremely high fatality rate of >80% to 90%, and dengue fever, which carries a relatively low rate of fatality at 0.8% to 2.5%, but can manifest in more severe forms of the disease (Rathish et al., 2023).
  - *Signs and symptoms:* Fever, headache, malaise, arthralgia, retro-orbital eye pain, eye redness, vomiting, abdominal pain, and diarrhea. Additionally, they may present with major bleeding episodes, bleeding gums, epistaxis, and petechiae.

- *Interventions:* It is important to obtain a detailed history from patients where hemorrhagic fever viruses are a cause for concern. Travel, any new bites or scratches, or known exposures can help to narrow down otherwise nonspecific symptoms. Anticipate orders for lab tests to include a complete blood count (CBC), complete metabolic panel (CMP), type and cross, coagulation studies, a chest x-ray, a urinalysis, and a polymerase chain reaction (PCR) test for the concerning viruses. Results may indicate leukopenia, thrombocytopenia, and elevated liver enzymes. Although a vaccine is currently available in some countries, in the United States, treatment is based on supportive therapy and isolation to prevent further transmission. There is no current antiviral available (Rathish et al., 2023).

NERVE AGENTS

Among the most toxic substances known to humans are nerve agents, a subsection of organophosphates, classified into four categories. Although they are considered first-line agents in chemical warfare, these toxins are used in insecticides and contribute a great deal to modern agricultural practices (Rathish et al., 2023).

- *Causes:* When inhaled, the organophosphate compounds (OPCs), cross through the membranes of the skin and respiratory tract, binding to acetylcholine esterase, inhibiting hydrolysis of acetylcholine (a natural, and necessary, occurrence for homeostasis), leading to a cholinergic crisis. It is an irreversible process that, unless caught early, is fatal (Rathish et al., 2023).
- *Signs and symptoms:* Patients experience a cholinergic crisis, with the lungs and eyes absorbing the toxin the fastest. Patients may exhibit mitosis, productive cough, chest tightness, respiratory compromise, incontinence of urine, excessive salivation, vomiting, sweating, and abdominal pain, with seizures and significant altered mental status presenting in severe cases. **The 3 Bs—bradycardia, bronchospasm, bronchorrhea** (Rathish et al., 2023).
- *Interventions:* Because of its high transmission rate of liquid agents, healthcare workers and prehospital staff are at great risk of contamination. Don appropriate PPE (gown, gloves, face shield, mask, and eye protection) prior to interacting with contaminated patients. Decontaminate the patient by removing and containing clothing and jewelry, and wash with soapy water. Patients who are showing signs of severe poisoning, the 3 Bs, should be treated as soon as possible with a three-step system (Rathish et al., 2023).
    - *Step 1:* Atropine—5 to 10 mg IV/intraosseous (IO) every 5 minutes, titrated to desired effect (normal heart rate, improved airway capacity, and decreased production in cough)
    - *Step 2:* Pralidoxime—2 g IV/IO slow
    - *Step 3:* Appropriate support—airway management and anticonvulsants for those who do not improve with treatment

FAST FACTS

In the event of a nerve agent attack, atropine could quickly become scarce because of the volume needed for treatment. The advanced cardiovascular life support (ACLS) bradycardia protocol uses 1 mg every 3 to 5 minutes, whereas treatment for nerve agents is 5 to 10 mg every 5 minutes.

SUMMARY

Disaster scenarios and MCIs are something we as healthcare providers hope to never encounter. It can raise moral and ethical dilemmas that can cause significant stress on providers when having to allocate resources. When our norm of doing everything for one patient has to shift to doing the best we can for the greatest number of people, it creates a paradigm that can be challenging to accept. The importance of debriefing after these events cannot be overlooked. Healthcare professionals who triage patients in these situations can sometimes have difficulty with the decisions they had to make. Checking on ourselves and our coworkers, preparing for an event that we hope never comes, and being ready to establish that care if need be are resources that should never be underestimated.

REVIEW QUESTIONS

1) What is the recommended dose for atropine in the treatment of nerve agent exposure (i.e., organophosphate poisoning)?
   a. 0.5 mg every 3 to 5 minutes
   b. 1 mg every 3 to 5 minutes
   c. 5 to 10 mg every 5 minutes
   d. 1.5 mg every 5 minutes
2) Why is the smallpox vaccine no longer administered in the routine vaccination schedule?
   a. It was eradicated in 1980.
   b. The vaccine is no longer being produced; therefore, it cannot be administered.
   c. We have reached herd immunity, and it is no longer necessary.
   d. Studies showed it was useless in its endeavor to protect against the virus.

REFERENCES

Centers for Disease Control and Prevention. (2025, January 31). *About anthrax*. Centers for Disease Control and Prevention. https://www.cdc.gov/anthrax/about/index.html

Clarkson, L., & Williams, M. (2023, August 8). *EMS mass casualty triage*. In StatPearls [Internet]. StatPearls Publishing. Retrieved August 26, 2025, from https://www.ncbi.nlm.nih.gov/books/NBK459369/

Dillard, R. L., & Juergens, A. L. (2023, August 7). *Plague*. In StatPearls [Internet]. StatPearls Publishing. Retrieved August 26, 2025, from https://www.ncbi.nlm.nih.gov/books/NBK549855/

Jeffery, I. A., Nguyen, A. D., & Karim, S. (2024, November 24). *Botulism*. In StatPearls [Internet]. StatPearls Publishing. Retrieved August 26, 2025, from https://www.ncbi.nlm.nih.gov/books/NBK459273/

Peterson, J. K., Densley, J. A., Hauf, M., & Moldenhauer, J. (2024). Epidemiology of mass shootings in the United States. *Annual Review of Clinical Psychology, 20*(1), 125–148. https://doi.org/10.1146/annurev-clinpsy-081122-010256

Rathish, B., Pillay, R., Wilson, A., & Pillay, V. V. (2023, March 27). *Comprehensive review of bioterrorism*. In StatPearls [Internet]. StatPearls Publishing. Retrieved August 26, 2025, from https://www.ncbi.nlm.nih.gov/books/NBK570614/

Rathjen, N. A., & Shahbodaghi, S. D. (2021, October 15). *Bioterrorism*. American Family Physician. https://www.aafp.org/pubs/afp/issues/2021/1000/p376.html

Simonsen, K. A., & Chatterjee, K. (2023, July 23). *Anthrax*. In StatPearls [Internet]. StatPearls Publishing. Retrieved August 26, 2025, from https://www.ncbi.nlm.nih.gov/books/NBK507773/

Safety in the ED

Alexander Menard

> You must always remember that your safety is paramount. If you are not safe, you cannot do your job. Workplace violence (WPV) has been increasing for years. This chapter provides some background information and helpful tips to keep you safe in the ED.

In this chapter, you will learn to:
1. Discuss the safety concerns in the ED
2. Identify the signs of patient escalation in the ED
3. Review the interventions to de-escalate patients or families in the ED

WORKPLACE VIOLENCE

WPV is any act or threat of physical violence, harassment, intimidation, or other threatening behavior that occurs at work (Occupational Safety and Health Administration, 2025). Nurses are not immune to WPV, particularly working in the ED. According to the Bureau of Labor Statistics Census of Fatal Occupational Injuries (CFOI), of the 5,283 fatal workplace injuries that occurred in the United States in 2023, 740 were the result of violent acts. Homicides (458) accounted for 61.9% of violent acts and 8.7% of all work-related fatalities (Bureau of Labor Statistics, 2024). Violence against ED staff causes significant physical and mental distress and affects work productivity and patient care (Sachdeva et al., 2019).

FAST FACTS

Violence against ED staff causes significant physical and mental distress.

Signs of Patient or Visitor Escalation

The ability to recognize when a patient or visitor is escalating is essential. Intervening early, whether it be using de-escalation techniques or getting appropriate security or management teams, will be helpful. The majority of WPV incidents are not random and often have a set of behaviors that precede the incident. Signs of impending violence can manifest as pacing, restlessness, loud voices and excitability, erratic movements, or tense and/or angry facial expressions (Horn & Dubin, 2013; Koller 2016).

Preparation and Training

Evaluating your ED's physical environment is a good place to start. Security should be available around the clock and visible to staff, patients, and visitors (Cabilan et al., 2022). Panic buttons can be useful tools that allow staff to discreetly and emergently alert the appropriate people that a violent event is impending or occurring. Some facilities use physical barriers.

ED staff should be trained on the proper procedures to use in the event of a violent event. Simulations and drills should be done surrounding violent events and involving local responders, including police. Drills give nurses the opportunity to test their knowledge, ask questions of the experts, and identify gaps in their responses. A well-written policy for reporting, responding to, and debriefing violent events will assist staff when confronted with a violent event (Koller, 2016).

De-escalation Techniques

De-escalation techniques are designed as initial steps to address a potentially violent situation. These techniques include speaking to the person in a reassuring tone, communicating concern of personal safety to others, and using verbal reassurance (Demenchyan, 2018). Figure 24.1 provides resources for purposeful actions, verbal communications, and body language.

FAST FACTS

Safety is everyone's responsibility.

SUMMARY

In summary, WPV is increasing. Having a good understanding of the precursors to WPV and interventions to use to mitigate it is essential. Be informed about your local policies surrounding WPV, and when questions arise, ensure you are asking your leadership team. Remember: your safety is your priority—be involved in making your ED a safer place to give and receive care.

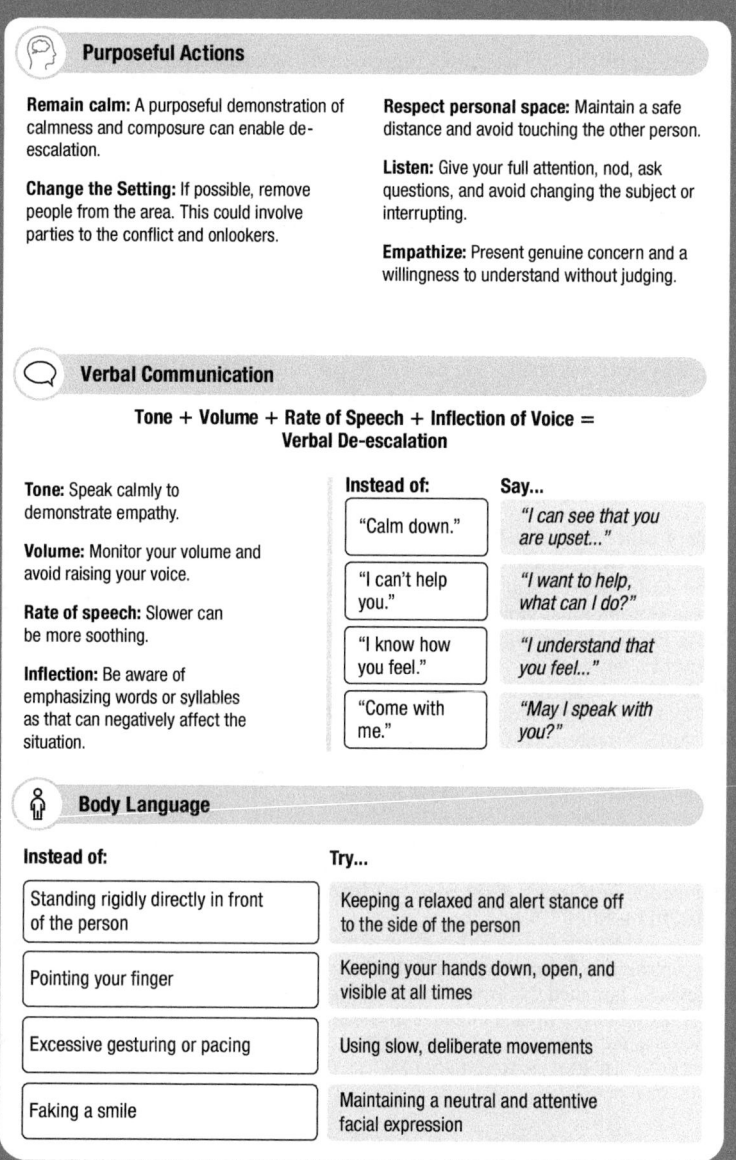

Figure 24.1 How to address or respond to escalating behaviors.

Source: Cybersecurity & Infrastructure Security Agency. www.cisa.gov/sites/default/files/2022-11/De-Escalation_Final%20508%20%2809.21.21%29.pdf.

REVIEW QUESTIONS

1) A patient in the ED becomes increasingly agitated and begins threatening staff. What is the first action the nurse can take?
   a. Prepare for physical restraint.
   b. Attempt verbal de-escalation and maintain a safe distance.
   c. Administer a sedative immediately per standing orders.
   d. Leave the patient alone to calm down.
2) A nurse in the ED is confronted by an aggressive patient who is yelling and making threatening gestures. What is the most appropriate initial nursing intervention?
   a. Speak in a calm, nonthreatening manner while maintaining a safe distance.
   b. Physically restrain the patient to prevent potential violence.
   c. Ignore the behavior and continue providing care.
   d. Threaten to call security if the patient does not calm down.

REFERENCES

Bureau of Labor Statistics. (2024). *National census of fatal occupational injuries in 2023*. U.S. Department of Labor. https://www.bls.gov/news.release/pdf/cfoi.pdf

Cabilan, C. J., Eley, R., Snoswell, C. L., & Johnston, A. N. B. (2022). What can we do about occupational violence in emergency departments? A survey of emergency staff. *Journal of Nursing Management*, 30(6), 1386–1395. https://doi.org/10.1111/jonm.13294

Dermenchyan, A. (2018). Addressing workplace violence. *Critical Care Nurse*, 38(2), 81–82. https://doi.org/10.4037/ccn2018389

Horn, A. E., & Dubin, W. R. (2013). Management of aggressive and violent behavior in the emergency department. In L. S. Zun, L. G. Chepenik, & M. N. S. Mallory (Eds.), *Behavioral emergencies for the emergency physician* (1st ed., pp. 170–176). Cambridge University Press. https://doi.org/10.1017/CBO9781139088077.028

Koller, L. H. (2016). It could never happen here: Promoting violence prevention education for emergency department nurses. *The Journal of Continuing Education in Nursing*, 47(8), 356–360. https://doi.org/10.3928/00220124-20160715-06

Occupational Safety and Health Administration. (n.d.). *Workplace violence*. U.S. Department of Labor. https://www.osha.gov/workplace-violence

Sachdeva, S., Jamshed, N., Aggarwal, P., & Kashyap, S. R. (2019, July–September). Perception of workplace violence in the emergency department. *Journal of Emergencies, Trauma, and Shock*, 12(3), 179–184. https://doi.org/10.4103/JETS.JETS_81_18. PMID: 31543640; PMCID: PMC6735201.

Tips for Success for ED Nurses

Sarah Berry

> *The cliches are true. "You can't pour from an empty cup," "Take care of yourself so you can take care of others," "Hug your loved ones a little tighter when you go home," "When you leave the house, wear underwear that you wouldn't be embarrassed about others seeing if you were in a car accident." Our careers are about taking care of others on what could be the worst days of their lives, and sometimes we carry that with us.*

Phew. Wow, that was a lot of information. How do you feel? Overwhelmed, saturated, dissociated. Maybe you feel good; a little more prepared. Preparation is everything. If you are prepared for anything, you can do anything, even if in that preparation it means you have a resource to turn to when you do not know something. It was stated at the beginning of the book that you are never expected to know *everything,* and even after a very thorough review, that still rings true.

Although there are a lot of things about being an ED nurse that one would assume to be obvious, it is very easy to get caught up in the environment. There have been several times where after you get the report, you get so consumed in the flow of the shift that before you know it, it is three o'clock, you have not had anything to eat or drink, and you have not gone to the bathroom since you left your house. As we take care of some of the sickest, most complex, most taxing, most rewarding populations, we forget to take care of ourselves. Much like in mass casualty management, resource allocation is almost exclusively lost on us and given to others.

Here are a few key reminders and little tidbits to think about as you perform your day to day activities and duties that may help to balance the need to care for yourself while caring for others.

- *Drink water:* Starting off strong with the "assume to be obvious." Many nurses will tell you they have gone an entire shift without getting a drink. This may be said out of humor, or even irritation. But it should not be said out of honor. Some ways to potentially increase your water intake would be to have a fun cup or jug. There are thousands of designs and colors out there. Pick one that appeals to you, fill it at the beginning of your shift, and sip on it throughout the day or night. Whenever you sit down to chart, take a gulp or two. If you are going to get water to give your patient nonemergent medications, take a few seconds at the water machine and get half a glass for yourself. "You can't pour from an empty cup," can be both literal and figurative in this sense, but if you are not meeting even your most basic needs, you are going to burn out taking care of someone else's.

- *Eat:* If this means stepping off the unit for 10 minutes for a snack when your patients are settled and do not have anything pressing or time sensitive, do it. You would never expect a car to run on an empty tank. Your body is the same thing. Even if you do not get to take a full lunch break, snacking on quick, healthy snacks that give you pops of energy throughout the shift can help.
- *Take breaks:* It is hard. It is hard to step away, especially if your assignment is sick or needy and ringing the bell every 5 minutes. Asking a coworker to watch your people might feel like you are asking too much or you are passing the buck. But taking care of patients requires you to take care of yourself and returning the favor to your coworker if they want it. Take a break and detach from the environment for a few minutes. A constant tax on your brain can cause situational saturation, and you might not be thinking as clearly. Allowing yourself a few minutes to step away from situations can refresh your eyes and your mind, letting you see or understand something in a way you may not have before.
- *Go to the bathroom:* You have a trauma alert coming in 10 minutes. Go to the bathroom. Even if you do not think you need to go. Our parents were right on the money growing up: "Go to the bathroom, we're leaving for the road trip soon," . . . "But I don't have to go!" . . . "Try anyway." Take a minute and go to the bathroom. You will thank yourself later when the "low-budget trauma alert" turns into a traumatic cardiac arrest with a mass transfusion, the operating room (OR) is delayed, and you are stuck in the trauma bay for 3 hours.
- *Establish a bedtime routine:* This becomes especially important if you are working night shift. Night shift can be very challenging, especially if you are not the best daytime sleeper. Establishing a routine can help to set the mood, train your brain to unwind, and prepare for sleep. Some people like to shower before bed. Watch an episode of your favorite show. Eat a light breakfast. Whatever it is, set it up, and be consistent. When it comes to daytime sleep, attempt to simulate nighttime as best you can. If this means getting room-darkening curtains or wearing a mask to cover your eyes, do what works for you. An app for white noise or a machine can help to block out daytime sounds. Your circadian rhythm is forced into reverse when you work nights. Every little bit of nighttime simulation may prove to make a big difference.

- *Establish a wake-up routine:* If you like your cup of coffee and scrolling or reading before work, set time aside to do those things. Shower before work. Take a short walk. Go the gym. Again, establish a routine that works for you and makes you happy. Nursing asks us to constantly give to others. We give our time, energy, empathy, knowledge, compassion, and advocacy. Be sure to fill your cup however makes you happy in order to pour it for others.
- *Rediscover your hobbies or discover new ones:* Nursing school is time consuming. Between classes, studying, clinicals, and maybe a job or family to tend to, we can sometimes lose the little things in life that brought us joy before. You are finished with school (for now, if you so choose), and now you are working. Finding "work/life balance" is your new challenge. It is time to rediscover your hobbies. Remember the things you used to love to do? Do them. Read, journal, play the guitar or piano that has been gathering dust. Break out your crafts or cookbooks. If you did not have a hobby or something you enjoyed before or you feel you have grown out of it, try something new. Take up baking or crocheting or a new sport. Take this newfound freedom and run with it.

All of these little things that you can do for yourself add up over time. Taking care of yourself outside of work makes it so that you can take care of others when you walk through the hospital doors. And once you are in those doors, it is time to take care of others, while being mindful of yourself and your license. Just like there are tips on caring for yourself outside of work, there are tips on caring for yourself inside of work. Some of these you have heard before because, generally, they are true. But here are a few things to think about integrating into your professional life to make the transition to the ED smoother:

- *Establish a start-of-shift routine:* You get to work, you get your assignment, you get the report. Suppose you have a few patients to see. Set a routine that allows you to lay eyes on all of your patients briefly, assess their acute needs, and introduce yourself. "Hi, my name is [your name]. I'm your nurse for today. I have a couple more patients to meet quickly, then I'll be back. Is there anything I can get for you right now?" Meet everyone, then get your game plan together. The sickest patient is first, then the easiest/fastest, then the longest. If you have an open room without a patient in it, make sure that you have all of your equipment and it is stocked and ready for whatever rolls in the door.
- *Document like you are going to court:* You have definitely heard this before. But it is true. There may come a time where, 3 years from now, you are subpoenaed to court regarding a patient you cared for in the ED. Something happened, one thing led to another, and BAM—you are sitting in the hot seat trying to remember who they were or what happened. Now does this mean you should write a narrative note for every single thing that happens on your shift? Not necessarily, because you would never leave the nurses' station. But document appropriately

on the basis of events or findings, especially if they are unusual. It may save you someday.
- *If you did not document it, it did not happen:* Another gold standard. Whether it is clicking boxes or writing short notes, document what happens. If the patient ambulates, if the team rounds, if there are physical therapy/occupational therapy visits, if the patient refuses to take their medication, document it. Do not rely on the notes of other teams or staff to account for your own documentation.
- *If you do not know the answer, do not lie—ask for help:* Someone asks you a question, and you are caught on the spot. If you do not know the answer, do not lie or try to fabricate one. Simply say "I don't know, but I'll find out. I'll ask someone who does know and get back to you." This is for anyone; patients, families, physicians, or other staff. Admitting a gap in knowledge is not a bad thing. It may even allow you to open a dialogue with another provider and learn something new.
- *You are never going to know everything. And that is okay:* There is no "I" in team; it is a cliché but true. Always be open to learning and being taught. Take opportunities to listen to physicians or other nurses teach and ask questions. You may learn a different way to do something or get the answer to a question you have been meaning to ask. Be a sponge, and soak up all the education around you.
- *It takes about a year:* Benner's theory on novice to expert model might ring a bell. Benner theorized that we all start as novices and advance through the stages of nursing development as time passes and experiences are acquired. According to this theory, it takes about a year to be considered "competent" in an area of study, like the ED. It may feel overwhelming at first but give yourself grace. Every shift gets you closer to competency. Take every opportunity to learn and to better yourself so you can do better for your patients.

Hopefully after the thorough review of knowledge and these few tips, you feel a little more ready to take on your new role.

So, take a deep breath and go make a difference!

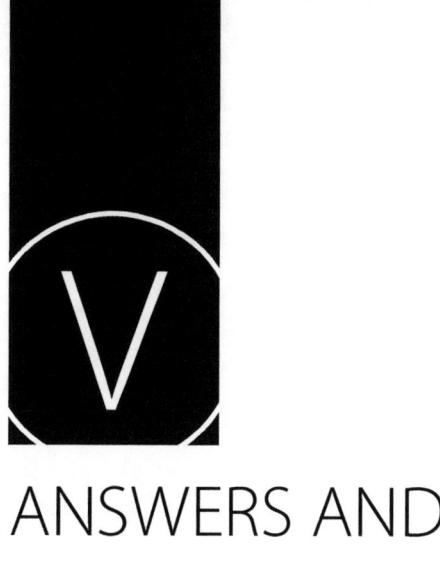

ANSWERS AND RATIONALES

Answers and Rationales

Chapter 1
1. Answer: B
   Rationale: The correct answer is to outline a patient's wishes regarding medical care. Advance directives can vary by state, but the purpose of an advance directive is to document the patient's wishes for their medical care.
2. Answer: C
   Rationale: The correct answer is closed-loop communication. Closed-loop communication is when the person receiving instructions or information repeats the information back to the speaker to ensure understanding.

Chapter 2
1. Answer: A
   Rationale: The correct answer is on an infant scale, after removing their clothes and diaper. For the most accurate weight, pediatric patients should be weighed this way until they are able to walk independently. All medications and fluids that are ordered are weight based, and thus an accurate weight is critical.
2. Answer: B
   Rationale: The correct answer is a 65-year old female with a history of coronary artery disease (CAD) and hypertension (HTN) presenting with crushing chest pain, diaphoresis, and nausea. Chest pain is a concerning chief complaint. With a history of CAD and HTN, in addition to the presenting symptoms the patient now has "high-risk situation" indications, upgrading their acuity level. Patients presenting to the ED with chest pain should receive an EKG within 10 minutes of arrival to rule out life-threatening conditions.
3. Answer: D
   Rationale: Triage should be able to be completed in about 2 to 5 minutes. The process of information gathering starts when the nurse lays eyes on the patient. The "assessment from the door" establishes the groundwork, then additional questions can be asked when the patient enters the triage space. If the nurse is not sure about which acuity level to assign, vital

signs can sometimes be the deciding factor to either maintain their acuity score or advance them.

Chapter 3
1. Answer: C
   Rationale: The correct answer is respiratory acidosis. The pH is less than 7.34, making this an acidosis. Next the $PaCO_2$ is greater than 45, making the acidosis being driven by the above normal $PaCO_2$.
2. Answer: B
   Rationale: Initiation of BiPAP to increase ventilation is the correct answer. The patient has a respiratory acidosis meaning too much CO_2). CO_2 can be reduced by increasing ventilation.

Chapter 4
1. Answer: C
   Rationale: The correct answer is potassium. Hyperkalemia can cause peaked T waves.
2. Answer: B
   Rationale: Magnesium follows calcium; thus, a low magnesium level should raise concerns over low calcium. The correct answer is calcium.

Chapter 5
1. Answer: C
   Rationale: Bell palsy is the most common condition in which there is a rapid and unilateral paralysis of cranial nerve VII, the facial nerve.
2. Answer: B
   Rationale: The patient is presenting with an acute neurological deficit. In this instance, the stroke protocol should be initiated, and the best next nursing intervention is to obtain IV access.

Chapter 6
1. Answer: C
   Rationale: This patient has a history of congestive heart failure (CHF) with edema present. Despite the fact that they are hypotensive, giving this patient a full volume resuscitation could potentially push this patient into fluid volume overload, leading to flash pulmonary edema. Relay concerns about this order before giving it. Discuss modified fluid resuscitation before looking to vasopressor support. Therefore, the correct answer is to clarify the order with the provider.
2. Answer: A
   Rationale: The correct answer is to obtain an EKG. This patient is exhibiting some classic signs of a myocardial infarction (MI), but it truly could be a multitude of things. The best first step in this case is to obtain an EKG while also getting vital signs to determine if they are having a heart

attack. Remember, the door-to-EKG time is 10 minutes, and time is muscle!

Chapter 7

1. Answer: D
   Rationale: Bacterial pneumonia is one of the leading causes of sepsis, accounting for about half of all sources of infection of sepsis.
2. Answer: A
   Rationale: The ideal oxygen saturation for a patient with chronic obstructive pulmonary disease (COPD) is 88% to 92%. Patients with COPD have a lower oxygen requirement because their baseline CO_2 is higher than normal. If the patient is provided too much oxygen, they may lose their hypoxic respiratory drive. This could lead to the patient decompensating and becoming confused.

Chapter 8

1. Answer: C
   Rationale: Acute mesenteric ischemia is a surgical emergency requiring urgent abdominal imaging. The correct answer, then, is to prepare the patient for emergency imaging and immediately notify the provider.
2. Answer: B
   Rationale: The correct answer is to obtain large-bore IV access and initiate fluid resuscitation. Upper gastrointestinal (GI) bleeding can lead to hypovolemic shock, making fluid resuscitation and appropriate IV access essential for the care of this patient.

Chapter 9

1. Answer: B
   Rationale: Milk is the best option to maintain the integrity of a tooth that has been dislodged from its socket. If milk is not available, you can have the patient place the tooth in the buccal pocket of their mouth and have their saliva maintain the tooth.
2. Answer: C
   Rationale: The correct answer is to visualize the tympanic membrane (TM) to ensure it is intact and not perforated. If the TM is ruptured, it can increase the risk of vertigo, hearing impairment, or worsening infection if not treated appropriately.

Chapter 10

1. Answer: C
   Rationale: A teardrop-shaped pupil suggests globe rupture, requiring immediate protection of the eye with a rigid shield, head elevation to reduce intraocular pressure, and nothing by mouth (NPO) status in the event surgical intervention is needed.

2. Answer: C
Rationale: Immediate and continuous irrigation **with** copious amounts of normal saline or lactated Ringer's solution is used to dilute and remove the chemical agent. Therefore, this is the correct answer.

Chapter 11

1. Answer: D
Rationale: Blood glucose level of <100 mg/dL is not a characteristic of diabetic ketoacidosis.
2. Answer: A
Rationale: A serum potassium level of <3.3 mEq/L should cause the nurse to pause and contact the provider prior to giving additional doses of IV insulin. Insulin pushes potassium into the cell, leading to hypokalemia, a serious electrolyte abnormality. This abnormality can lead to deadly arrythmias and needs to be monitored closely during treatment for diabetic ketoacidosis (DKA).
3. Answer: B
Rationale: The patient's Glasgow Coma Score (GCS) and mentation should be of highest consideration when correcting hypoglycemia. If the patient is able to participate in glucose correction such as participating in oral (PO) intake, encourage the patient to consume a simple carbohydrate such as juice or milk, followed by a complex carbohydrate like a sandwich. If the patient is unable to participate in treatment, consider IV dextrose or intramuscular (IM) glucagon to improve hypoglycemia.

Chapter 12

1. Answer: B
Rationale: Pyelonephritis is a serious bacterial infection of the kidneys that can lead to urosepsis if not promptly treated. Obtaining blood and urine culture and starting IV fluid and antibiotics are the next best interventions and the correct answer.
2. Answer: B
Rationale: Epididymitis is an infection or inflammation of the epididymis. Pain relief with scrotal elevation helps differentiate this presentation from testicular torsion, making epididymitis likely. Obtaining a urine sample for urinalysis and culture and then anticipating empiric antibiotic therapy are the next reasonable interventions.

Chapter 13

1. Answer: B
Rationale: Tumor lysis syndrome results from the rapid breakdown of malignant cells releasing intracellular contents into the bloodstream. This can result in hyperphosphatemia, hyperkalemia, hyperuricemia, and hypocalcemia.

2. Answer: B
Rationale: The correct answer is petechiae and oozing from IV sites. Disseminated intravascular coagulation (DIC) often presents with signs of bleeding because of clotting factor consumption, including petechiae, ecchymosis, hematuria, and bleeding from puncture sites.

Chapter 14

1. Answer: D
Rationale: The patient's symptoms are concerning for impairing blood flow and compartment syndrome. The next best intervention is to loosen any restrictive dressings or splints to reduce pressure and immediately notify the provider.
2. Answer: A
Rationale: Rhabdomyolysis results from muscle breakdown, releasing myoglobin and other cellular contents into the bloodstream, which can manifest as elevated creatine kinase (CK) levels and dark-colored urine. Aggressive IV fluid resuscitation is needed.

Chapter 15

1. Answer: C
Rationale: *Clostridioides difficile* requires the use of soap and water to cleanse the hands prior to leaving patient rooms. Because the spore is protected by an enteric coating, alcohol-based hand sanitizer is not sufficient to penetrate the outer layer of the germ. Soap and water allows for the spore to be washed down the drain, decreasing the risk of transmission.
2. Answer: A
Rationale: Scabies-infested objects that cannot be cleaned in the washing machine should be sealed for at least 72 hours and kept in an area where the temperature does not rise above 70°F to allow the scabies to die.

Chapter 16

1. Answer: B, C, D
Rationale: Although a fever frequently accompanies patients in septic shock, requirements for diagnosis are lactic acid level >2 mmol/L, hypotension despite adequate fluid resuscitation, and vasopressors.
2. Answer: D
Rationale: Beck triad is the correct answer. This is a phenomenon sometimes exhibited by patients as fluid gathers in the pericardial sac around the heart. Low blood pressure, jugular venous distention (JVD), and muffled heart sounds are the angles of the triad.

Chapter 17

1. Answer: A
Rationale: The primary survey follows the ABCDE approach (**A**irway, **B**reathing, **C**irculation, **D**isability, and **E**xposure). The correct answer is to assess airway patency and prepare for possible intubation.

2. Answer: D
   Rationale: This patient is showing signs of hemorrhagic shock. The next best nursing action is to ensure adequate IV access and be ready to transfuse blood products.

Chapter 18
1. Answer: B
   Rationale: Anticholinergic toxidrome is characterized by dry skin and mucous membranes, mydriasis (dilated pupils), urinary retention, hyperthermia, and altered mental status.
2. Answer: C
   Rationale: Naloxone is the opioid antagonist of choice for reversing opioid-induced respiratory depression. It works by competitively binding to opioid receptors, displacing the opioid molecules.

Chapter 19
1. Answer: B
   Rationale: Falls are a leading cause of injury in older adults, often resulting in hip fractures, head trauma, or spinal injuries. A focused musculoskeletal assessment is necessary, and the provider is likely to order imaging studies.
2. Answer: B
   Rationale: In older adults, urinary tract infections (UTIs) frequently present with confusion. The priority action is to obtain a urine sample for urinalysis and culture to evaluate for a possible infection.

Chapter 20
1. Answer: A
   Rationale: A delayed cord clamping in the stable infant of 30 to 60 seconds or until the cord is no longer pulsatile allows for the remaining blood that is circulating in the placenta to be delivered to the infant. This decreases the risk for a need for neonatal transfusion.
2. Answer: B
   Rationale: An ectopic pregnancy is defined as a gestational sac that implants in a location that is not the uterus.

Chapter 21
1. Answer: B
   Rationale: The patient is exhibiting warning signs. A thorough suicide risk assessment, including intent, plan, and access to means, needs to be completed.
3. Answer: B
   Rationale: De-escalation techniques are the first-line approach for an agitated patient. This includes speaking calmly, maintaining a

nonthreatening stance, offering personal space, and using therapeutic communication.

Chapter 22
1. Answer: C
   Rationale: The correct answer is 10 mL/kg. Much like fluid resuscitation in those with sepsis, patients experiencing diabetic ketoacidosis (DKA) may require aggressive fluids to combat impending cardiovascular collapse. Be sure to have an accurate weight in kilograms and verify the calculation of the fluids prescribed to avoid fluid volume overload. If the calculations do not match, inquire with the ordering provider to be sure the patient is receiving appropriate fluids.
2. Answer: D
   Rationale: Neglect is the most common form of abuse, but other forms should not be discounted in the presenting patient.

Chapter 23
1. Answer: C
   Rationale: A dose of 5 to 10 mg every 5 minutes is recommended for treatment of severe organophosphate poisoning to combat the 3 Bs—bradycardia, bronchospasm, and bronchorrhea.
2. Answer: A
   Rationale: Smallpox was eradicated in 1980, and the vaccine is no longer administered in the vaccination schedule in the United States.

Chapter 24
1. Answer: B
   Rationale: Attempting de-escalation techniques is a reasonable initial step.
2. Answer: A
   Rationale: De-escalation techniques are first-line interventions when dealing with an aggressive patient.

INDEX

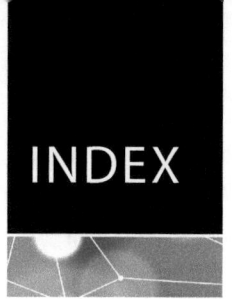

ABCs. *See* airway, breathing, and circulation
abdominal trauma
   liver laceration, 196
   pelvic fractures, 196
   splenic injuries, 195–196
abruptio placentae, 236–237
ACEs. *See* adverse childhood experiences
acid–base imbalances
   common acid–base disorder patient presentations, 28, 29
   interpreting values from ABG, 28, 29
   metabolic acidosis, 30–31
   metabolic alkalosis, 31
   oxyhemoglobin dissociation curve, 27, 28
   respiratory acidosis, 29–30
   respiratory alkalosis, 30
ACLS. *See* advanced cardiovascular life support
active listening, 5–6
acute arterial occlusion, 58
acute cholecystitis, 93–94
acute compartment syndrome, 153–154
acute ischemic stroke, 44–45
acute leukemia, 142–143
acute myocardial infraction
   NSTEMI and STEMI, 54, 56
   patient's history, 53, 55
acute otitis externa, 104–105
acute otitis interna, 108
acute otitis media, 105–106
acute respiratory distress syndrome (ARDS), 70–71, 165
acute stroke, 43

advanced cardiovascular life support (ACLS), 240, 277
adverse childhood experiences (ACEs), 232
advocacy
   advance directives, 7
   coworkers, 8
   for families, 7–8
   nurse-to-patient ratio, 6
airway, breathing, and circulation (ABCs), 193
airway obstructions, 71, 72
airway, with restriction of c-spine motion, breathing, circulation, disability, and exposure (ABCDEs), 189–190
allergies and reactions, medications past illnesses pregnancy status, last meal, and events/environment (AMPLE) related to injury, 190, 191
Alzheimer disease, 224
amputation, 153
anemia, 137–139
anxiety, 250
aortic injuries and dissection, 60–61
appendicitis, 92, 93
ARDS. *See* acute respiratory distress syndrome
arrhythmias
   supraventricular tachycardia, 62–63
   symptomatic bradycardia, 61–62
   ventricular fibrillation or pulseless ventricular tachycardia, 63–65
asthma, 82, 83

Bartholin cyst, 228–229
basilar skull fracture, 197–198
bedbugs, 174–175
Bell palsy, 48
bioterrorism
   anthrax, 273
   botulism, 273–274
   hemorrhagic fevers, 275–276
   plague, 274
   smallpox, 274–275
   tularemia, 275
blunt ocular trauma, 116
bowel obstruction, 91–92
bradykinin-mediated angioedema, 74
brain attack, 43
bronchiolitis, 259
burns, 154–156

cardiac tamponade, 59–60, 182–183
cardiogenic shock, 181–182
cardiovascular emergencies
   acute arterial occlusion, 58
   acute myocardial infraction, 53–56
   aortic injuries and dissection, 60–61
   arrhythmias, 61–65
   cardiac tamponade, 59–60
   endocarditis, 59
   heart failure, 57–58
   post cardiac arrest, 66–67
   pulseless electrical activity, 65
caries, 101
central retinal artery occlusion, 113–114
cerebrovascular accident, 43
cerumen impaction, 103–104
child maltreatment, 262–263
chronic obstructive pulmonary disease (COPD), 81–82
closed-loop communication, 5–6
concussion, 202
condylomata acuminate. *See* genital warts
conjunctivitis/pink eye, 115
contusion, 199–200
COPD. *See* chronic obstructive pulmonary disease
corneal abrasions, 114
coronavirus-19, 168–169

croup, 72, 259–261
Cullen sign, 124, 125

DAI. *See* drug-assisted intubation
deep venous thrombosis (DVT), 168
dehydration, 35, 223
dementia, 224
dental abscess, 99–100
dental emergencies
   caries, 101
   dental abscess, 99–100
   fractured tooth, 100–101
   tooth avulsion, 102
depressed skull fracture, 198
depression, 250–251
detached retina, 115
DI. *See* diabetes insipidus
diabetes insipidus (DI), 128
diabetic ketoacidosis (DKA), 120–121
diaphragmatic injuries, 194
DIC. *See* diffuse intravascular coagulation
diffuse intravascular coagulation (DIC), 168
disaster management
   bioterrorism, 273–276
   immediate response to walk-in patients, 269–271
   mass casualty incident triage, 271–272
   mass shooting, 272–273
   nerve agents, 276–277
dislocations and subluxations, 153
displacement, obstruction, pneumothorax, and equipment (DOPE), 80–81
disseminated intravascular coagulation, 140–141
distributive anaphylactic shock, 184
distributive septic shock
   neurogenic shock, 185–187
   symptoms based on system, 185, 186
diverticulitis, 92
DKA. *See* diabetic ketoacidosis
DOPE. *See* displacement, obstruction, pneumothorax, and equipment

drug-assisted intubation (DAI)
   intubation medications, 75, 78, 79
   paralytics, 79–80
   premedications, 78–79
   preparation checklist, 75, 76
   troubleshooting, 80–81
DVT. *See* deep venous thrombosis

ear emergencies
   acute otitis externa, 104–105
   acute otitis interna, 106
   acute otitis media, 105–106
   cerumen impaction, 103–104
   foreign objects, 102–103
   Ménière disease (MD), 106–107
   ruptured tympanic membrane, 106
eclampsia, 238–239
ectopic pregnancy, 233
elder maltreatment, 221–222
electrolyte abnormalities
   hypercalcemia, 38
   hyperkalemia, 36–37
   hypermagnesemia, 39
   hypernatremia, 36
   hypocalcemia, 37
   hypokalemia, 36
   hypomagnesemia, 38
   hyponatremia, 35–36
emergency department (ED) nurse
   ability to focus, 4–5
   acid–base imbalances, 27–31
   active listening, 5–6
   advocacy, 6–8
   cardiovascular emergencies, 53–68
   closed-loop communication, 5–6
   compassion, 4
   dental emergencies, 99–102
   disaster management, 269–277
   ear emergencies, 102–107
   endocrine emergencies, 119–128
   flexibility, 4
   fluid and electrolyte emergencies, 33–39
   gastrointestinal emergencies, 89–96
   genitourinary emergencies, 131–135
   geriatric emergencies, 221–225
   hematologic emergencies, 137–145
   infectious disease emergencies, 159–175
   mental health emergencies, 249–253
   musculoskeletal and wound care emergencies, 149–156
   nasal emergencies, 107–109
   neurological emergencies, 43–50
   OB/GYN emergencies, 227–244
   ocular emergencies, 113–117
   pediatric emergencies, 255–264
   problem-solving and troubleshooting, 5
   respiratory emergencies, 69–85
   safety in, 279–280
   shock emergencies, 179–187
   substance abuse and toxicologic emergencies, 203–216
   teachability, 4
   therapeutic silence, 5
   therapeutic touch, 5
   throat emergencies, 109–110
   tips for success for ED nurses, 283–286
   traumatic emergencies, 189–200
   triage, 11–24
emergency medical service (EMS), 189, 269
Emergency Medical Treatment and Active Labor Act (EMTALA), 12, 21
emergency severity index (ESI), 13
EMS. *See* emergency medical service
EMTALA. *See* Emergency Medical Treatment and Active Labor Act
endocarditis, 59
endocrine emergencies
   pancreatic-related, 119–125
   thyroid-related, 125–128
endometriosis, 227–228
epididymitis, 133
epidural hematoma, 199
epiglottitis, 72–73, 258
epistaxis, 107–108
ESI. *See* emergency severity index
esophageal obstruction, 94–95
esophageal varices, 95

falls, 222
flail chest, 194
fluid balance
  common IV fluid compositions, 33, 34
  dehydration, 35
  overhydration, 34
foreign objects, ear emergencies, 102–103
fractured tooth, 100–101
fractures, 151–153

gastritis, 90
gastroenteritis, 90–91
gastroesophageal reflux disease (GERD), 91
gastrointestinal emergencies
  abdominal assessment, 89–95
  gastrointestinal bleeding, 95–96
genital warts, 135
genitourinary emergencies
  epididymitis, 133
  genital warts, 135
  penile fracture, 134
  priapism, 135
  pyelonephritis, 132
  renal calculi, 132–133
  testicular torsion, 134
  urinary retention, 134–135
  urinary tract infection, 131–132
GERD. *See* gastroesophageal reflux disease
geriatric emergencies
  Alzheimer disease, 224
  dehydration, 223
  dementia, 224
  elder maltreatment, 221–222
  falls, 222
  pneumonia, 224–225
  syncope, transient loss of consciousness, 222–223
  urosepsis, 225
gestational hypertension
  eclampsia, 238–239
  preeclampsia, 237–238
  prolapsed cord, 239–240
glaucoma, 114

head trauma
  basilar skull fracture, 197–198
  concussion, 198
  contusion, 199–200
  depressed skull fracture, 198
  epidural hematoma, 199
  increased intracranial pressure, 200
  linear skull fracture, 196–197
  subarachnoid hemorrhage, 199
  subdural hematoma, 198–199
headache, 49–50
heart failure, 57–58
HELLP. *See* hemolysis, elevated liver enzymes, and low platelets syndrome
hematologic emergencies
  acute leukemia, 142–143
  anemia, 137–139
  disseminated intravascular coagulation, 140–141
  hemophilia, 141–142
  sickle cell anemia, 139–140
  tumor lysis syndrome (TLS), 143–145
hemolysis, elevated liver enzymes, and low platelets (HELLP) syndrome, 241
hemophilia, 141–142
hemorrhagic stroke, 45–46
hemothorax, 193–194
hepatitis, 171
HHS. *See* hyperosmolar hyperglycemic syndrome
histamine-mediated angioedema, 74
human immunodeficiency virus/acquired immunodeficiency syndrome, 165–173
hypercalcemia, 38
hyperkalemia, 36–37
hypermagnesemia, 39
hypernatremia, 36
hyperosmolar hyperglycemic syndrome (HHS), 121–123
hyperventilation, 30
hyphema, 116
hypocalcemia, 37
hypoglycemia, 123–124
hypokalemia, 36

hypomagnesemia, 38
hyponatremia, 35–36
hypovolemic shock, 180–181

ICH. *See* intracerebral hemorrhage
increased intracranial pressure, 200
infectious colitis, 160–161
infectious disease emergencies
   coronavirus-19, 168–169
   environment of care, 175
   food and drinks at workstations, 175
   hepatitis, 167
   human immunodeficiency virus/
      acquired immunodeficiency
      syndrome, 165–173
   infectious colitis, 160–161
   influenza, 163, 165
   meningitis, 161–163
   parasitic and insect infestations,
      174–175
   tick-borne illnesses, 169–172
   tuberculosis, 172–173
influenza, 163, 165
intracerebral hemorrhage (ICH),
   45–46
intussusception, 264
ischuria. *See* urinary retention

labyrinthitis. *See* acute otitis interna
lacerations *vs.* cuts, 154
linear skull fracture, 196–197
liver laceration, 196
lower gastrointestinal bleeding, 96
Ludwig angina, 73–74, 102

manic behavior, 253
mass casualty incident (MCIs),
   271–272
mass shooting, 272–273
MCIs. *See* mass casualty incident
MD. *See* Ménière disease
Ménière disease (MD), 106–107
meningitis, 161–163
mental health emergencies
   anxiety, 250
   depression, 250–251
   manic behavior, 253

   posttraumatic stress disorder, 250
   psychosis, 253
   suicide, 251–252
   violent or aggressive behavior,
      252–253
mesenteric ischemia, 94
metabolic acidosis, 30–31
metabolic alkalosis, 31
MG. *See* myasthenia gravis
multiple sclerosis, 49
musculoskeletal and wound care
   emergencies
   acute compartment syndrome,
      153–154
   amputation, 153
   burns, 154–156
   dislocations and subluxations, 153
   findings with palpation, 150
   fractures, 151–153
   lacerations *versus* cuts, 154
   osteomyelitis, 156
   rhabdomyolysis, 156
   sprains, 150–151
   strains, 150
myasthenia gravis (MG), 48
myxedema coma, 126–128

nasal emergencies
   epistaxis, 107–108
   nasal fracture, 108–109
   periorbital cellulitis, 111
nasal fracture, 108–109
nephrolithiasis. *See* renal calculi
nerve agents, 276–277
neurological emergencies
   acute ischemic stroke, 44–45
   acute stroke, 43
   Bell palsy, 48
   headache, 49–50
   multiple sclerosis, 49
   myasthenia gravis (MG), 48
   seizures, 47
   transient ischemic attack, 46
new-onset type 1 diabetes mellitus,
   265–266
non-ST elevation myocardial infarction
   (NSTEMI), 53, 54, 56

NSTEMI. *See* non-ST elevation myocardial infarction
nursemaid's elbow (radial head subluxation), 263

obstetrical (OB) and gynecological (GYN) emergencies
  abruptio placentae, 236–237
  Bartholin cyst, 228–229
  delivery in ED
    Apgar score, 243
    concern for impending birth, 242
    postpartum hemorrhage (PPH), 243–244
    target neonatal room air oxygen levels postdelivery, 242, 243
  ectopic pregnancy, 233
  endometriosis, 227–228
  pelvic inflammatory disease (PID), 229–230
  placenta previa, 234, 236
  pregnancy-induced hypertension, 237–240
  sex or human trafficking, 232–233
  sexual assault, 230–232
  spontaneous abortion (miscarriage), 233–235
  trauma during pregnancy, 240–241
  vaginitis, 229
obstructive shock
  cardiac tamponade, 182–183
  pulmonary embolus, 183–184
  tension pneumothorax, 183
ocular burns, 116–117
ocular emergencies
  central retinal artery occlusion, 113–114
  conjunctivitis/pink eye, 115
  corneal abrasions, 114
  detached retina, 115
  glaucoma, 114
  ocular burns, 116–117
  ocular trauma, 115–116
ocular trauma, 115–116
osteomyelitis, 156

overhydration, 34
pancreatic-related emergencies
  diabetic ketoacidosis (DKA), 120–121
  hyperosmolar hyperglycemic syndrome, 121–123
  hypoglycemia, 123–124
  pancreatitis, 124–125
pancreatitis, 124–125
parasitic and insect infestations
  bedbugs, 174–175
  scabies, 174
PAT. *See* pediatric assessment triangle
pediatric assessment triangle (PAT), 18
pediatric emergencies
  bronchiolitis, 259
  child maltreatment, 262–263
  croup, 259–261
  epiglottitis, 258
  fever, 256, 258
  intussusception, 264
  new-onset type 1 diabetes mellitus, 261–262
  normal pediatric vital signs, 256, 258
  nursemaid's elbow (radial head subluxation), 263
  sudden infant death syndrome (SIDS), 263–264
pelvic fractures, 196
pelvic inflammatory disease (PID), 229–230
penile fracture, 134
perimortem cesarean delivery (PMCD), 240
periorbital cellulitis, 109
peritonsillar abscess, 109–110
pharyngitis/tonsillitis, 109
PID. *See* pelvic inflammatory disease
placenta previa, 234, 236
PMCD. *See* perimortem cesarean delivery
pneumonia, 84–85, 224–225
pneumothorax, 193

postpartum hemorrhage (PPH), 243–244
posttraumatic stress disorder, 250
PPH. *See* postpartum hemorrhage
preeclampsia, 237–238
pregnancy-induced hypertension
    eclampsia, 238–239
    preeclampsia, 237–238
    prolapsed cord, 239–240
priapism, 135
PRICE. *See* protect, rest, ice, compression, elevate
prolapsed cord, 239–240
protect, rest, ice, compression, elevate (PRICE), 150
psychosis, 253
pulmonary embolus, 183–184
pulseless electrical activity, 65
pyelonephritis, 132

rapid sequence intubation (RSI)
    intubation medications, 75, 78, 79
    paralytics, 79–80
    premedications, 80–81
    preparation checklist, 75, 76
    troubleshooting, 80–81
renal calculi, 132–133
respiratory acidosis, 29–30
respiratory alkalosis, 30
respiratory emergencies
    acute respiratory distress syndrome (ARDS), 70–71
    airway obstructions, 71, 72
    angioedema and anaphylaxis, 74–75
    asthma, 82, 83
    chronic obstructive pulmonary disease, 81–82
    croup, 72
    drug-assisted intubation (DAI), 75–80
    epiglottitis, 72–73
    escalation of oxygen delivery, 69, 70
    Ludwig angina, 73–74
    pneumonia, 84–85
    rapid sequence intubation, 75–80
    spontaneous pneumothorax/tension pneumothorax, 84
    status asthmaticus, 83
return of spontaneous circulation (ROSC), 65
rhabdomyolysis, 156
RMSF. *See* rocky mountain spotted fever
rocky mountain spotted fever (RMSF), 169
ROSC. *See* return of spontaneous circulation
RSI. *See* rapid sequence intubation
ruptured tympanic membrane, 106

scabies, 174
seizures, 47
sex/human trafficking, 232–233
sexual assault, 230–232
shock
    cardiogenic, 181–182
    category of, 180
    distributive anaphylactic, 184
    distributive septic shock, 184–187
    hypovolemic, 180–181
    obstructive, 182–184
    stages of, 179
sickle cell anemia, 139–140
SIDS. *See* sudden infant death syndrome
SIRS. *See* systemic inflammatory response syndrome
spinal cord injuries, 194–195
splenic injuries, 195–196
spontaneous abortion (miscarriage), 233–235
spontaneous pneumothorax/tension pneumothorax, 86
sprains, 150–151
status asthmaticus, 83
ST-elevation myocardial infarction (STEMI), 182
STEMI. *See* ST-elevation myocardial infarction
strains, 150
subarachnoid hemorrhage, 199

subdural hematoma, 198–199
substance abuse and toxicologic emergencies
  acetylcholinesterase inhibition (cholinergics), 203
  alcohol abuse, 203
  anticholinergic overdose, 203–204
  anticoagulants-oral, 205
  anticoagulants-parenteral, 206
  benzodiazepines, 206
  beta-blockers, 207
  caffeine powder/capsules, 207
  calcium channel blockers, 207
  carbon monoxide poisoning, 207
  cardiac glycosides, 208
  DXM, 208
  ethylene glycol (antifreeze), 208
  factor Xa inhibitor, 205
  GHB acid, 209
  hallucinogens, 209
  insulin, 209
  iron, 210
  marijuana concentrates, 210
  MDMA, 211
  narcotics (opioids), 211
  neuroleptics, 212
  salicylates, 212
  stimulants (sympathomimetics), 213
  synthetic cannabinoids, 213
  synthetic cathinones, 214
  Tylenol (acetaminophen) overdose, 215
  vaping devices, types of, 216
  venom of rattlesnakes, cotton mouth/water moccasins, and copperheads, 215
sudden infant death syndrome (SIDS), 263–264
suicide, 251–252
supraventricular tachycardia (SVT), 62–63
SVT. *See* supraventricular tachycardia
swimmer's ear. *See* Acute otitis externa
symptomatic bradycardia, 61–62
syncope, 222–223
systemic inflammatory response syndrome (SIRS), 185

T1DM. *See* type 1 diabetes mellitus
tension pneumothorax, 183
testicular torsion, 134
therapeutic silence, 5
therapeutic touch, 5
thoracic trauma
  diaphragmatic injuries, 194
  flail chest, 194
  hemothorax, 193–194
  pneumothorax, 193
  spinal cord injuries, 194–195
thyroid storm, 126
thyroid-related emergencies
  diabetes insipidus (DI), 128
  myxedema coma, 126–128
  thyroid storm, 126
TIA. *See* transient ischemic attack
tick-borne illnesses, 169–172
TLS. *See* tumor lysis syndrome
tooth avulsion, 102
transient ischemic attack (TIA), 46
traumatic emergencies
  abdominal, 195–196
  head, 196–200
  penetrating trauma, 192–193
  primary survey, 189–190
  road burn or road rash, 191–192
  secondary survey, 190–191
  thoracic, 193–195
  trauma triad of death, 191, 192
triage
  acuity systems
    across-the-room assessment, 14
    age-specific normal vital signs, 15, 16
    comparing triage systems, 13, 14
    elicit chief complaint, 15
    focused physical assessment, 15
    multitasking, 15
    patient interviewing, 15
    resources vs. nonresources, 17
  common pitfalls of, 22–24
  interventions
    age of child, 21
    environmental interaction, 20
    pediatric assessment triangle (PAT), 18

tone, interactivity, consolability, look or gaze, and speech or cry (TICLS), 19–20
legal issues, 21–22
patients safety, 12–13
tuberculosis, 172–173
tumor lysis syndrome (TLS), 143–145
type 1 diabetes mellitus (T1DM), 265

upper gastrointestinal bleeding, 95
urinary retention, 134–135
urinary tract infection, 131–132
urosepsis, 225

vaginitis, 229
ventricular fibrillation (VF), 63–65
ventricular tachycardia (VT), 63–65
VF. *See* ventricular fibrillation
violent/aggressive behavior, 252–253
VT. *See* ventricular tachycardia

workplace violence (WPV)
    de-escalation techniques, 280, 281
    preparation, training, 280
    signs of patient, visitor escalation, 279–280
WPV. *See* workplace violence

FAST FACTS FOR YOUR NURSING CAREER

Choose from 50+ Titles!

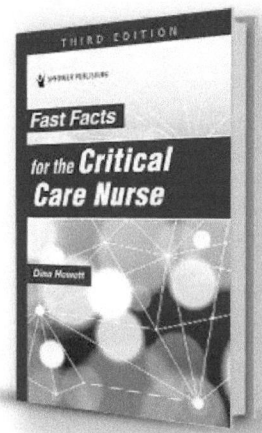
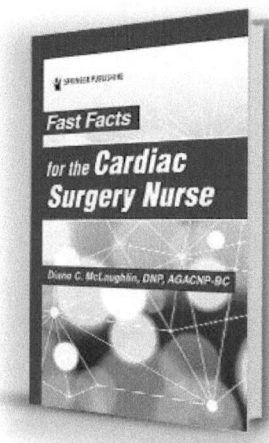
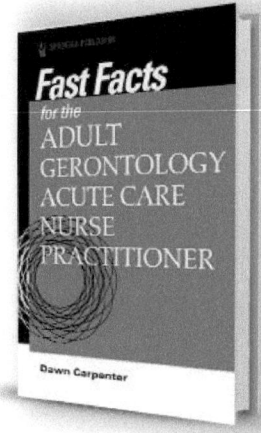
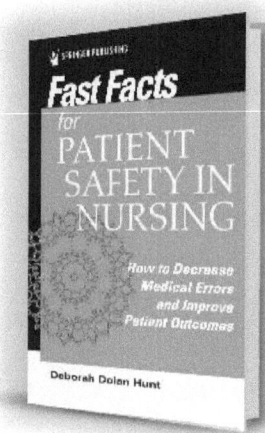

These must-have reference books are packed with timely, useful, and accessible information presented in a clear, precise format. Pocket-sized and affordable, the series provides quick access to information you need to know and use daily.

springerpub.com/FastFacts